T0261028

CIVIL WAR
MEDICINE

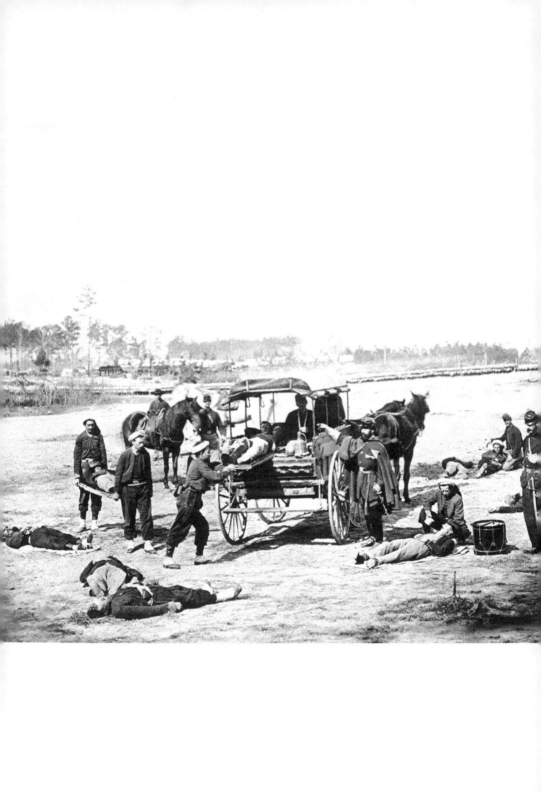

EDITED BY
ROBERT D. HICKS

CIVIL WAR MEDICINE

A SURGEON'S DIARY

INDIANA UNIVERSITY PRESS

This book is a publication of

Indiana University Press
Office of Scholarly Publishing
Herman B Wells Library 350
1320 East 10th Street
Bloomington, Indiana 47405 USA

iupress.indiana.edu

Manufactured in the United States of America

Library of Congress Cataloging-in-Publication Data

Names: Hicks, Robert D., [date] editor.
Title: Civil War medicine : a surgeon's diary / Robert D. Hicks.
Description: Bloomington, Indiana : Indiana University Press,
   2019. | Includes bibliographical references and index.
Identifiers: LCCN 2018049706 (print) | LCCN 2018050670
   (ebook) | ISBN 9780253040084 (e-book) | ISBN
   9780253040077 (cl : alk. paper)
Subjects: LCSH: Fulton, James, (U.S. Civil War surgeon)—
   Diaries. | United States—History—Civil War, 1861-1865—
   Medical care. | United States. Army—Surgeons—Diaries. |
   United States. Army. Pennsylvania Infantry Regiment, 143rd
   (1862-1865)
Classification: LCC E621 (ebook) | LCC E621 .H53 2019 (print) |
   DDC 973.7/75—dc23
LC record available at https://lccn.loc.gov/2018049706

1 2 3 4 5   24 23 22 21 20 19

For

ROB LUKENS,

President, Chester County Historical Society

and

GARRETT G. HOLLANDS,

who made this book possible

CONTENTS

ACKNOWLEDGMENTS

IN DECEMBER 2012, I PRESENTED A TALK ON CIVIL WAR MEDICINE at the Worcester Historical Society in Massachusetts. A portion of the presentation concerned a letter written by Henry S. Huidekoper to Dr. S. Weir Mitchell, one of the country's most famous nineteenth-century physicians. Huidekoper, during the Civil War a lieutenant colonel with the 150th Pennsylvania Volunteers, received the Medal of Honor for his actions at Gettysburg on July 1, 1863, which resulted in the amputation of his wounded arm. At the conclusion of the talk, a man in the audience raised his hand to say that Huidekoper was mentioned in the diary of his ancestor, Assistant Surgeon James Fulton of the 143rd Pennsylvania, which fought alongside the 150th. This man, Garrett G. Hollands, immediately offered to share what turned out to be an exciting discovery. Conversations and correspondence followed, and Garrett and Brenda Hollands provided me with a digital version of Fulton's unpublished diary, along with a bundle of information concerning family genealogy, service records, and their own transcript of the diary. The Hollands family had also visited the locations of Fulton's camps and battlefields. Without their generosity and early research, this book would not have been possible. They are due profuse thanks for their own extensive research, their recognition that the Fulton diary has significance, and their willingness to share it with the world.

This volume required a new, definitive transcript for scholarly purposes, and the usual business of tracking sources, obtaining illustrations and permissions, and correspondence with custodians of other collections with illuminating materials. Alex Tonsing, a Haverford College student, had the first go at transcribing the diary. Mary Ellen Donatelli, Wood Institute Associate,

The College of Physicians of Philadelphia, was an indefatigable and enthusiastic assistant in all essential tasks, particularly editing the transcript. Retired literature professor Kathleen R. D. Sands tirelessly collaborated in producing the definitive transcript and in proofreading text. Kerry Bryan, a Wood Institute Research Associate and a diligent researcher, sallied forth to the Pennsylvania archives in Harrisburg to locate relevant Fulton records.

Many colleagues in the universe of archives and libraries extended a helping hand. The roll call includes F. Michael Angelo, University Archivist and Head of Historic Collections, Thomas Jefferson University; Constance Carter, Science Reference Services, and Kenneth Johnson, Duplication Services, both of the Library of Congress; Pamela Powell, Photo Archivist, Chester County Historical Society; Tabitha Cary, Carl A. Kroch Library, Cornell University; Natalie Shilstut, Presbyterian Historical Society; Denise P. Gallo, Daughters of Charity, Emmitsburg, Maryland; and at my own institution, the Historical Medical Library of The College of Physicians of Philadelphia, Caitlin Angelone, Chrissie Perella, and Emily Snedden Yates. David Smith, another Fulton descendant, shared images from a century-old, privately printed family history. Theresa M. Altieri Taplin, Archivist, The Foundations of The Union League of Philadelphia, opened her rich collection, one that deserves huge promotion for its Civil War value. Barbara Franco, Founding Director, Seminary Ridge Museum, Gettysburg, furnished leads to the identities of doctors mentioned in the diary by surnames only. Her own compilation of all physicians, Confederate and federal, who served at Gettysburg, will be a boon to scholarship when completed. I am most grateful to Diane Wendt, Deputy Chair and Curator, Medicine and Science, Smithsonian Institution, for allowing me to study the diary of Fulton's colleague, Surgeon M. A. Henderson of the 150th Pennsylvania. Oberlin College student Sophie Everbach contributed help at an early stage of this project. Bill Nelson's wonderful maps give the topographic context to make the diary comprehensible. Tim Korba of RichArt Graphics enhanced and improved the photographs wonderfully.

I owe a huge debt to an A-list of scholars for their willingness to engage with the diary and provide the analysis and context requisite to circumscribing Fulton's experience during the war. A huge shout-out to Shauna Devine, Margaret Humphreys, Randall M. Miller, James M. Edmonson, Guy R. Hasegawa, and Barbra Mann Wall. I hope that they found the Fulton diary a rewarding discovery. Their essays were critical to producing this book. Two anonymous reviewers made important criticisms that resulted in significant revisions and reorganization of material. Gold-star thanks to Indiana University Press for taking on the project. Ashley Runyon, Trade and Regional Acquisitions Editor, and Peggy Solic took the book in hand and ably ushered it forward. Nancy Lila Lightfoot, project manager, and Maya Bringe of Amnet, who oversaw copyediting and typesetting, drove it home. Their careful stewardship of the project speaks to the academic presence of Indiana University Press on the Civil War bookshelf.

I thank George M. Wohlreich, MD, President and CEO, The College of Physicians of Philadelphia, for his interest, advice, support, and encouragement.

CIVIL WAR
MEDICINE

Introduction

Becoming a Military Doctor

DR. FULTON GOES TO WAR

During the first half of 1862, only a year into the Civil War, twenty-nine-year-old James Fulton, MD, of Chester County, Pennsylvania, applied for an appointment as an assistant surgeon in a Union army volunteer regiment. He had obtained an unused pocket diary for the year 1862, and on traveling to Philadelphia to sit for an examination at the University of Pennsylvania in August, he transformed it into a diary of his experiences in the army, written in either daily or every few days until shortly before his resignation in spring of 1864. Possibly before his resignation, while the army prepared for what became known as the Overland Campaign and the Battle of the Wilderness, Fulton began a second narrative, an incomplete attempt to give form and structure to his experience at the Battle of Gettysburg, clearly the signature experience of his military career. The diary hints at his motives for joining the fight and only briefly notes why he decided to resign. Despite capture by Confederates at Gettysburg and the confiscation of his medical tools, Fulton apparently kept the diary on his person at all times.

Why did Fulton join the war effort a year after fighting began? We cannot know his motivation, but his marriage only a month after the war began might have tempered his patriotic ardor. Possibly the precipitating event was President Lincoln's June 30, 1862, order for troops, his first call for enlistments since the initial call for seventy-five thousand soldiers during spring 1861. Perhaps Lincoln's public appeal persuaded him:

> The capture of New Orleans, Norfolk, and Corinth by the national forces has enabled the insurgents to concentrate a large force at and about Richmond, which place we must take with the least possible delay . . . With so large an

army there, the enemy can threaten us on the Potomac and elsewhere. Until
we have reestablished the national authority, all these places must be held,
and we must keep a respectable force in front of Washington ... To accomplish the object stated we require without delay 150,000 men.[1]

During the war, Fulton served as assistant surgeon with the Bucktail
Brigade, formed of the 143rd, 149th, and 150th Pennsylvania Volunteer Infantry Regiments. He passed the army examination requisite to an appointment
as assistant surgeon and mustered in at Pennsylvania's key organizing center
for volunteer regiments, Camp Curtin in Harrisburg. Initially assigned to the
150th Pennsylvania, within two months, he transferred to the 143rd, where
he remained for the rest of his army service.

Upon resigning, Fulton returned home and resumed the management
of his household. He subsequently raised a family, several members of which
remained at the Fulton residence or nearby, established a private practice,
maintained professional relationships with other physicians in his region,
and ran a farm. He apparently never traveled and so did not venture abroad
to the key medical centers of Europe, but plied a career as a country doctor
in a part of Chester County, Pennsylvania, that to this day retains much of
its rural ambience.

Members of the 150th created their own regimental history decades after
the war, in which Fulton receives brief mention, but veterans of the 143rd
did not. Fulton's diary supplies the voice of one member of the command,
and a distinctive one as well, given Fulton's status as an assistant surgeon.
Fulton's diary reveals him to be an articulate and intelligent observer of
events, particularly the Gettysburg battle, with an acute eye for landscape
and environment.

PLAN OF THIS BOOK

This book is divided into two parts. Following this introductory chapter, in
part 1, Fulton's diary occupies chapters 1 through 5. The chapters reflect the
editor's subdivision of the diary into roughly equal components. Fulton's
spelling and punctuation have been retained, and footnotes serve to identify
people or places he mentions. Chapter 6 sketches Fulton's experiences following his departure from federal service in 1864 and his subsequent career as a
country doctor while he and his wife, Anna, raised a family. Part 1 concludes

with commentary on the diary (chapter 7). Part 2 consists of scholarly essays (chapters 8 through 13) that address and amplify the diary. All contributing authors consider Fulton within his own time and circumstances, thus avoiding ahistorical comparisons between Fulton's medical world and ours.

This book may be read as an anthropological history. It furnishes an opportunity for the reader to experience the war through Fulton's eyes, to survey the war from a surgeon's (all physicians in Union army service were called surgeons) perspective. The invocation of anthropology in what appears historians' territory—the presentation of a nineteenth-century text—requires justification. A half century ago, British cultural historian Keith Thomas published an essay arguing why historians should examine anthropological scholarship:

> One great incentive for historians to read anthropology, therefore, is that the anthropologists can offer detailed analyses of phenomena roughly comparable to those which the historians are endeavouring to reconstruct with a good deal less evidence ... From the union of techniques derived from social anthropology and social psychology there could arise a whole new world of historical investigation which might illuminate so much of what is most baffling and most crucial to human existence.[2]

Thomas gives examples of fruitful collaborations of anthropology and history, including studies of pain, drunkenness, and "the nervous and mental life of society as reflected in dreams." Many of these topics have been addressed in recent scholarship (of the Civil War and other periods and cultures), thanks to recent trends in multi- and interdisciplinary studies. A scholarly work on dreams in the Civil War now exists.[3]

By framing the Fulton book as an anthropological history, the diary can be read as a transcribed oral history in an ethnography of the Union army medical subculture. The essence of anthropological fieldwork (although no longer unique to anthropology) is participant observation. The anthropologist may exercise this technique to elicit insight and understanding through interviews with cultural participants in constructing an ethnography. An ethnography studies a culture intensively via observation and interviews with informants who are members of that culture, which can be a professional one, such as medical doctors.[4] We have Fulton's narrative, but we cannot ask him questions about his actions, choices, and beliefs, the "detailed analyses of phenomena" Thomas describes.

We can envisage Fulton in his cultural environment where he exercises opinions, writes reports, attends to ill or wounded soldiers, eats with colleagues, huddles in the snow on picket duty, or packs up the camp to move. How can we build on Fulton's own words to investigate his activities within a broader culture of military doctors? The essays in this volume were solicited to investigate Fulton's medical culture through his experience. The contributors were asked to study the diary and write essays in response to specific questions intended to examine Fulton as an actor within his military medical culture. Some essays necessarily visit extant scholarship (often by the essayists themselves), but all scholars have oriented their observations to Fulton's narrative. The essays offer insight into Fulton's activities, especially where essays extrapolate Fulton's actions to explore contexts barely mentioned or hinted at in the diary, but not explicitly discussed—women nurses, for instance. Taken as a whole, then, this book suggests a profitable way to read diaries or other first-person accounts, not singly as individual narratives but collectively as cultural informants to construct an ethnography.

If Fulton can be read as an ethnographic informant, then his and other surgeons' diaries or compilations of correspondence can be read collectively as ethnographic data. Although the literature of first-person accounts by Civil War soldiers is abundant and growing as long-hidden or overlooked diaries and correspondence come to light, accounts by physicians represent a subgenre to this literature (discussed below). Most scholars comb diaries and correspondence for new evidence to illuminate major battles, campaigns, or notable personalities, or to capture the experience of the common soldier or civilian. That most diaries and correspondence were not subject to censorship heightens scholarly interest. Others read the same accounts to elicit insights about motivations, responses to events, and relationships with other soldiers, civilians, and their families to construct the wartime social milieu. Literature and American studies professor Daniel Aaron has observed, "The noble and shoddy story of those 'convulsive' days still lies buried in newspapers, magazines, diaries, memoirs, and official records."[5]

Historian James McPherson's study of why soldiers fought the war, based on an analysis of thousands of letters they wrote, prizes correspondence because of its immediacy, with none of the retrospection and reworking of personal narratives that veterans published as memoirs and regimental histories decades later, which "suffer from a critical defect: they were written for publication. Their authors consciously or subconsciously constructed their narratives with a public audience in mind."[6] Diarists may have had other audiences in mind, such as their families and descendants. Fulton's diary apparently does not suffer from this "critical defect," but he may have intended it as an *aide memoire* to create a later narrative, possibly for his young, new wife.

Exclusive of doctors' war memoirs written years after the fact, Fulton's diary keeps company with approximately thirty-five published diaries or collections of wartime letters by doctors. These books have been edited by scholars, descendants, amateur historians, or physicians with a Civil War interest. Most contain a thumbnail sketch of the military campaigns in which the diarist or correspondent participated. None of these books examines the physician within his (invariably *his*) cultural and professional milieu. Some books include implicit or explicit biases about the Civil War medical realm that, ironically, may denigrate the achievements of the diarists themselves by dismissing wartime medical practices as prescientific and not worthy of serious study.[7]

Taken singly, surgeons' diaries may disappoint some historians who expect them to feature explicit medical discussions. Certainly, in common with other soldiers, surgeons miss their homes and families and complain about camp conditions, but taken collectively as ethnographic data, their diaries and correspondence say much about the military medical culture. They reveal surgeons' observations about their lives, work, relationships, and values. Their diaries, for instance, reveal freedom of movement in and around camps that soldiers do not enjoy. Doctors have access to resources that soldiers do not, including hygienic oversight of entire campsites, the location and construction of sinks (latrines), and the location and preparation of cooking fires. Surgeons can command resources and people in ways that soldiers cannot. Surgeons can determine medical discharges and remove soldiers from duty. Surgeons enjoy liberal fraternization across the ranks. Their chain of command differs from that of soldiers: they report both to a military commander and to a medical director. They can, under some circumstances, legitimately address officers of high rank within or without their chain of command for medical purposes. They alone have the prerogative to invade bodies with tools or to require soldiers to consume possibly poisonous substances. No other edited, published diary or compilation of correspondence of federal surgeons explores these matters within a cultural perspective, analyzing these sources collectively and comparatively. Analyzing physicians' diaries as collective informant accounts may not present "a whole new world of historical investigation," as Thomas wrote, but doing so creates a thorough world of historical investigation.

SCHOLARLY ESSAYS

The ethnographer strives to share the experience of the informant. Surgeon Frederick Winsor, 49th Massachusetts Volunteers, captured the essence of participant observation: "To realize the surgeon's experience you must not only see with his eyes and hear with his ears, you must *feel* with him; for he and his patients are all *feeling*; they feel the suffering; he feels with the sense of touch, the skilled touch."[8]

To feel with Fulton requires a thought experiment. Readers are challenged to imagine the surgeon's role within America's worst health crisis. As close as the diary may bring the reader to feeling his experience, Fulton leaves some important matters largely unsaid, such as the presence of women in a medical context and relief efforts for the troops. Other matters, such as Fulton's relationships with other doctors and the medical hierarchy, may not be easy for most modern readers to grasp without interpretive help. To thus bring the reader closer to Fulton's world and experience, leading scholars have written the essays in part 2 to amplify aspects of his wartime work.

In chapter 8, Shauna Devine, medical historian and author of *Learning from the Wounded: The Civil War and the Rise of American Medical Science*, examines the professional and educational culture of physicians in army service. Her essay places Fulton within a professional medical community and elucidates how the war profoundly influenced his evolution as a medical practitioner. She illuminates the infrastructure innovations introduced by Surgeon General William A. Hammond, which shaped Fulton's career. Fulton learned medicine through medical college instruction and apprenticeship in an era with no prescribed standards for training and practice and no licensing. The army furnished the most rigorous system for standardization and supervision. This chapter also illuminates the nature of treating prevalent and challenging diseases among soldiers, such as typhoid and smallpox, diseases that Fulton discusses.

The two emblems of the physician's work are medicines and instruments. In chapter 9, Guy R. Hasegawa, a pharmacist and historian of Civil War pharmacy, illuminates the military doctor's management of medicines. The Union army Standard Supply Table carried about two hundred substances that could be compounded to make hundreds more. Fulton, in common with other physicians, probably administered medicines the army way and his own way. Hasegawa discusses the medical recipes that appear in the diary and speculates that they represented departures from standard medicines and may not have been administered during wartime. He also examines the text sources of the medicines named and links Fulton's ideology of *materia medica* (medicines) to his training at Jefferson Medical College. The actual preparation and administration of medicines must have occupied considerable time for both Fulton and his steward. What were the medicines most commonly prescribed during regimental sick call for common maladies? What medicines might Fulton have had the most confidence in prescribing? What medicines, therefore, best express Fulton's professional identity and function to sustain his authority? How were Fulton's prescriptions written and filled, and who compounded the medicines? Importantly, while we expect many medicines today to cure diseases, Fulton's aim was not to cure but, as Hasegawa states, "to reduce symptoms and correct imbalances in the body until the patient improved through nature taking its course."

In the diary, Fulton had little reason to mention his tools except to say that they were stolen in Gettysburg. In chapter 10, historian and Senior Curator James M. Edmonson of the Dittrick Medical History Center in Cleveland, Ohio, finds comparable Civil War medical instruments in his collection that speak to how they not only mended bodies but signified status and professional authority. Edmonson examines the organization and diversity of the surgeon's medical tools in relation to personal idiosyncrasy and habit, the tools used most often and retained close to hand, tools that were surely extensions of the surgeon's *feel*. What "tool skills" were required of Fulton? How did his tools augment the authority and prestige of his military rank? What did his tools signify to other soldiers about the expertise and abilities of the surgeon who may work on their bodies? Who made and sold instruments, where were they made, and how did surgeons procure them? Both Hasegawa's and Edmonson's essays help the reader realize Fulton not just as a diarist, but as a type character to most army soldiers: the doc, Sawbones, or sometimes "the butcher." We can see the doctor with his instruments and medicines not strictly as a professional whose paraphernalia served only utilitarian and prescribed purposes, but as a whole man, bound up with the uniform, his personality, his abilities, and his accessibility as a dispenser of wisdom about health.

Fulton says little about the presence of women in military medicine or in relief efforts such as the United States Sanitary Commission. In chapter 11, historian of nursing and registered nurse Barbra Mann Wall constructs the world of women in military health care that Fulton experienced. When Fulton tried to manage two makeshift hospitals in Gettysburg churches, he negotiated with and was aided by several townswomen, whom he named. If we could accompany Fulton during the Gettysburg battle, what other women would we see? Soldiers in one of the hospitals, St. Francis Xavier Catholic Church, widely praised nursing by Catholic nuns, although Fulton apparently did not encounter them during the battle. Fulton acknowledges the Catholic center of learning in Emmitsburg, Maryland, through which soldiers marched to Gettysburg, but who were these women, and how did Fulton admit them within his professional medical milieu? Wall offers a fascinating glimpse into the organization of battlefield first aid by women. How might Fulton have observed, interacted with, and benefitted from relief organizations and women as medical assistants?

Author of two major studies of the medical Civil War, *Intensely Human: The Health of the Black Soldier in the American Civil War* and *Marrow of Tragedy: The Health Crisis of the American Civil War*, physician and historian Margaret Humphreys examines Fulton's role in managing the nutrition of soldiers in chapter 12. Outside of his fruitless quest to have bread baked during the Gettysburg battle, Fulton does not discuss diet in detail. Diet, however, was medicine, and camp cooking fell within the surgeon's purview. How did Fulton understand the nutritional needs of the body? How did nineteenth-century physiology inform what foods were provided by the army to soldiers? What was the common diet of soldiers during the campaigns of Fulton's regiment? What part of his therapeutic regimen for sick or wounded soldiers concerns diet? How effective might Fulton have been in ensuring that soldiers ate healthily? Humphreys helps the reader imagine the demands on armies to stay fed. Civil War soldiers did not expect the army to supply all of their food. Soldiers had to forage, and they and their officers formed informal alliances with other soldiers to procure, store, and prepare meals, activities that required a great deal of time. Finally, Humphreys examines the army diet within the context of 1860s biochemistry.

To illuminate Fulton's world beyond the administration of wartime medicine, we must consider other matters on his mind that found their way into the diary. Historian Randall M. Miller, who has published widely on the Civil War and the political history of the United States, explores Fulton's political, ethical, and moral thinking in chapter 13. Fulton's frequent paeans to landscape and countryside say much about his Republican views, tied to beliefs about manliness, courage, loyalty, and a providential view of American destiny. His rapturous moments with nature's vistas reflect views shared by many who embraced the Union cause: free-soil ideology and an implicit promise that honest farm labor underpins the country's prosperity and hence its place as a refuge for freedom under divine guidance. Fulton had no sympathy for the secessionists whom he met in Virginia, especially when they complained about their ungrateful slaves. The war nevertheless tried Fulton's standards of Christian forbearance and generosity, particularly when he turned a blind eye to foraging and theft of rebel property. Miller's close reading of the diary, taken in context with the essays by the medical historians, sculpts a full man, professionally able within a complex moral universe.

WRITING AND READING THE DIARY

To record his wartime experience, Fulton obtained "Clothbound Clayton's Octavo Diary" for 1862, published by E. B. Clayton's Sons, Printers and Stationers, No. 157 Pearl Street, New York. Each page is headed by a single date and day of the week, followed by twenty-two ruled blank lines for personal information. The diary's small size permitted Fulton to write between three and seven words per line. His first entry is August 18, 1862, beginning on the diary page printed for January 1, 1862. Here he records the passing of his examination at the University of Pennsylvania for assistant surgeon and the first days of his mustering in at Camp Curtin. The last diary entry, for January 20–29, 1864, written in winter quarters in Virginia, concluded on the calendar page for November 4, 1862. From the first to last entry, Fulton clearly labeled the beginning of each day. Many pages carry inscriptions vertically in the margin to denote the subject of the entry, an attempt to create a reference system to locate topics. In the diary transcript chapters, the vertical label for a given page is enclosed within a pair of virgules (/ ... /).

Following the printed diary page for December 31, 1862, the diary contains forty-three blank, ruled pages. The next eighteen pages include Fulton's second narration of his Gettysburg experience. Three more blank pages follow, then eight pages of medical recipes (prescriptions, in our medical parlance). Considering the diary's age and the brittle, acidic pages characteristic of inexpensive nineteenth-century printing, it is remarkable that the diary is as intact as it is. It suffers from a damaged region about midspine, possibly a scorch from a flame. Something caused a burn or hole at the spine, which has not much affected the text, but some words on some pages are missing or indecipherable because of this wound.

The diary has remained with Fulton's family to the present, at this writing possessed by Fulton's great-granddaughter Brenda Hollands of Boylston, Massachusetts. The diary apparently has not been studied by scholars and has never been cited, although the Seminary Ridge Museum in Gettysburg, which opened in 2013, has exhibited it as a long-term loan with additional paraphernalia owned by Fulton (and still in possession of the Hollands family), a then-antique pistol (a flintlock upgraded to a percussion-cap mechanism) and a plate.

Fulton's handwriting challenges the reader with its lack of consistent punctuation and capitalization. He wrote in an idiosyncratic manner of staccato note-taking. Upper- and lowercase words alternate in see-saw fashion. In writing rapidly, he frequently struck the page with his pen tip. This habit of writing resembles tapping a telegraph key, alternating words with dots. The diary transcript presented in this volume retains Fulton's idiosyncrasies, except that the short lines demanded of the small pages are not retained. Indecipherable words are indicated, missing words are shown in brackets, and question marks within brackets indicate best guesses. Dots that may represent punctuation are shown, but other dots are not. Paragraph breaks represent the editor's discretion in segmenting the text for readability.

Whereas correspondence is addressed to an external audience, a diary is a dialogue with the self. Fulton's voice when the army is in camp touches on administrative issues and occasionally the maladies (and treatments) of his officer colleagues and soldiers. When his brigade experiences combat,

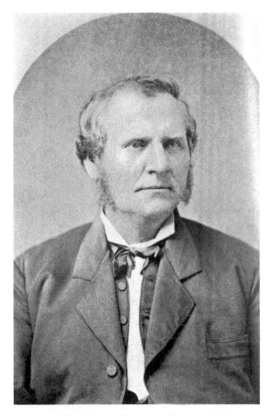

Figure 0.1. This image of James Fulton probably
dates to the 1870s. From Hugh R. Fulton, ed.,
Genealogy of the Fulton Family, Lancaster, PA, 1900.
Courtesy David Smith.

Fulton writes in a different voice, one concerned with describing the larger
environment of war, circumscribing his role within a narrative that he real-
izes is much larger than himself. He evidently wished his diary to record not
quotidian matters but memorable events and circumstances. He rarely struck
out a name or phrase; written in ink, the diary reflects his unedited thoughts.

The diary contains six distinctive features. First, the July 1–3 battle
marked Fulton's signal experience of the war. His brigade participated in
the opening actions of the battle west of Gettysburg at the McPherson farm.
Over the course of hours, the brigade fought an increasingly desperate battle
against an overwhelming Confederate force. Virtually all brigade officers
were killed or wounded. Before the brigade was ordered to conduct a fighting

retreat eastward to Seminary Ridge and then to Cemetery Hill immediately southeast of Gettysburg, Fulton was ordered to leave his regiment and make his way a mile east into the town to assume control over makeshift hospitals at Catholic and Presbyterian churches. The town itself became a chaotic battlefield as rebel forces entered and fought the federal troops street by street. Fulton's diary records his observations of the confusion, the movements of frightened civilians and retreating soldiers, and his engagement with townspeople who risked injury or death to help wounded troops. Fulton devoted the most words to these experiences on July 1, 1863. As a measure of the importance of his actions on July 1, decades later, Fulton published an account of the day for a veterans' newspaper, apparently drawing from his diary.

Second, Fulton wrote another narrative of the same Gettysburg experience. One is the diary itself and the other, written back to front (and upside down), seems intended as a fluent narrative of his Gettysburg experience on July 1, 1863. In this narrative, Fulton took care with sentence structure and punctuation, unlike the diary entries. Most likely, he wrote this in the months between his last entry in January 1864 and before he resigned in April. The narrative differs very little from the diary itself, but Fulton wrote retrospectively, effectively creating a memoir while the experience was fresh. This narrative aims to order the larger events in which Fulton participated. By the time he wrote the second account, he had had opportunity to reflect and discuss events with fellow soldiers. In it, he cited an article about Gettysburg from an English magazine published in 1863.

The third distinctive feature is an eight-page section at the end of the diary that records medical recipes. These recipes may have been written for specific soldiers in Fulton's regiment, or he may have recorded commonly used recipes in the diary for ease of reference. His frequently mentioned hospital steward (assistants to physicians who had pharmaceutical experience), Josiah L. Lewis (usually referred to as "Joe"), would have supervised the regimental pharmacy and prepared prescriptions as directed. The recipes are probably contemporary with the diary. For example, Fulton named Sergeant William S. Leach, Co. G, 143rd Pennsylvania, in connection with one recipe. Leach mustered in on September 18, 1862, but owing to disease or illness was invalided to the Veterans Reserve Corps on November 15, 1863. When Fulton was first assigned to the 150th Pennsylvania, after beginning his diary, he evidently flipped to the end to create separate pages headed by names of soldiers in the regiment. Perhaps he intended to record prescriptions for medicines under the names of the men for whom he prescribed them. Perhaps he intended to keep informal notes on the health of these men, which would have made the diary very unusual. Some recipes may have been written in the pocket diary by others, perhaps Lewis. Other surgeons recorded recipes in their diaries, but doing so was rare (because they would have recorded such information on official reports), and Fulton's list is longer than most.

The fourth distinctive feature is two hand-drawn maps showing the highlights of the Gettysburg battle (see maps 6, 7, 8, and 9). Fulton asked, or his commanding officer, Colonel Edmund L. Dana, 143rd Pennsylvania and commander of Second Brigade, volunteered to draw maps summarizing the events of the three days of fighting. Sketches in soldiers' diaries or correspondence are not rare, but the fact of Fulton engaging his commanding officer to draw one highlights the facility with which surgeons could communicate with senior officers. One sketch shows the position of Dana's troops and those of the enemy at roughly midafternoon on July 1 at McPherson's farm west of Gettysburg. The second sketch shows the town of Gettysburg and the area to the south along Cemetery Ridge extending to Little Round Top, where much of the decisive fighting occurred on July 2–3. By the end of July 1, Fulton had been ordered to leave the 143rd troops who were still fighting from a defensive position and enter Gettysburg to assume control over makeshift hospitals. From this time until July 4, when the battle ended, he was effectively a prisoner of the rebel army, unable to communicate with the rest of his brigade, which had reformed on Cemetery Hill south of town. Dana noted the locations of specific events such as the deaths of Major General John F. Reynolds (on July 1 close to where the 143rd took position) and Confederate Brigadier General William Barksdale. He also showed the locations of rebel forces on the second and third days. Dana's sketches, presumably drawn soon after the battle, appear within the very long diary entry for July 1. Fulton may have flipped several blank pages ahead and handed the diary to Dana for the sketches, and then written his diary entry around them. Dana's sketches are roughly accurate, given the circumstances under which he evidently drew them. The sketches show topography, roads, shifting positions of rebel troops, a few prominent landmarks, headquarters for Gens. George G. Meade and Robert E. Lee, and the deaths of Gens. Reynolds and Barksdale. Dana tried to show a dynamic tactical picture with troops on the move, so evidently he sketched (in ink) while describing his version of the battle to Fulton. The sketches, apparently done as a courtesy, were probably intended to give Fulton a comprehensive overview of the battle, most of which he was not able to observe.

Fifth, Fulton observed and commented on the environments through which he campaigned. Virginia's countryside interested him, not only because he compared the Virginia landscape with his home in Chester County, but because he was interested in farming. His frequent comments about the weather, however, can also be read as important to managing soldiers' health. Until recently, most scholars have treated the casual observations about weather and countryside in letters and diaries "as background rather than objects of analysis."[9] For the common soldier, however, the environment governed how he understood and managed his own mental and physical health. For the physician, these considerations may have mediated therapies for ill soldiers. Further, army regulations directed medical officers to observe and record meteorological phenomena, a task not required of other officers. As a farmer, Fulton may have recorded his observations as a matter of personal interest, but he also noticed how changing environments affected health. Fulton and his fellow soldiers "connected the visible changes in nature, which governed planting and harvesting, to the invisible worlds of their bodies and minds," as historian Kathryn Shively Meier has shown.[10] By observing different natural environments, Fulton and other soldiers, both Union and Confederate, disclosed cultural insights. For instance, Confederates marching into Pennsylvania were impressed with the small patchwork of fenced farms denoting individually owned domains, in contrast to the very large landholdings characteristic of Southern plantations. They may have envied their enemy's comparative autonomy as small property owners.[11]

The sixth feature is Fulton's recording of the first public memorialization of the Gettysburg battle, the Gettysburg Address of President Abraham Lincoln and the dedication of the National Cemetery. On November 19, 1863, while he was camped at Warrenton Junction, Virginia, Fulton recorded the dedication of the National Cemetery as "a step highly to be commended as a testimonial of Respect to the Many departed heroes that fell" and expected that "it will be Something to attract visitors from Every Nation Every clime to the great Battlefield of America—And there do homage to the heroism of her Departed great." Although Fulton expresses his views within the sentimental

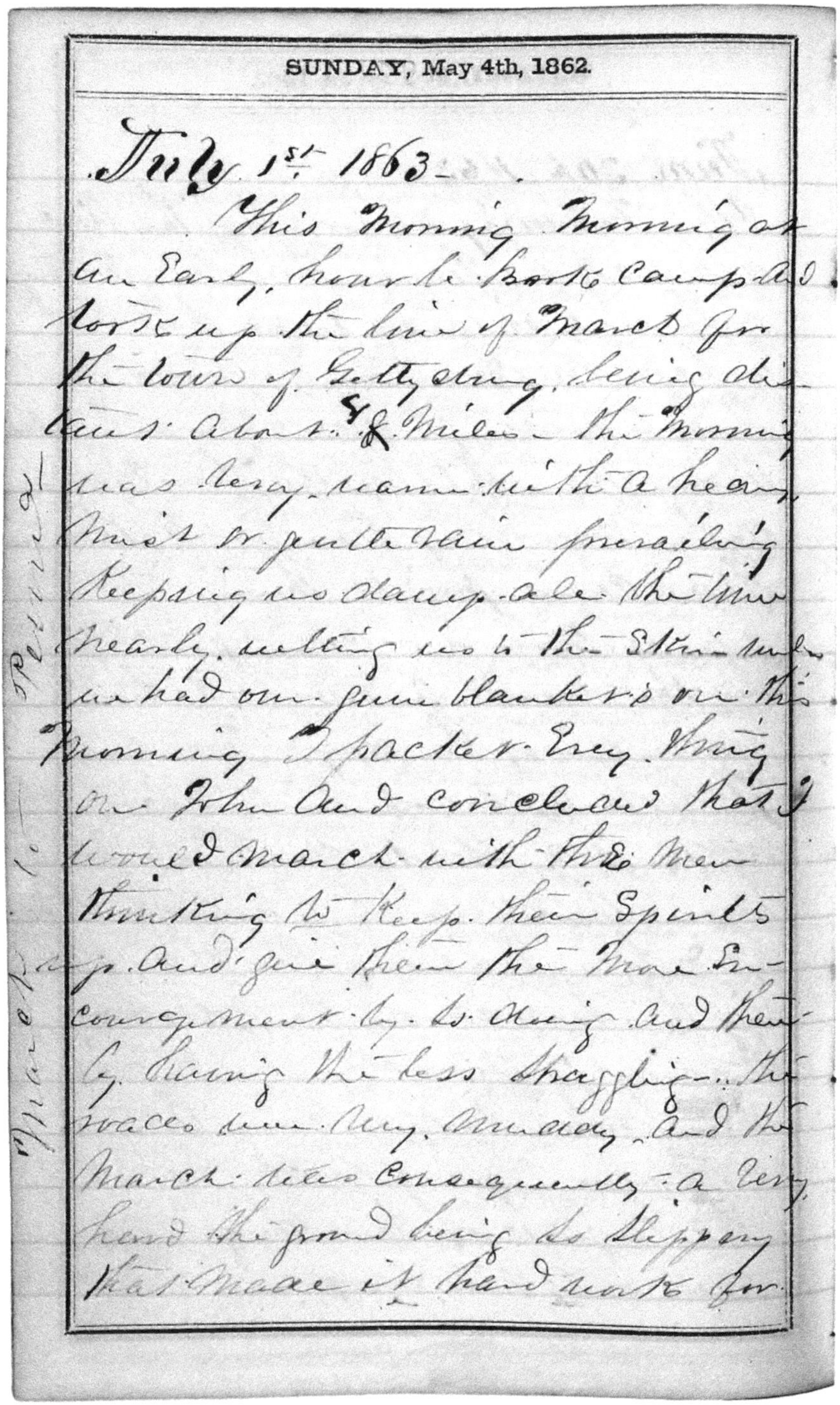

July 1st 1863 –

This morning morning at
an early hour be broke camp and
took up the line of march for
the town of Gettysburg, being di-
tance about ... Miles – the morning
was very warm with a heavy
mist or gentle rain prevailing
keeping us damp all the time
nearly, wetting us to the skin unless
we had our gum blankets on this
morning I packed every thing
on John and concluded that I
would march with the men
thinking to keep their spirits
up and give them the more encouragement by so doing and there
by having the less straggling the
roads were very muddy and the
march tedious consequently a very
hard the ground being so slippery
that made it hard work for

Figure 0.2. The beginning of Fulton's diary entry for the Gettysburg battle, July 1, 1863.

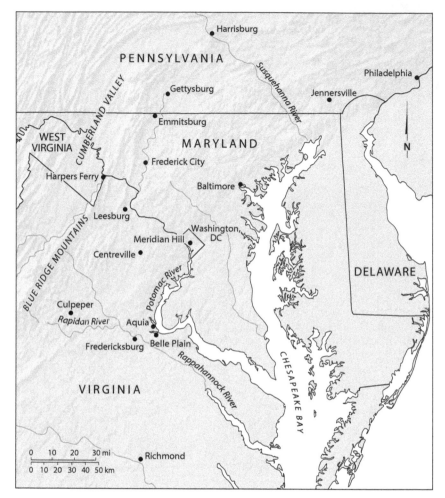

Map 0.1. Overview map: Virginia, Maryland, Pennsylvania

parlance of the time, it is remarkable that within the same diary pages, he experiences pivotal and momentous events and later records the first memorialization of the same events and reflects on them.[12]

Unlike his contemporary Union army doctors, as expressed in their correspondence or diaries, Fulton rarely criticized others or engaged in ad hominem thoughts. He did not express ambition for higher rank, although he readily assumed extra responsibilities and duties when assigned. He presented no portraits of other personalities, yet a reader can infer that he enjoyed the camaraderie of brigade officers, not just those of his own regiment. Views he expressed about patriotism may strike modern readers as sentimental and even trite, but such expressions were common within wartime discourse at this time and should not be read as insincere. For instance, while in Washington in late 1862, Fulton derogated critics and Southern sympathizers:

> It seems that men can go to any length with their treasonable declarations— and use [every] means to injure the cause of the Union—I only hope hard soon such Men May be silenced And go sneaking to their dens of infamy unnoticed—and unheeded their names handed down to posterity an Everlasting disgrace not only to themselves but their posterity—Our nation is certainly tried as by fire ... it certainly will not be long untill there will be something decisive known in regard to our countrys future—it is to be hoped that our nation punished Enough for her many transgressions—And that the good time is not far distant when peace Shall again bless this people—[13]

By comparison, Union Surgeon Thomas S. Hawley, MD, wrote to his mother sentiments that Fulton might have shared:

> This great Civil War has ... opened a new field for heroism and pure self-sacrificing patriotism which is in my opinion one of the greatest virtues of an honorable citizen of this great free and glorious republic. ... The sunny hours of happy youth are past, never to be recalled. The sun advancing rapidly to the zenith of my manhood arouses me from the pleasant fanciful dreaming life of youth and loudly calls to action. The stern battles of life must be fought and won.[14]

The diary reveals Fulton as curious, sociable, eager to perform competently and with a professional demeanor, conscientious, and acutely observant. His diary sometimes reads as a travel account by turns wry and ironic, at other moments a naturalist's notebook. Comments about family and home are virtually absent: presumably, Fulton reserved family matters for private correspondence, none of which apparently survives. Readers should not expect substantive medical discussions in the diary: army surgeons were required to complete and submit to higher authority daily, monthly, and quarterly reports of the sick and wounded, requisitions, accounts of the employment and pay of hospital stewards, nurses, and matrons, and records of food purchased and dispensed.[15] It is not surprising, then, that his diary records what Fulton's reports do not: impressions of friendships and frustrations with other army doctors, military strategy, and civilians with whom he came in contact. He wrote observations about military leaders and repeated political gossip probably overheard around the campfire.

James Fulton does not assume much dimension in the historical record until he entered a prestigious school. In terms of receiving an education, Fulton was fortunate to live in a rural zone between growing Philadelphia and the Delaware border that featured a predominant Quaker community. The Society of Friends established many schools there; the primary business of local meetings was to set up schools. Apart from schooling and Fulton's war service, he remained close to the family's first abode in Chester County, which included a farm that saw the unsettled era leading to American independence, to the Civil War, and into the twentieth century.

Fulton's ancestor, John Fulton (b. 1713), a Scot, emigrated in 1753 to America and settled in Chester County in 1762. His grandson, James J. Fulton, married Nancy Ramsey and fathered several children, including James, who was born on November 12, 1832. James, the eldest, had three brothers, William T., Joseph M., and Hugh R., and two sisters who died in infancy, Rachel and Jane. The 1850 census for East Nottingham, Chester County, lists the Fulton household as consisting of parents James and Nancy, son James, the eldest, at sixteen years; William at fourteen; Joseph at ten; and Hugh at six. A relation of Nancy's, Sarah Ramsey, age forty-two, also was part of the household. Throughout the lifetime of James Fulton and his later family, his household typically numbered many people, including family, servants, and others. As the children reached adulthood, some remained in the Fulton household for years, while others moved to other small townships nearby. The townships within which the Fulton family flourished—East and West Nottingham, Penn, New London—are contiguous at the southwest corner of the county and border both Maryland and Delaware. Before and during the war, this border was crucial to the enforcement of the Fugitive Slave Act, with African Americans fleeing enslavement coming into the county pursued by both federal authorities and slave owners or their representatives.[16]

James's brother William, who was born in West Nottingham in the house his grandfather had lived in, worked as a farmer, blacksmith, schoolteacher, and lawyer. He read law with Thaddeus Stevens, already a famous lawyer and abolitionist. Likely the law instruction occurred after Stevens' first term (and re-election) in the House of Representatives but before he returned to the House in 1858. William may have studied with him when Stevens practiced in Lancaster. Stevens had defended men who fought and killed a slave owner trying to recover a runaway slave, so his notoriety may have become national. James Fulton and his brothers appear to have supported abolitionism, if passively. During the war, William was recruited into Company E, Purnell Legion Maryland Infantry, and rose to the rank of major until dismissed from the army for a physical disability. He resumed his practice of law until the Confederate army invaded Pennsylvania in 1863, when he re-entered military service as a first lieutenant, Company A, 29th Pennsylvania (state militia). He and his brother James met occasionally during the war.

Younger brothers Hugh and Joseph also participated in the war. All brothers held the view in common that loyalty to the United States was paramount. They were Presbyterian and worked in socially acceptable middle-class roles, from storekeeper to attorney to physician. Hugh worked in house construction and in the "chrome [chromium] banks [mines]" before the war. In June 1863, having come of age, he enlisted in Company G, Pennsylvania Six-Month Volunteers (later the 187th Pennsylvania), and upon discharge joined the Fifth United States Artillery of the regular army. Achieving the rank of sergeant, he saw combat at the battles of the Wilderness and Spotsylvania Courthouse, and later at Cold Harbor, Petersburg, and Sailor's Creek, all in Virginia. Joseph, too, entered the army, as a corporal, in 1863, also joining the 29th Pennsylvania, and mustered out in August 1863, after the invasion scare had ended.

Scant records allow us to pick up the thread of James's life during the 1850s. A family history privately published for the Fulton family in 1900 includes a poem by brother Hugh in honor of "Dr. James Fulton 50th Birthday," and if it can be trusted, presents the boy James as a budding farmer who learned stonemasonry until an eye injury turned him to teaching following a stint at Delaware College.[17] James and his brothers attended "common schools" (a nineteenth-century term for public schools) during their early years. Later, James and William attended the Jordan Bank Academy in East Nottingham, directed by Evan Pugh from 1847 to 1853. Raised in the nearby township of Oxford, Pugh (1828–1864) was a successful education leader and agricultural chemist, and left his school to attend German universities, where he obtained the degree of Doctor of Physical Science from Goettingen University before returning in 1859 to become president of the Agricultural College of Pennsylvania. This institution transformed, partially with Pugh's leadership and political advocacy, into Pennsylvania State University. Pugh's wife, Rebecca, operated the Pleasant Valley Seminary for Girls next door to Jordan Bank.

An advertisement for Jordan Academy promises that its teaching "embraces all the branches of a thorough English education, including the art of phonographic reporting and chemical analysis." The advertisement also promised courses in mineralogy, geology, and botany.[18] Local newspapers in later years reported recollections of former Jordan Bank students, but an anonymous poem titled "Education" (and sung to the tune of "Uncle Sam's Farm," a popular song about westward expansion), attributed to the Jordan Bank Academy and published in March 1853, extols the virtues of learning.[19] Probably written by a student to display his mastery of language and form, the poem charmingly conveys an adolescent's attempt publicly to profess his love of knowledge with a hint of school spirit:

> Of all important subjects, in the East or in the West,
> The theme of Education, is the greatest and the best;
> It treats of all creation, and its banners are unfurled,
> With a general invitation, to the people of the world.
> *Chorus:* Then come along, come along, don't stay away;
> Leave the roads to Ignorance—leave them all to-day;
> Our benches are long enough, O don't you hear the call?
> For Jordan Bank is ready now, to educate you all.[20]

A program for the Academy's public semiannual exhibition on March 12, 1852, lists orations, performances, and other presentations by students, including "capital punishment," "Mexican War," and "Ossian's Address to the Sun." James Fulton appears twice, first for an oration on "Union of the States" and second as one of three students performing a dialogue on "Doctoring."[21] Perhaps this exhibition attests not only to Fulton's patriotic sentiments but also to an early interest in medicine. After Jordan Bank, Fulton attended Delaware College in Newark, Delaware, precursor to the University of Delaware. The Delaware connection may have had Chester County roots, as the college's precursor was a Presbyterian "free school" (public school) in New London Township, founded in 1743 to educate clergy. Fulton's postwar life included active participation in the Presbyterian church, so perhaps religion dictated this choice of school in Delaware. The free school relocated to Newark in 1843 and became Delaware College, later a land-grant institution.[22]

While Fulton's curriculum at Delaware College and his tenure there remain unknown (although brother Hugh's poem about Fulton says that he studied Latin and Greek), he evidently sustained an interest in medicine and entered Jefferson Medical College in Philadelphia for the 1856–57 course, followed by a year's break, and returned for a second year, 1858–59, and received his MD degree. During his medical study, his home community became a political fire zone between North and South. Antagonisms between unionists and those with Southern sympathies—who were numerous in Pennsylvania—fueled ostracism, riots, vandalism, and worse. Events in Fulton's region received national attention, such as the Christiana Riot of September 11, 1851, involving armed resistance to the Fugitive Slave Law, which not only permitted slave owners to hunt escaped slaves anywhere, but *required* citizens to participate in returning people to slavery.

A party of slave catchers tried to recover four former slaves and encountered violent resistance at a farm in Christiana, Sadsbury Township, in adjacent Lancaster County. A few years later, in 1855, Passmore Williamson, a radical abolitionist and member of the Pennsylvania Anti-Slavery Society, arranged to hide Jane Johnson, an enslaved woman traveling with her children through Pennsylvania with her owner. Johnson was duly hidden beyond her owner's reach, although Williamson did not know her whereabouts. He was removed from Chester County to stand trial in Philadelphia, where he was imprisoned for refusing to disclose Johnson's whereabouts. While serving one hundred days in Moyamensing Prison in Philadelphia, he famously received celebrity visitors, including Frederick Douglass and Harriet Tubman. Williamson's guest book for his prison visitors is now a treasured artifact in the collection of the Chester County Historical Society.[23]

Fulton and his family certainly followed these events with apprehension. That their community did not share proslavery views was evident in a local news filler that slyly hints that such views were not welcome, especially immediately after Fort Sumter in April 1861:

JENNERVILLE.—A correspondent informs us that there are a few tories in that neighborhood and that one "Minister of the Gospel" takes occasion to show his secession proclivities in the pulpit. We should suppose that such a minister would be left to preach to very sparse congregations.[24]

The newly doctored James Fulton could not ignore such stresses, because even Jefferson Medical College and other local medical schools experienced battle lines drawn between students from North and South. Contemporary medical student and later assistant army surgeon William Williams Keen began to carry a concealed pistol in fear of bullying from Southern students.[25] In response to an offer from the nascent Confederate states to fund medical training for its students ensconced in Northern schools and in anticipation of a military need, in 1859, hundreds of students left their Philadelphia medical schools and paraded en masse to a train to Richmond, Virginia, to be taken to Southern schools, a widely publicized event.[26]

Although Fulton had received his medical doctor degree and was working with an established physician, he had another concern on his mind: courtship and marriage. The 1860 census lists him as living in Jennerville (also Jennersville) in Penn Township at the home of elderly Daniel and Albina Johnson; their son Hoopes Johnson and his wife, Hannah; daughter Anna M. Johnson, age eighteen; two other women; and two other men. Fulton's first medical practice was based here, in a town named for the discoverer of vaccination, Edward Jenner.[27] On May 16, 1861, in New London, James and Anna married.[28] Their first child, a daughter, was born on September 25, 1862, a month after James reported for military duty.

ANSWERING THE CALL TO THE HEALING ARTS

James Fulton may have sat in the audience at Jefferson Medical College on October 17, 1856, to hear Dr. Samuel D. Gross give an inaugural address to faculty and students at the beginning of the course in surgery. Gross's image remains well known today because he occupies a divinely illuminated position at the center of a surgical amphitheater in the 1875 painting by Thomas Eakins, *The Gross Clinic*. Gross (1805–1884) had become a nationally renowned teacher and surgeon by this time, having published the first treatise on pathological anatomy in the United States, and he also helped found the American Medical Association. By the time Fulton received his MD, Gross had published his monumental *System of Surgery*, which was consulted into the twentieth century.[29] In his lecture, Gross urges his listeners to avoid compartmentalizing surgery as a mechanical activity divorced from medicine as philosophy and science. Thus, he emphasizes "the indispensable importance of a thorough knowledge of the principles of medicine to the successful practice of surgery":

> My object will be to make surgeons of you in the true sense of the term; not mere operators, artists, mechanics, or hewers of flesh, or, to use a felicitous modern expression, mere knife-men; but rational, philosophical practitioners, physicians as well as surgeons, men qualified for every emergency involving human suffering and human life . . . Surgery should at all times be conservative, but especially should it be so at the present day, when our minds are so much enlightened by the march of science. Its aim should be to preserve, not to mutilate and destroy, and yet it should always be ready and willing to obey the mandate of the intelligent and conscientious practitioner.[30]

A pre-eminent educational institution during Fulton's day and now, Jefferson Medical College was the first to open a clinic, but at the time did not feature a hospital, library, or laboratory. It did, however, showcase some of Philadelphia's brightest medical minds. At the same lecture possibly sat Thomas D. Mütter, MD, in 1856 an emeritus professor of surgery, later founder of the Mütter Museum of The College of Physicians of Philadelphia, and a pioneer of plastic surgery. His colleague, Joseph Pancoast, MD, may also have heard the lecture. A professor of "General, Descriptive, and Surgical Anatomy," Pancoast had been physician-in-chief of Children's Hospital in Philadelphia, the first hospital in the country to specialize in children's health. Robley Dunglison, MD, dean of Jefferson Medical College, had studied in Edinburgh and Paris (where he met Thomas Jefferson) and reputedly exercised a mind that "preferred to analyze the researches of others, and base his conclusions on accumulated evidence," according to a history of the college. John K. Mitchell, MD, another faculty member known for his "original thought and thorough research," taught the practice of medicine. His son, S. Weir Mitchell, MD, who had begun to practice medicine before the war, became a contract army surgeon and later helped found American neurology. Franklin Bache, MD, whose province was chemistry at Jefferson, was a great-grandson of Benjamin Franklin and served as a surgeon during the War of 1812, "a man of absolute precision." Finally, Charles D. Meigs, MD, specialized in obstetrics, and Robert M. Huston, MD, taught "Materia Medica and General Therapeutics."[31]

W. W. Keen described Gross as "tall and handsome, with a fine presence and a fine address." Pancoast he found to be "one of the most brilliant, self-possessed, daring surgeons" he had ever seen. Dunglison was "encyclopedic in his knowledge," and Meigs's "vivid scientific imagination saw what was revealed to colder minds only after many years." Despite this luminous faculty, Keen found that Jefferson's students were a mixed lot, some having had, like Fulton, a substantial education, while others "came directly from the plough or the anvil." During the academic session, students were expected to attend all lectures for one year and then repeat the sequence. Still, outside of chemistry experiments and the twice-weekly clinic with patients, Keen said that "[t]here was no demonstrative teaching."[32]

In 1859, when Fulton received his degree, Charles Darwin's *On the Origin of Species* appeared, and Jefferson Medical School matriculated more students (630) than any other medical school anywhere in the country. At this time, dramatically for the country, John Brown and a few followers tried to incite a slave uprising at Harper's Ferry, Virginia, only to be caught, tried, and executed. Brown had become a cause célèbre who excited much political debate nationally. In December, provoked by Brown, Hunter H. McGuire, MD, who had graduated from the Medical College of Virginia and was furthering his education in Philadelphia, organized and led the mass exodus of about two hundred medical students from Jefferson and the University of Pennsylvania to the Southern states. Jefferson lost half of its medical students overnight. McGuire himself joined the Confederate army and saw much action at Gettysburg and other battles. He amputated General Thomas J. "Stonewall" Jackson's arm in 1863. Fulton was doubtless aware of these matters, although he had received his MD degree before Brown's raid.[33]

After receiving his MD, Fulton returned home to run a farm and a medical practice, still under his preceptor, Thomas H. Thompson, but he must have considered the probable impact of war—which many people predicted as inevitable—on his country, community, and family. Once he had applied for an examination to be an army surgeon, events happened quickly. Under the tenure of Surgeon General William Hammond, the examination process was daunting. Sitting for the examination required both oral and written components over the course of several days. Applicants had to show knowledge of current thinking about sanitation and hygiene, broad knowledge of history, geography, languages, and natural philosophy, and take a written examination in the various branches of medicine, including *materia medica,* surgery, anatomy, and chemistry.[34]

Army medical regulations required an examining board of not fewer than three medical officers, all appointed by the Secretary of War. The board was charged with examining candidates between ages twenty-one and twenty-eight to assess their "moral habits, professional acquirements, and physical qualifications."[35] The army also authorized the Secretary of War to select a noncommissioned officer to serve as hospital steward known "to be temperate, honest, and in every way reliable, as well as sufficiently intelligent, and skilled in pharmacy."[36] William Mervale Smith, surgeon, 85th New York, recalled the examination. On March 23, 1863, Smith took a four-hour examination on hygiene and anatomy but found the questions "often more abstract than practical." The next day, he was examined for four hours on practice and felt exhausted at the end. The next day's four hours were on surgery, with specific questions touching on fractures, treatment of the hydrocele (watery fluid accumulation around the testicles), and hemorrhage following amputation. The penultimate, fourth day "of this tedious examination" included the questions, "What were the causes of the last war with Great Britain; in what year did it commence; in what year was the treaty of peace signed, and who were the commissioners who signed the treaty?" and "Describe one species in each class of the vertebrate animals."[37]

Appendix A lists the questions Fulton was likely asked. Having passed the examination, Fulton was thrust into a military world.

THE MILITARY MEDICAL CULTURE

Per army regulations, a surgeon was "charged with the whole sanitary care of his corps." Surgeons served as the commanding officer's key counsel on where to encamp, how to organize a camp, and how best to realize good health through diet. When in battle, they quickly and carefully attended to incoming patients at field stations, promoted triage to manage cases, and arranged for ambulance transportation for the severe ones. The army's handbook for surgeons states:

> [The surgeon] is not to suppose that he is to sit in his tent, and when called
> upon to see a patient, he is to repair to the bedside of the sick, prescribe
> and retire, as in civil life. On the contrary, he is most valuable when having

carefully reflected upon the laws of Hygiene, so that he has them at fingers'
ends, he is ready to apply them to the emergency before him, so as to afford
the troops under his immediate charge, the greatest possible security against
the invasion of disease. Nothing so much embarrasses operations in a campaign, as a large sick report.[38]

Surgeons in the United States Army differed in status and organizational
relationships from line officers and soldiers, the ones who did the fighting.
Army surgeons wore uniforms and participated in most army rituals, such
as appearance on parade for inspection, but owing to their profession, they
managed soldiers' lives in intimate ways. Surgeons respected two chains of
command, one administrative, one operational. Surgeons reported to their
regimental commanders (operational) but also negotiated an administrative chain of command that extended to the surgeon general. The surgeon's
supplies, for instance, were procured through medical purveyors, doctors
tasked with buying medical items on the market or from designated facilities
(government-run laboratories in which standardized medicine production
was a wartime innovation). Division or brigade surgeons supported and
tasked regimental medical staff, but the regimental commander had paramount authority. Army quartermasters met nonmedical supply needs.

Each year of the war witnessed innovations in medical management. An
ambulance corps developed; a medical cadet system was established, a precursor status to assistant surgeon. Bureaucracy became more bureaucratic.
"Red tape" was an expression well understood during the Civil War. By 1865,
the medical hierarchy had become diverse and specialized. The regular army
had its surgeons and assistant surgeons; the volunteer regiments, which
contributed most of the soldiers, had surgeons and assistant surgeons; state
governors sometimes appointed regimental surgeons and their assistant surgeons; acting assistant surgeons and civilian contractors were appointed to
remedy the chronic shortage of doctors; and the Veterans Corps had its own
medical personnel. Outside of this structure, the quasi-governmental relief
organization, the United States Sanitary Commission, hired its own physicians, who evaluated and reported on the military management of medical
affairs and extended direct aid to relieve battlefield suffering, particularly in
the form of paid and volunteer women nurses.[39]

Union army assistant surgeons carried the rank of lieutenant, while surgeons, including brigade surgeons or those assigned to division hospitals,

generally wore the rank of major. Relatively few doctors earned the rank of lieutenant colonel, colonel, or above. The attribution of rank, however, did not necessarily mean that medical officers commanded soldiers. They were empowered to assign soldiers to hospitals, determine fitness for duty, or recommend discharges for medical disability. Hospital stewards assisted doctors, noncombatants whose rank was equivalent to noncommissioned officers (sergeants). Ideally, the steward was a pharmacist because of the primary responsibility to prepare prescriptions of medicine, administer the drug supply, supervise hospital wards and camp cooking and cleanliness, and assist the surgeon in treating ill or wounded men. Medical orderlies and ambulance personnel rounded out the medical retinue, except for nurses. To a soldier at the beginning of the war, "nurse" connoted a soldier, untrained in medical skills, physically unfit to participate in combat, assigned to provide general help in a hospital setting. By the end of the war, the word connoted a woman, paid or volunteer, who performed paraprofessional and administrative services in hospitals (see chapter 11).[40]

Because surgeons and assistant surgeons were officers, they were expected to make friends and alliances within this social stratum. Although their fellow officers, with few exceptions, worked at drill to cement their leadership with their troops and evolve a common standard of performance in combat, all officers participated in a common social arena. Surgeon James D. Benton, 111th and 98th New York, wrote to his father that he was acquainted with many surgeons in different regiments, and "in camp some of them are men of the best education and some just the other way but in general they are a fine set of men."[41] Other doctors contended with a lonelier existence. Surgeon William Mervale Smith found "no mind to mate with mine among the officers of the regiment. There are most excellent men among them, but none with whom my mind can hold that communion & fellowship for which I so much long. I walk in restless idleness the grounds in front of my quarters every evening—lonely & weary of the slowly passing hours."[42]

Social bonding was deepened by living and mess arrangements. Doctors shared tents with fellow officers. Tent mates tried to establish some homely comforts if time permitted: they might forage for furniture from abandoned homes, construct a fireplace, or "liberate" fence rails to make a floor. Fulton refers to several social functions (such as a Christmas party in 1863), and he, in common with other doctors, participated in a mess, a small group of officers who shared common cooking and eating arrangements and jointly paid for food and its preparation. Hospital Steward and later Surgeon Thomas S. Hawley wrote to his parents about his comfortable messing situation:

> Dr. R. and myself commenced messing at our tents last week and have had so far a pleasant time. We have a good mess with teapot and all the necessary [items] for nutrition for cooking. Also stoneware plates & tea cups. All in order. We must purchase all the victuals but can live for $2.00 or $2.50 per week. The mess charges $4.00 for week. Bill of fare for breakfast—coffee, sugar, light bread . . . We now procure fruits, etc., from the Sanitary Commission as there is a depot there.[43]

At the beginning of the war, citizens could consult physicians of multiple philosophical approaches to human health. The Union army exclusively selected physicians with a common ideology of medical practice. Under Surgeon General Hammond, the army desired allopathic or "regular" physicians (those who prescribed medicines that produced symptoms opposite to those produced by the disease), as opposed to homeopaths, Thomsonians, or eclectics. Army surgeons, all regulars, likely trained at common institutions, and a loose fraternity existed, as it did in the Confederate medical service. Union and Confederate surgeons shared a consensus about clinical practice and promoted common therapies. Of the other philosophies, homeopaths understood disease symptoms to be evidence of the body's attempt to regain equilibrium of its "vital force," and accepted the principle that like cures like. In this view, a medicine that produces given symptoms in a healthy person can be effective when used on a sick person with the same symptoms. Thomsonians, named for herbalist Samuel Thomson, eschewed allopathic and homeopathic remedies and promoted botanical medicines. Eclectics fused Native American plant-based and European traditions of healing.[44] The Surgeon General's Office irregularly issued circulars that prescribed various practices and techniques and even published its own medical handbooks.[45] Although Fulton did not mention any such activities in his diary, Union army physicians were encouraged to perform scientific studies in addition to keeping soldiers healthy. Among the war's scientific achievements were the increasing emphasis placed on autopsies, the use of microscopy, and photomicrography of cellular tissue.

At encampments when soldiers experienced days of discipline and drill, doctors maintained a different schedule of holding sick call, attending to hospital patients, or handling administrative duties such as paperwork and the procurement of supplies. The general orders book of a regiment raised in Pennsylvania at roughly the same time as Fulton's brigade was organized, the 124th Pennsylvania Infantry, offers a glimpse at the daily routine that must have been familiar to Fulton. This nine-month regiment organized during summer 1862, recruited in Chester County and Delaware, and received initial training at Camp Curtin in Harrisburg. It saw action at Antietam in September 1862, and Chancellorsville in early 1863, after which its soldiers mustered out.[46] The extant orders book of the 124th Pennsylvania, issued by Headquarters, Second Brigade, First Division, XII Corps, contains fifty-seven directives, of which only six explicitly address medical matters, from the assignment of surgeons to transportation of medical supplies to camp cleanliness. All orders issued by the commander of the 124th that pertain to medical matters were intended to integrate the organization and management of medical matters into military routine so that the lading and unlading of medical stores on the march corresponded to the movement of all other materiel and its deployment as necessary.

General Order Four mandated the following daily schedule, weekends excepted:

Reveille at daybreak
[?] at 5 ½ am
Morning roll call
Squad drills, 6–7am
Surgeon's call, 6 ½ am
Breakfast 7am
Morning report 7 ½ am
Inspection of qtrs.
Mount guard 9m
Squad drill 10 ½–11 ½
Noon call and Division 12
Drill of officers 1 ¼ pm to 4 ½ pm
Dress parade, first call 5
Second call 5pm 10 mins
Supper 6
School of instruction 7 ½
Tattoo 8 ½
Roll call immediately after
Taps 9pm[47]

This schedule enforced the discipline of a military day with limited leisure and much emphasis on mastering drill and enforcing discipline and the
authority of the chain of command. While doctors did not participate in drill,
their relationship with soldiers began when performing physical examinations of prospective recruits in a volunteer regiment. Army regulations were
explicit about how surgeons were to conduct examinations, even if in practice
surgeons could be superficial:

> In passing a recruit the medical officer is to examine him stripped; to see that
> he has free use of all his limbs; that his chest is ample; that his hearing, vision,
> and speech are perfect; that he has no tumors, or ulcerated or extensively
> cicatrized legs; no rupture or chronic cutaneous affection; that he has not
> received any contusion, or wound of the head, that may impair his faculties;
> that he is not a drunkard; is not subject to convulsions; and has no infectious
> disorder, nor any other that may unfit him for military service.[48]

Surgeons' relationships with the bodies of soldiers continued through
sick or surgeon's call. Surgeon's call required all soldiers who considered
themselves unfit for duty to report to the medical tent. Fulton and his assistants examined each soldier and made a determination about whether the
soldier was fit to return to duty, required hospitalization, or needed medicine.
This evolution may have taken several hours, depending on the number of
troops who reported themselves ill. Chronic complaints such as diarrhea,
constipation, muscular aches, or breathing difficulties constituted the routine problems. Doctors wrote certificates for soldiers too ill to perform duties
as their ticket of admission to hospitals. Fulton would not have had absolute
discretion in this work: issuance of an excessive number of certificates, in a
regimental commander's view, could become the basis for disciplinary action
against the doctor. Accidents and disease constituted the maladies common
to military camps. Some surgeons gained a reputation for conservatism and
even lack of human feeling by returning most self-declared sick soldiers to
duty, while other soldiers feigned illness in order to avoid it. How did Fulton
manage this essential daily duty? In the only known memoir by a member
of the 143rd Pennsylvania Volunteers, Corporal Avery Harris, Company B,
recounted an anecdote about Fulton at sick call during February 1864:

> I was weak ... and I laid down along the tent of the dispensary to await my
> turn and while lying there an idea came into my head. After the last man had

been served, I got up slowly and went in. Hello corporal! Thought I was all through. See your tongue please. I stuck out my tongue, and Fulton turned to the steward with the same old prescription, when I said to him, doctor, can you not by a change of treatment get me out of this? I don't want to die like a dog here in my quarters.

No! said he, we are not allowed such treatment as you need and if I had you home in civil life, I could cure you, but there is one thing I can do for you corporal, I am going to order an ambulance for a fellow in another company and I will send you with him to the general hospital. By your life doctor, I would prefer to stay in camp. There was some starring [*sic*] at me by both Surgeon Fulton and [Josiah] Lewis the steward who was a rough fellow and exclaimed that's a hell of an idea. There isn't another man in camp but would jump at the chance to go to the general hospital. Fulton asked me why I objected to going to the general hospital and I told him my reasons were private or at least personal, but that I thanked him for the offer to send me when he said, 'I can't excuse you from duty unless you report at the sick call.' I then said to him that if the other corporals did not object to doing my duty I would be compelled to go. And thus the matter ended. I believe today that I am thankful I did not go to the general hospital, though not one man in a thousand suffered what I suffered during the following campaign.[49]

The anecdote represents the negotiation that must frequently have taken place between doctors and soldiers. It speaks to the necessity for surgeons to think quickly on their feet not only to prescribe a therapy for a malady but to get a psychological gauge on a soldier the doctor was likely to see again. These interactions also served as an assertion of the surgeon's prerogative to supersede the authority of line officers in controlling the soldier's body. In a letter to his parents, Surgeon James D. Benton wrote, "The authority of a surgeon over sick men is supreme and when either officer or man is excused from duty by them no one however high in military authority can with safety interfere with it."[50]

Some maladies seemed so common that doctors at sick call offered some medicines in assembly-line fashion, as remembered by Union soldier John D. Billings:

The proverbial prescription of the average army surgeon was quinine, whether for stomach or bowels, headache or toothache, for a cough or for lameness, rheumatism or fever and ague. Quinine was always and everywhere prescribed with a confidence and freedom which left all other medicines far in the rear.[51]

Doctors were the experts of last resort in matters pertaining to animals, mainly horses and mules. Veterinary surgeons were sparse, and surgeons were expected to pull a bad tooth, apply salve or bandage to a wound, or perform some minor surgery. Diseases could also consume hoofed animals, perhaps necessitating their killing and burial. Approximately one million horses and mules died in wartime service: their large corpses appear in numerous wartime photographs, poignant evidence of combat's rapacious and random killing. The rigors of the campaign and combat entailed a high body count for animals. Surgeon William Mervale Smith recorded the loss of one horse, his own, which attests to the close relationships between soldiers and camp animals. After a battle, he dismounted and noticed that "Kit" was ailing.

> [S]he hung her head as I had never seen her before. I sent for a farrier [and] the man done all he could for her, but she grew rapidly worse and died . . . Poor Kit—dear Kit—good Kit, how much I shall miss you. She was the superior of any horse I ever owned, and the equal of any I have known in the service, where both man & beast are tried to the utmost limits of their endurance. With this tribute to thy worth & excellence, and lying between and near to, two rebels slain in their flight from the battlefield . . . I leave thee forever— peace to thy ashes![52]

Fulton and his regimental surgeon, fellow assistant surgeon, steward, and medical orderlies constructed the sick call tent and created temporary medical depots when the regiment was preparing to enter combat. Regulations specified how tents were to be arranged and what type of tent could house how many soldiers. The depot functioned both as a way station for medical supplies and a first aid center. Beyond immediate treatment, ailing or wounded soldiers were moved to hospitals serving the brigade or division, which would transfer Fulton's regimental soldiers to the purview of other doctors. Other physicians in the larger system made treatment decisions on their own authority: Fulton's authority did not reach beyond his immediate treatment of soldiers. Doubtless, as the junior doctor, Fulton spent much time, when not seeing patients, ordering supplies from purveying depots (or negotiating with the quartermaster when supplies could not be obtained through the medical system) and completing paperwork. The administrative tasks required diverse record-keeping, including the maintenance of requisitions, a register of patients, a prescription book, diet book, case book, meteorological register, quarterly reports of the sick and wounded, a letter and order book, muster rolls and payrolls, and a morning report of the day's sick.[53]

Hospital management also necessitated Fulton's involvement in both medical and administrative capacities. A letter written by William W. Potter, MD, surgeon, 57th New York Volunteers and later the 49th New York, describes the intricacy and cunning of managing hospital funds, a responsibility that Fulton likely handled similarly:

> I have been to City Point today where I ordered a bill of goods, through the medical purveyor, from Baltimore for the hospital, amounting to $1,200. This will give the patients canned fruits, oranges, lemons, and many other luxuries not furnished by the commissary department, which will be paid for out of the hospital fund. This fund accrues from the savings in the rations on the march and in an active campaign, when we cannot use all we are entitled to. Such as are not drawn each day are passed to the hospital as a cash credit, and against this fund we can draw for the purchase of whatever we need not furnished in the supply tables of the several departments, medical, commissary, or quartermasters.[54]

Doctors jealously guarded and disbursed hospital funds. These funds met shortfalls in the army logistics system, and their management was held as a matter of pride, attesting to the maturity of the doctor as a military officer, an emblem of having learned to work the system.

The degree to which surgeons were required to participate in military rituals of parade (inspection) varied with the regimental commander. Surgeons were generally excluded from parade appearances and thus were not integrated with the line officer corps. Fulton's diary includes a mildly comic moment when he and his fellow assistant surgeon, Dr. David L. Scott, were required to appear for inspection:

> [T]o day at two o Clock we had inspection. Dr. Scott And Myself were—the Col would not Excuse us I guess he wanted to have some fun at our Expense for when we advanced then he ordered us to right Dress And we were So green that we did not Know how it should be done—For My part I care but little as Military outside of our particular Duties And of Course get but little attention—[55]

When on the march, surgeons and their staff appeared at the end of the column, so they were less likely to be noticed by commanders for their military deportment. Nevertheless, even within an exclusively medical environment such as the hospital, military ritual was observed. Surgeon William Child, Fifth New Hampshire, wrote to his wife that he had been designated hospital Officer of the Day, a rotated duty among doctors. "The officer of the Day's duty is to look after the whole hospital. We have now 587 patients and nurses. It is no small work to attend to the whole duty of officer of the Day. You are to run to everybody's call and see that all things are right."[56] Nevertheless, regimental officers occasionally subjected medical officers and their subordinates and materiel to inspection. Major William Watson, surgeon, 105th Pennsylvania, wrote to his father that "[t]he Colonel just informed me that tomorrow there will be a rigid inspection of the Medical Dept. of his Regt. by a board appointed by [General] Birney. My records, prescription Book, Hospital instruments and all cases reported sick will be examined."[57]

In combat, surgeons shared the apprehension, fear, and emotional intensity of frontline soldiers. Surgeon Winsor's metaphor succinctly describes the doctor's role: "His place is in an eddy of the mighty current of battle where the wrecks sweep in, and his business is to mend them as he may."[58] Despite not being part of an attack force, surgeons risked wounding and death and conducted their lifesaving work within the full environment of terror that is battle. Surgeon of the 19th Massachusetts Jonah Franklin Dyer took advantage of a lull in fighting to write home that the very room in which he was composing his letter, "and in which all our surgeons sleep, is used as an operating room, and for six days the tables have been occupied from morning until late at night." The hours of intense work in the operating room probably precluded introspection until much later, but a day or two after Antietam, Surgeon Child reflected in a letter to his wife that battle "seems so strange. Who permits it. To see or feel that a power is in existence that can and will hurl masses of men against each other in deadly conflict slaying each other by thousands—mangling and deforming their fellow men is almost impossible. But it is so." Daniel M. Holt, assistant surgeon, 121st New York, communicated similar thoughts in a letter to his wife but with more eloquence; it was atypical for a soldier to write with such honesty to an anxious spouse.

> You must stand as I have stood, and hear the report of battery upon battery, witness the effect of shell, grape and canister—you must hear the incessant discharge of musketry, see men leaping high in air and falling dead upon the ground—others without a groan or a sigh yielding up their life from loss of

blood—see the wounded covered in dirt and blackened by powder—hear their groans—witness their agonies, see the eye grow dim in death, before you can realize or be impressed with its horrors. Notwithstanding all this, you do not see it in its true light. You become excited, enraged, and the only feeling is that of retaliation and revenge. You will scarcely believe me when I say, that during that awful conflict I forgot that my office and duty was to care for the wounded—that I longed to be in the fray and unnecessarily exposed myself to dangers such as I now shrink from . . . But when cool reflection comes—when exhausted nature gives place to repose—when reason resumes her throne, you begin to realize the awful tragedy.[59]

Surgeon General Hammond issued periodic circulars to all medical directors that provided guidance on a variety of administrative or practical matters. Circular No. 2, which mandated the reporting of explanatory information in monthly reports of the sick and wounded, also required the collection of "all specimens of morbid anatomy, surgical or medical, which may be regarded as valuable" along with related bullet or shell fragments that "may prove of interest in the study of military medicine or surgery" (see chapter 8). Thus laying the foundation of the Army Medical Museum, Circular No. 5 required the cooperation of all medical officers in furnishing data for the publication of the *Medical and Surgical History of the Rebellion*.[60] Fulton participated in military medicine at a time when the army's surgeon general required doctors to observe a scientific orientation to their work: they were required to attend to the ill and wounded and also document their treatments and results, conduct autopsies, and collect and forward specimens of interest to a central repository and information clearinghouse, the new Army Medical Museum in Washington, DC. While Fulton did not mention these requirements in his diary, he doubtless read the circulars and must have cooperated with his medical supervisors in this work.

Physicians observed and meditated on the psychology of men at war when psychology as an intellectual endeavor did not yet exist. Thomas T. Ellis, post surgeon of New York and medical director of Virginia (supervising Union hospitals in that state), noticed one Pennsylvania soldier who had been brought in to the field hospital with the wounded. He "had become a raving and violent maniac from fright. The shock to his nervous system was more than he could bear. His exclamations of terror were piteous and heart-rending, and caused such discomfort to the other sufferers that I sent him on shore to the hospital."[61] At other times, doctors marveled at how soldiers relieved stress. At the Gettysburg battle, Surgeon Dyer noticed a group of soldiers sitting by the roadside and discovered that they were "quietly playing poker, while shells were bursting frequently and unpleasantly near. They sought mental occupation to divert their attention from more serious subjects."[62] Assistant Surgeon John Gardner Perry, 20th Massachusetts, had a similar experience: "I noticed a man near me in the ranks at this time singing a hymn with all his might and main. His head was thrown back, his mouth wide open, and he seemed completely absorbed in the emotion called forth to the hymn, which made him oblivious of all surroundings. I watched him curiously, and understood that it was an instinctive impulse on his part to try to hold his senses together and to steady himself under the well-nigh unendurable strain."[63]

What did soldiers think of their surgeons? Abundant caricatures of them—satirical or buffoonish representations in print or image—may have masked fear of the grim work that only surgeons could do in repairing torn bodies. In the main, however, soldiers respected and relied on what surgeons could do for them. Assistant Surgeon Perry records that before battle, soldiers came to him "asking [him] to take charge of watches and personal effects, and to deliver messages to friends at home, of which [he] made careful memoranda, and begging [him] to promise to send everything to their families if they were killed."[64] And what of the physician left in possession of personal items owned by a soldier who had just died? Contract surgeon John Vance Lauderdale, aboard a hospital ship, wrote, "Letters are sent back to the friends from where they came, with a line stating the circumstances of the death of the person. The baggage is generally delivered over to the lieutenant whose business it is to send anything valuable to his friends. But the knapsack, gun, and other accoutrements are turned over to the government."[65]

Assistant Surgeon Holt felt a deep kinship with the soldiers of his regiment who "good naturedly" call him "old doctor." He cultivated an avuncular relationship with soldiers and adopted a particular mien and deportment. "It does no man good to wear a long, mournful face and in a mood of despondency to hear from the Surgeon that his case is desperate and that death will probably result. Better tell him that *nothing* is the matter—that *imagination* is the disease and dismiss him . . . I have cured many a man who was really unwell by simply making him believe that his sickness was all in his mind."[66]

All soldiers who experienced combat meditated on the meaning of it all. Physicians at war did the same, but they also philosophized about what good they felt they could do, lamenting their powerlessness when confronting wounds and disease that their tools and methods were inadequate to address. Surgeon Child wrote to his wife about the strangeness of men:

> [W]e are born—we live—we labor—we seek pleasure—we get pain—we strive for power and wealth—we excite commotion—we differ in opinions— we quarrel—we become angry—have heart burnings—have wars—we live a life of constant anxiety and turmoil only to die—our body food for worms— our ashes to mingle with our mother earth, leaving nothing behind except a new generation to enact the same scenes. Only He who rules all things knows why man exists.[67]

Assistant Surgeon Perry occupied the same environment of death and suffering and took inspiration: "My respect for human nature grows every day that I am here. I see its littleness, but its greatness makes far the deeper impression. The fortitude with which these men bear their hard lot is wonderful, but they are not the only heroes; I am constantly brought in contact with such courage in so many of the men, and such magnanimity, that I am fairly awed."[68]

CIVIL WAR MEDICAL HISTORY AND FULTON'S DIARY

The medical dimension of the Civil War has received peculiar treatment by historians. Those who write eloquently and with insight about the war's cultural, economic, political, or military dimensions may ignore, dismiss, or marginalize the medical discussion by invoking the ahistorical tendency to contrast Civil War medical practices with those of the next century. Even the best historians repeat canards about its medical dimension, highlighting the apparent uselessness of available medicines, lack of antisepsis and knowledge of bacteria and viruses as causes of disease, and excessive amputations. In short, these judgments are ahistorical for their implicit or explicit condemnation of Civil War physicians for not practicing medicine to twenty-first-century standards. True, accounts by the war's participants of the agonies of the wounded and diseased betoken a frightful picture of a battlefield aid station or general hospital. Nevertheless, most historians evaluate Civil War doctoring according to what it could *not* do, explicitly or implicitly highlighting its miseries.[69]

Historians judge the culture of Civil War medicine by asking of its therapies, Did they work? To historian of medicine Charles E. Rosenberg, "the
generally unquestioned criterion for understanding pre-nineteenth century
therapeutics has been physiological, not historical: did a particular practice
act in a way that twentieth-century understanding would regard as efficacious?" Surgeons and soldiers shared an ideology about how contagion happened, what remedies did or did not work, and what to expect of healing.
Civil War surgeons ran hospitals, supervised pharmacies, managed the medical supply system, conducted autopsies, reported anomalies, tried to keep
current with medical literature, and wrote and delivered papers. Medical
knowledge accrued during the war, but most historians have not engaged
with it as a respectable intellectual activity that existed within a wider scientific and social context. According to Rosenberg, "historians have not only
failed to delineate this change [the transformation of medical therapeutics in
the nineteenth century in relationship to social change] in detail, they have
hardly begun to place it in a framework of explanation which could relate
it to all those other changes which shaped the twentieth-century Western
World."[70]

Recent popular and scholarly writing minimizes the war's medical dimension and sometimes ignores it altogether.[71] Many historians, perspica-
cious about the war's social, economic, and political dimensions, apparently
do not read the literature produced by the doctors themselves, who were
unquestionably creating medical knowledge. Lack of attention to surgeons'
own writings diminishes the opportunity to engage with the culture of military doctors. Continued assertions that Civil War doctors were ignorant of
germ theory, antisepsis, or other later practices and therapies is ahistorical.
Historians diminish an assessment of what surgeons accomplished by mea-
suring them against the standard of what they did not know at the time. Some
writers' brisk dismissals of Civil War medical practices must be re-examined
for lack of evidence.[72]

Recent scholarship has penetrated the haze of the rote repetition of such
generalizations by examining the production of knowledge by Union army
doctors, particularly the research conducted in specialty hospitals. Civil War
doctors doubtless contributed to their own bad press by derogating their
own ignorance when reflecting on the war years later following the introduction of aseptic practices and the recognition of bacterial and viral contagion.

In the early twentieth century, Keen reminisced, "Only too sharply do we remember the dreadful things that we did do and the good things that we did not dare to do".[73] Nevertheless, much clinical writing of wartime doctors displays an orientation to a future time, arguing that continued investigations may eventually solve problems unresolved during the war. The encyclopedic *Medical and Surgical History of the War of the Rebellion*, published by the federal government a decade after the war's end, attests to the innumerable medical challenges doctors faced and presents the best scientific statement of what they knew and did not know, and how they managed to save lives. This work was intended to furnish a platform for further research and refinement of techniques. Fulton completed daily forms to account for his work and documented lists of the sick and their disposition. His reports became absorbed into the summary observations found in the *Medical and Surgical History*, although none of his cases is specifically cited.

In locating Fulton within his milieu of military medicine, the diary is most fruitfully read without the filter of common biases about Civil War medicine described above. James Fulton's diary is not a technical record of medical labor. It is a rounded account of travel, observations on colleagues, reflections on political and military events, and, of course, many observations on health, wounds, and illness. The late Harvard American literature professor Daniel Aaron wrote that "[o]ur untidy and unkempt War still confounds interpreters."[74] Fulton's diary is also untidy and may confound generalizations about the medical Civil War. His diary and his first attempt to round his experiences into a narrative would have presented, if published during his day, another "story of the civil war as daily emergency and liberty's crucible."[75] These characteristics are present in the diary, but we can read it in wonder that he left a pregnant wife and a new career to answer the call of national duty and in so doing coped with the unimaginable and somehow kept "faith in the ideals or motives that had impelled them to go to war."[76]

Fulton was not, and should not be, faulted for not being a seasoned writer, philosopher, or journalist. Taking him all in all, Fulton was one doctor among many in military service who endured frightful and brilliant moments under fire, long and tiresome marches, and the building and dismantling of camps. He attended to his duties, and unlike soldiers who left the army to pursue other careers, returned to medicine in civilian life, certainly having learned much about wounds, illnesses, and the behavior of men under extreme stress.

That Fulton was not a pioneering surgeon, nor rose to high military rank and responsibility, nor befriended the elite does not diminish his account. His diary becomes the more historically valuable *because* Fulton's experiences may have been widely shared by other doctors. The diary communicates freshness and immediacy and a lack of self-consciousness not found in later memoirs reworked for publication. For that, it is a comparatively rare gem.

NOTES

1. Abraham Lincoln, "Executive Order—Call for Troops," June 30, 1862, online by Gerhard Peters and John T. Woolley, *The American Presidency Project*, at https://www.presi dency.ucsb.edu/documents/executive-order-call-for-troops, accessed October 22, 2018.

2. "History and Anthropology," *Past and Present* 24 (1963): 3–24; quotations at 12, 15.

3. See Jonathan W. White, *Midnight in America: Darkness, Sleep, and Dreams during the Civil War* (Chapel Hill: University of North Carolina Press, 2017).

4. Many works outline the process of ethnographic fieldwork: Benjamin F. Crabtree and William L. Miller, eds., *Doing Qualitative Research*, second edition (Newbury Park, CA: Sage, 1999); H. Russell Bernard, ed., *Handbook of Methods in Cultural Anthropology* (Walnut Creek, CA: Alta Mira, 1998); W. Penn Handwerker, *Quick Ethnography* (Walnut Creek, CA: Alta Mira, 2001); and Jeffrey J. Johnson, *Selecting Ethnographic Informants* (Newbury Park, CA: Sage Publications, 1990).

5. Daniel Aaron, *The Unwritten War: American Writers and the Civil War* (New York: Alfred A. Knopf, 1973), 334; James M. McPherson, *For Cause and Comrades: Why Men Fought in the Civil War* (New York: Oxford University Press, 1997), 334.

6. McPherson, *For Cause and Comrades*, 11.

7. Some of the original diaries no longer exist but were edited by the authors themselves in subsequent years for publication or for private circulation. Thomas P. Lowry, ed., *Swamp Doctor: The Diary of a Union Surgeon in the Virginia & North Carolina Marshes* (Mechanicsville, PA: Stackpole Books, 2001) presents the best comparison with Fulton's diary. The diary's author is William Mervale Smith, MD, Surgeon, 85th NY. Alas, the book is poorly edited and the editor, an MD, makes dismissive ahistorical observations about Smith's era of medicine.

8. Frederick Winsor, "The Surgeon at the Field Hospital," *Atlantic Monthly* 46 (August 1880): 186.

9. Kathryn Shively Meier, *Nature's Civil War: Common Soldiers and the Environment in 1862 Virginia* (Chapel Hill: University of North Carolina Press, 2013), 2.

10. Ibid., 16. The requirement to record meteorological conditions is found in *Regulations for the Medical Department of the Army* (Washington, DC: Government Printing Office, 1861), 38ff, online at https://babel.hathitrust.org/cgi/pt?id=hvd.32044089268627;view=1up;seq=7, accessed October 22, 2018.

11. Allen C. Guelzo, *Gettysburg: The Last Invasion* (New York: Alfred A. Knopf, 2013), 70.

12. Historian Frances M. Clarke has analyzed similar rhetoric among Union soldiers, which she characterizes as an idealization of suffering: "Holding up white Union soldiers as exemplary sufferers, and pointing to white Northern volunteers' more extensive and automatic response to men in pain, in other words, were some of the major ways that Northern whites

constituted national identity during the war." Clarke, *War Stories: Suffering and Sacrifice in the Civil War North* (Chicago: University of Chicago Press, 2011), 22.

13. James Fulton, Diary, 1862–1864, entry for January 16, 1863.

14. Hawley letter, February 20, 1863, in *"This Terrible Struggle for Life": The Civil War Letters of a Union Regimental Surgeon* [Thomas S. Hawley, MD], ed. Dennis W. Belcher (Jefferson, NC: McFarland & Company, 2012), 92.

15. *Regulations for the Medical Department of the Army.*

16. Fulton family data comes from three sources: Hugh R. Fulton, ed., *Genealogy of the Fulton Family* (Lancaster, PA: privately printed, 1900), 42, 97–125, online at https://archive.org/stream/genealogyoffultooofult#page/100/mode/2up, accessed October 22, 2018; J. Smith Futhey and Gilbert Cope, *History of Chester County, Pennsylvania* (Philadelphia: J. B. Lippincott, 1881), 306–10, 555–7; and United States Federal Census returns for 1850 (East Nottingham, Chester, Pennsylvania, Roll M432_764, p. 23B; 1860 (Penn, Chester, Pennsylvania, Roll M653_10094, p. 12).

17. *Genealogy of the Fulton Family*, 101–2.

18. *Village Record*, West Chester, March 22, 1853.

19. For the history of the song, see *Voices Across Time*, a music history website maintained by the University of Pittsburgh, online at http://www.library.pitt.edu/voicesacrosstime/come-all-ye/ti/2006/Song%20Activities/03MedvicUncleSam.html, accessed October 22, 2018.

20. Folder, Jordan Bank Boarding School for Boys, newspaper references, box 88, Chester County Historical Society.

21. Folder, Jordan Bank Academy exhibition programs 1852–1853, East Nottingham. Chester County Historical Society.

22. University of Delaware website http://www.udel.edu/about/history/, accessed October 22, 2018.

23. Chester County Historical Society website http://www.chestercohistorical.org/historys-people-chester-countys-passmore-williamson-famed-abolitionist, accessed September 1, 2016.

24. *Chester County Times*, May 25, 1861.

25. W. W. Keen James, ed., *The Memoirs of William Williams Keen, M.D.* (Doylestown, PA: privately published, 1990), 153–4.

26. "John Brown's Body," 1859: Philadelphia's Medical Schools Rebellion Against Its Presence in the City." *Hidden Histories* blog, Historical Society of Pennsylvania, https://hsp.org/blogs/hidden-histories/john-browns-body-1859-philadelphias-medical-schools-rebellion-against-its-presence-in-the-city, accessed October 22, 2018; Jedidiah H. Adams, *History of the Life of D. Hayes Agnew* (Philadelphia: F. A. Davis, 1892), 91–2.

27. Edward Pinkowski, *Chester County Place Names* (Philadelphia: Sunshine Press, 1962), 131–2.

28. *Chester County Times*, May 25, 1861.

29. Gross's former student and eventual colleague, William Williams Keen, MD, recapitulated his mentor's achievements in a delightful memoir, "Samuel David Gross: The Lesson of His Life and Labors," a eulogy given at the 85th annual commencement ceremony at Jefferson Medical College on June 6, 1910. Jefferson Biographies, Paper 5, online at http://jdc.jefferson.edu/jeffbiographies/5, accessed October 22, 2018.

30. *An Inaugural Address Introductory to the Course on Surgery in the Jefferson Medical College of Philadelphia* (Philadelphia: Joseph M. Wilson, 1856), 20–1.

31. George M. Gould, *The Jefferson Medical College of Philadelphia* (New York: Lewis Publishing Company, 1904), 1:121–46. Quotations at 122, 134, and 146.

32. W. W. Keen, "Some Reminiscences of Student Days at Jefferson," reprinted from *Jeffersonian* (November 1905): 68–71, online at http://wellcomelibrary.org/item/b22401416 #?c=0&m=0&s=0&cv=2&z=0.1219%2C0.842%2C0.8342%2C0.4867, accessed September 16, 2016.

33. "Part I: Jefferson Medical College 1855 to 1865," in *Thomas Jefferson University— A Chronological History and Alumni Directory, 1824–1990*, Frederick B. Wagner Jr. and J. Woodrow Savacool, eds. (Thomas Jefferson University, 1992), 104, online at http://jdc .jefferson.edu/wagner1/17, accessed October 22, 2018.

34. George Worthington Adams, *Doctors in Blue: The Medical History of the Union Army in the Civil War* (Baton Rouge: Louisiana State University Press, 1996), 49.

35. Regulations 14, *Regulations for the Medical Department of the Army*.

36. Regulations 16, *Regulations for the Medical Department of the Army*.

37. Lowry, *Swamp Doctor*, 138–9.

38. Chas. Tripler and George C. Blackman, *Hand-Book for the Military Surgeon* (Cincinnati: Robert Clarke, 1861), 1.

39. Adams, *Doctors in Blue*, 48.

40. In addition to Adams, several recent books outline the organization and management of Union army medicine, including Frank R. Freemon, *Gangrene and Glory: Medical Care during the American Civil War* (Champaign: University of Illinois Press, 2001); Ira M. Rutkow, *Bleeding Blue and Gray: Civil War Surgery and the Evolution of American Medicine* (New York: Random House, 2005); Margaret Humphreys, *Marrow of Tragedy: The Health Crisis of the American Civil War* (Baltimore: Johns Hopkins University Press, 2013); and Shauna Devine, *Learning from the Wounded: The Civil War and the Rise of American Medical Science* (Chapel Hill: University of North Carolina Press, 2014.) On the presence of women and the work of the Sanitary Commission, see Jane E. Schultz, *Women at the Front: Hospital Workers in Civil War America* (Chapel Hill: University of North Carolina Press, 2004); Judith Giesberg, *Army at Home: Women and the Civil War on the Northern Home Front* (Durham: University of North Carolina Press, 2009); and Giesberg, *Civil War Sisterhood: The United States Sanitary Commission and Women's Politics in Transition* (Lebanon, NH: Northeastern University Press, 2000).

41. Benton letter, November 4, 1862, in *A Surgeon's Tale: The Civil War Letters of Surgeon James D. Benton, 111th and 98th New York Infantries 1862–1865*, ed. Christopher E. Loperfido (Gettysburg, PA: Ten Roads, 2011), 27.

42. Smith diary, August 4, 1862, in Lowry, *Swamp Doctor*, 30.

43. Hawley letter, December 7, 1862, in Belcher, *This Terrible Struggle for Life*, 69.

44. See discussion of medical training in Devine, *Learning from the Wounded*, 5ff.

45. See Joseph Janvier Woodward, *The Hospital Steward's Manual* (Philadelphia: J. B. Lippincott, 1863); Woodward, *Outlines of the Chief Camp Diseases of the United States Armies* (Philadelphia: J. B. Lippincott & Co., 1863); Roberts Bartholow, *A Manual of Instructions for Enlisting and Discharging Soldiers* (Philadelphia: J. B. Lippincott, 1863); and Tripler, *Handbook for the Military Surgeon*.

46. Samuel P. Bates, *History of Pennsylvania Volunteers, 1861–5* (Harrisburg: B. Singerly, 1870), 4:90–2.

47. 124th PA Vols Order Book, Archives of the Union League of Philadelphia, 1805.040.

48. Regulation 11 in *Regulations for the Medical Department of the Army* (Washington: Government Printing Office, 1861).

49. Peter Tomasak, ed., *Avery Harris Civil War Journal* (Luzerne, PA: Luzerne National Bank, 2000), 106. Harris (1840–1938) composed his memoir of the 143rd around 1902–10 based on a diary that no longer exists. The 143rd did not create its own regimental history.

50. Benton letter, March 6, 1864, in *A Surgeon's Tale*, 73.

51. John D. Billings, *Hardtack and Coffee or The Unwritten Story of Army Life,* reprint of 1887 edition (Lincoln, Nebraska: Bison Books, 1993), 176.

52. Smith diary, December 19, 1862, in Lowry, *Swamp Doctor*, 98.

53. Regulations 5, 10, 12 in *Regulations for the Medical Department of the Army.*

54. John Michael Priest, ed., *One Surgeon's Private War: Doctor William W. Potter of the 57th New York* (Buffalo, NY: White Mane, 1996), 124.

55. Fulton, November 19, 1863.

56. Child letter, October 22, 1862, in *Letters from a Civil War Surgeon: The Letters of Dr. William Child of the Fifth New Hampshire Volunteers,* ed. Merill C. Sawyer, Betty Sawyer, and Timothy C. Sawyer (Solon, ME: Polar Bear, 2001), 59.

57. Watson letter, February 2, 1863, in *Letters of a Civil War Surgeon* [Major William Watson], ed. Paul Fatout (Purdue, IN: Purdue Research Foundation, 1961), 54.

58. Winsor, "The Surgeon at the Field Hospital," 183.

59. The Dyer letter was written near Falmouth, Virginia, on December 18, 1862, in *The Journal of a Civil War Surgeon* [J. Franklin Dyer], ed. Michael B. Chesson (Lincoln: University of Nebraska Press, 2003), 53; Child's letter was written October 7, 1862, in Sawyer et al., *Letters from a Civil War Surgeon,* 47; Holt's letter is dated May 15, 1863, in Greiner et al., *A Surgeon's Civil War: The Letters and Diary of Daniel M. Holt, M.D.,* ed. James M. Greiner, Janet L. Coryell, and James R. Smither (Kent, OH: Kent State University Press, 1994), 101.

60. Surgeon General's Office, Circular No. 2, May 21, 1862 (http://resource.nlm.nih .gov/101534229); Circular No. 5, June 9, 1862 (http://resource.nlm.nih.gov/101534562, accessed October 22, 2018); Devine, *Learning from the Wounded,* 29–38.

61. Thomas T. Ellis, *Leaves from the Diary of an Army Surgeon* (New York: John Bradburn, 1863), 71.

62. *The Journal of a Civil War Surgeon* [J. Franklin Dyer], 97.

63. Perry letter, May 3, 1864, in *Letters from a Surgeon of the Civil War* [John Gardner Perry], comp. and ed. Martha Derby (Boston: Little, Brown, and Co.), 169.

64. Perry letter, December 3, 1863, in ibid., 144.

65. Lauderdale letter to sister, July 19, 1862, in *The Wounded River: The Civil War Letters of John Vance Lauderdale, M.D.,* ed. Peter Josyph (East Lansing: Michigan State University Press, 1993), 101.

66. Holt letter, April 10, 1863, in Greiner et al., *A Surgeon's Civil War* [Daniel M. Holt], 89.

67. Child letter to wife, November 2, 1864, in Sawyer et al., *Letters from a Civil War Surgeon* [William Child] 290.

68. Perry letter dated July 21, 1862, in Derby, *Letters from a Surgeon of the Civil War* [John Gardner Perry], 15.

69. See Devine, *Learning from the Wounded,* and Humphreys, *Marrow of Tragedy.*

70. Charles E. Rosenberg, "The Therapeutic Revolution: Medicine, Meaning, and Social Change in Nineteenth-Century America," *Perspectives in Biology and Medicine,* 20 no. 4 (Summer 1977): 485. As an example of a resurrected wartime study about smallpox vaccination, see Joseph Jones, "Researches upon 'Spurious Vaccination' or the Abnormal Phenomena Accompanying and Following Vaccination in the Confederate Army during the Recent American Civil War, 1861–1865" (Nashville: University Medical Press, W. H. F. Printer, 1867).

71. For instance, books aimed at wide general readership to commemorate the 150th anniversary of the war say little about the medical realm. Harold Holzer's *The Civil War in 50 Objects* (New York: Viking, 2013) includes no medically related object. Similarly, Neil Kagan, ed., *Smithsonian Civil War: Inside the National Collection* (Washington, DC: Smithsonian, 2013), tells the story of the war through 150 objects, only three of which have any medical relevance. Two of the objects are medicines and the third involves medical photography. The object descriptions give minimal context. The companion book to the Ken Burns television series on the Civil War, Geoffrey C. Ward's *The Civil War: An Illustrated History* (New York: Alfred A. Knopf, 1990), while highlighting the huge number of battle casualties and the demands on hospitals, states, "Medical care was primitive, at best, in both armies" (p. 184). Primitive in comparison with the present century? In the book's sidebar interview with writer Shelby Foote, he is asked, "Someone once remarked that the Civil War occurred during the medical middle ages. What was it like?" (p. 265). He responded: "I'm sure they did the best they could . . . They not only didn't subscribe to the germ theory: they didn't suspect that it existed. Blood poisoning, erysipelas, pneumonia, even measles was a big killer. They did not know how to treat them, let alone not having penicillin. It was just a question of a crisis and surviving or a crisis and dying. It's a wonder they did as well as they did" (p. 266). The statement minimizes Civil War physicians by claiming that they did not know how to treat serious illnesses, they did not possess a twentieth-century innovation, and they did not suspect that a germ theory existed.

A popular overview history, Peter J. Parish, *The American Civil War* (New York: Holmes & Meier, 1975), states that "the medical services represent one of the Civil War's most dismal failures" (p. 147). James M. McPherson's Pulitzer Prize-winning history, *Battle Cry of Freedom* (New York: Oxford University Press, 1988), quotes Parish on the same point. McPherson describes the reputation of doctors as "quacks" and "butchers" and the "generally low repute of the medical profession." He then gives an extensive list of innovations not yet available to wartime physicians. "The Civil War was fought at the end of the medical Middle Ages," says McPherson, and cites Louis Pasteur, Joseph Lister, the postwar science of bacteriology, and the link between mosquitos and yellow fever. "Civil War doctors knew none of these things . . . They were not aware of the exact relationship between water and typhoid, between unsterilized instruments and infection, between mosquitos and malaria. The concept of asepsis and antisepsis in surgery had not been developed" (p. 486). He also repeats a canard that the wartime shortage of medicines in the Confederacy "sometimes required soldiers to be dosed with whiskey and literally to bite the bullet during surgery" (p.487). No evidence yet exists that doctors North or South required pain-ridden, supine, wounded soldiers, going in and out of consciousness, to retain a lead bullet in their mouths to chomp on should anesthesia be unavailable, and not accidentally swallow it.

72. For instance, the Union army medical supply cabinet contained about two hundred substances that could be combined to form hundreds more compounds. This cabinet included mercury- and antimony-based medicines, now judged poisonous and deleterious to human health, plus many others now dismissed as useless. The Confederate project to inventory all southern plants to determine medicinal applications, Dr. Francis Peyre Porcher's *Resources of the Southern Fields and Forests* (1863), suggests a number of plants and trees that could have medicinal value, yet to date many have not been pharmacologically investigated. Even mercury, long a mainstay of the medicine cabinet, while no longer available in drugstores, continues to support some specific medical applications. On the pharmacological properties, known and unknown, of plants during the Civil War, see Michael Flannery, *Civil*

War Pharmacy: A History of Drugs, Drug Supply and Provision, and Therapeutics for the Union and Confederacy (New York: Haworth Press, 2004), 277–9. For example, Flannery lists several plants or trees that were identified by Confederate authorities as having medicinal value. Under the category of "symptomatic activity," several are listed as "possibly" or "likely," but pharmacological research into their medicinal value remains wanting. The editor of one wartime diary by a physician, himself a psychiatrist, equates the medical knowledge of the Civil War doctor to that of ancient Egyptians and dismisses most nineteenth-century therapies (see *Swamp Doctor*). On mercury medicines, see Bonnie Brice Dorwart, *Death is in the Breeze: Disease During the American Civil War* (Frederick, MD: NMCWM Press, 2009), 133.

73. See Devine, *Learning from the Wounded* and Humphreys, *Marrow of Tragedy*. Quotation is from Keen's wartime memoir, "Surgical Reminiscences of the Civil War," reprinted in William Williams Keen, *Addresses and Other Papers* (Philadelphia: W. B. Saunders, 1905), 433.

74. Aaron, *The Unwritten War*, 340.

75. Kathleen Diffley, ed., *To Live and Die: Collected Stories of the Civil War, 1861–1876* (Durham, NC: Duke University Press, 2002), 7.

76. Earl J. Hess, *The Union Soldier in Battle: Enduring the Ordeal of Combat* (Lawrence: University of Kansas Press, 1997), ix.

PART I

ONE

To Virginia, Measles, and Typhoid

Diary, August 18, 1862, to February 19, 1863

JAMES FULTON'S DIARY STARTS BY DESCRIBING HIS ENTRY INTO THE ARMY. His military career began with his appointment as assistant surgeon after passing an examination before medical faculty at the University of Pennsylvania. How Fulton was directed to appear for examination at the University of Pennsylvania remains obscure. In 1862, Jefferson Medical College and the University of Pennsylvania were the preeminent Philadelphia medical schools. At the outset of war in 1861, Southern medical students in Philadelphia left en masse to Southern medical schools or the Confederate Army, an event that caused the closure of Philadelphia's smaller medical schools and harmed the two remaining larger ones.

[diary front matter]
Jaˢ Fulton MD. Assistant Surgeon
In the 143ʳᵈ Regiment Bucktail Brigade

[Title page for Clayton's Octavo Diary for 1862]
Jaˢ Fulton Asst. Surg. 143ᵈ Reg. Pennᵃ Vols
Notes And Views of the war from the time of leaving home until

Jennerville¹ August 18ᵗʰ [1862]

Received orders from Surgeon General H[enry] H[ollingsworth] Smith to report to Dr. Nelson [unidentified] at Harrisburg as Soon as possible. packing up in All haste took the 3.40 train at Penn Station. Arrived in Phila at 7 o clock—at

August 19ᵗʰ 62

Took the cars at 11.30 for Harrisburg passing up the Pa Road the most prominent object of attraction on the way being the great Chester Valley the broad Expanse of highly cultivated and fertile land Stretching for Miles before the Entranced Vision of the beholder—the highly cultivated farms with Excellent buildings finely fenced making me feel if possible still more [ap]preciative [of] my native Country—in the Evening at 3.30 we arrived in Harrisburg went to Herrs Hotel deposited our Baggage—left immediately for camp Curtain [Curtin] in a [illegible word] the dust rising in cloud[s] And being almost insupportable—but not being any worse on the way than it was at camp. I have often Seen the roads dusty but never in My life have I Seen Anything to this. Bodies of Men continually on the March and counter March Kept the [dust] flying in clouds all the time—we soon found Dr. Wilson² And Reported to him—he appointed Dr. [Lewis R.] Kirk³ to the 131ˢᵗ Regiment Pa Vol. And told him to go to the Depot And see his Reg. off for the Seat of War. he and I went. A fine body of men they were—After this we went back to the Hotel taking our supper walked round town—the first time in My life that I Ever Saw [the] market at night—the Capitol of the State is quite a fine looking [buil]ding though not what [I ex]pected to See—the Court House and insane asylum are fine buildings—

after looking round untill nine o clock we came back to the Hotel where there was an order [a]waiting me from Dr. Smith to meet him at the Beuhler House doeing So he appointed me to the 143ᵈ regiment Bucktail Brigade to Report to Col Rough⁴ Phila to be mustered into service—

August 20ᵗʰ

This morning I took the cars at Harrisburg at 6.30 for Philᵃ— Arriving here at ten I immediately reported to D̶r̶. Col Rough and was Sworn in to the US Service—And at once Reported to Col Wister⁵—there being no duty for me to perform to day I am to call tomorrow at nine o clock the corner of 5th and c[hest (text torn)]

nut to Examine me[n]—for the Service—the remainder of the day
I Spent in reading and walking round—went to the depot of the
Phil[a] and West-Chester R R. and gave to Tho[s] Mackey[6] a package for
home—

Phil[a] August 21st 62

To Day I have been Engaged in Examining men for the Service—
Cap[tain William S.] Pine Cap[tain William A.] Elsegood Capt
[Benjamn F.] Janey. Capt [Henry W.] Gimber[7] are the only four
companys recruiting in the City for the Bucktails—the Recruiting is
not very brisk—Capt McDowl[8] has been at the Commercial Hotel
all week carrying on pretty [str]ong—To Day Col. [Cor]coran.[9]
Made his appearance in town and had a hearty reception—well
Showing the respect the country has for those who do and suffer
in its defence he looks much worn and fatigued, he has seen much
hardship—and privation—

/Meridian Hill/
Washington
Monday October 14th 1862

To Day I have been to the Sol[diers] home seeing the sick in Comp[s]
[Companies] D & K[10] typhoid Fever Seems to be the prevailing disease[11]—For the past six weeks we have been Encamped on Meridian
Hill—I have visited the public buildings or at least those belonging
to the Go[v]. the Capitol is the Finest building that I have Ever Seen
the ma[rble] work is truly magnify[cent] but the Idea of putting so
much Labor on marble dressing it and then painting it is something
that I cannot—understand—the paintings in the Capitol are fine
one of Gen [l] Washington the father of his country.

The Dome of the Capitol is Certainly the Most Magnificent
piece of Architecture the imense hollow dome the outside being
Constructed of Iron with such profusion of glass that Light is admitted in such a manner that the whole dome is [illegible word] lighted
with the farigated [variegated] colors.

/Meridian Hill Washington-D C/
Jan 2ond 1863

This is a fine day not much like winter—I am now Assistant Surgeon to the 143d Regiment—And have been acting with this Regiment since the 18th of December—I acted with the 150th Regiment until the 18th of October at which time the Authorities decided that properly I Belonged to Col[onel] E[dmund] L Danas 143d I made two pilgrimages to Harrisburg. The first—time Dr. King [unidentified] ordered me to Report to the 143d For duty but on goeing to the war department I was told that Dr. King had no Authority to order me there I then went to ~~Dr. King~~—Col H Puleston[12] for advice he told me to state my case I did so and he sent it to Dr King with remarks Dr King Denied ordering me to the 143d Reg. but stated that he requested me to go there to settle an Existing difficulty Col E H Puleston advised me to go to Col.[space] of the Pay Department for further advice. he told me to go to the war department for authority to join my Regiment—but they positively refused to act—Stating that the difficulty Existed with the State authorities and it was their duty to settle it—and I was accordingly compelled to visit Harrisburg—after getting there D King after considerable trouble the Adj general decided that I belonged to the 143d Reg. Penna Vols—

Col E L Dana—upon Returning to Washington I immediately Reported for duty to the Regiment and went to work being Located at Fort Slocum[13]—the men working on the Fort—the Fort is being greatly Enlarged—it Now Mounts Sixteen guns—when completed will mount Seventy-five—on Dec 31st 1862—we were Mustered for pay. The Reg. Made a fine appearance the Reg. is certainly a fine one—it was raised in Luzerne County—a great many of the men being from Wilkes-Barre—Dr. [Francis C.] Reamer is the surgeon Dr. D[avid] L Scott assist. Surgeon—The sick list is not very heavy there being no serious cases of disease of any consequence— Hospital Stewart is Jos [Josiah L.] Lewis.[14]

January 7th 1863

—Yesterday was wet and very unpleasant in Camp but the war news from Tenessee being of a character to dispel gloomy feelings. Rosencranz has just fought the greatest battle of the war And gained the greatest Victory—I hope this not a Mere flash but Something real and Lasting[15]—that will go on until the great Southern Rebellion Shall be known only in Story—To day is fine and clear with a fresh Sharp breeze from the North west for the past two or three weeks. the weather has been More like spring than winter—we have as yet had little of the wet and damp Expected in a climate like This—to day we had but Little news to day from Vicksburg—why we do not Know—the news from Rosencranz being good Enough for one day—

For some time the Col E L Dana has been trying to get the Reg^t into heavy Artillery but as yet has failed In the undertaking it will be quite pleasant to get rid of Marching and carrying the Knapsacks— The men are not working on the Fort to day, it being too cold for that purpose—My old horse is doeing fine having a tent for a Stable it protects him from the weather—and makes him in a better condition for duty when needed—

January 12th 1863.

To day was truly a beautiful day—this Morning was Spent in Examining the Sick at Morning call this afternoon. I took a walk goeing by the Soldiers Home and down by the Harewood Hospital[16]—and on until I came to Glenwood Cemetery—passing through the grounds viewing with pleasure the different walks and Lots—Elegantly Laid out with cariage Road and walk. Many of the Monuments are neat and Elegant presenting Some Elegant specimens of Workmanship—There were two of the finest tombs that I have Ever seen one was Marked Douglas + Rigs[17]—and had a grand door through which could be seen the Nich[e]s in which are placed the coffins there were two of them filled—

After looking round here and seeing all of interest I went across to 7th Street to See the 150th I found them in camp in the Swamp—being very unpleasantly situated indeed. I found A Letter here from Wm Wm[18] stating that he is slowly improving he is not as yet released from duty—his Resignation not as yet being accepted. to day we went into meet Capt. [William A.] Tubbs[19] And his lieutenant[20] with Chas. Cook[21] Dr Scott + Myself—they procured a cook stove to day for Six dollars and carried it up from town—I stayed with the 150th untill 5 oclock then started back by Harewood stopping awhile with Capt Smith—their is a contraband camp[22] doeing the Hos Washing—

/Camp Slocum—/
Jan 16th.

Last night was very stormy the wind blowing a gale the rain coming down in torrents—the night before Capt—Tubbs tent took fire and made quite a conflagration—they Lost nothing but one blanket and their Boots—On Monday Last we went into mess Capt Tubbs his Lietenants and Corporal. Dr. Scott + myself—we Live quite well—So far. Mrs. Sinclair [unidentified] thinks it a great privilege to have privilege [sic] to have the opportunity of [inviting] her friends. we do not consider it in a light So favorable—as yet we have had no pay and do not know how soon we will get it there was 26 deserters from company B—in one day—things Look bad at this time for the country the Democrats as a party doeing all in their power to cripple the administration in putting down the Rebellion—had it not been for the tories in the north the war would have been well nigh Ended by this time—The south are Encouraged by them all the time thinking that there is a strong party their that favor them and will ultimately divide the North—and thus in the End cause them to gain their independence—Old Valandingham[23]—made a speech in the house the 15th throwing out his treason such never have injury beyond calculation[24]—it seems that men can go to any length with their treasonable declarations—and use Ey. means to injure the cause of the Union—

I only hope hard soon such Men May be silenced And go sneaking to
their dens of infamy unnoticed—and unheeded their names handed
down to posterity an Everlasting disgrace not only to themselves
but their posterity—Our nation is certainly tried as by fire—there
is a large amount of money due the soldiers—and it appears no
money to pay them—it now becomes the duty of Congress to make
provision for the payment of the Army—to do so in such a way that
our Currency will not be Entirely worthless the Nation seems to be
undergoeing a great Struggle and a it certainly will not be long untill
there will be something decisive known in regard to our countrys
future—it is to be hoped that our nation [has been] punished
Enough for her many transgressions—And that the good time is not
far distant when peace Shall again bless this people—

Feb 17ᵗʰ 1863—

To Day packed up papers and took up the line of march for
Washington—it commenced Snowing about [10] oclock in the
Morning—Snowed on us All the way to the Landing—Many of the
Men were wet to the Skin—on getting to the Landing we all went
aboard of boat My old horse was not for goeing on the Boat but by
being blindfolded So that he could not see where he was goeing
went on—without Any trouble—the Boat Laid at the Wharf until
next morning at six oclock—it continued Storming throughout the
Day—the men while on the boat were protected from [the] Storm
though having but little protection from the cold—our Sick we put
in the Cabin

/Potomac River passage/
Feb 18ᵗʰ

—this morning the boat left her mooring at the wharf and started
for her destination passing down the Potomac, there was but little of
interest to meet the Eye, the Barren hills of Virginia

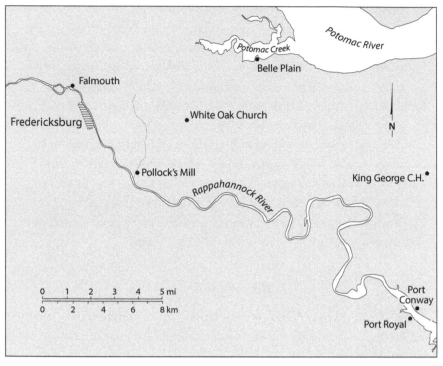

Map 1.1. Belle Plain, Virginia

on the right—those of the Maryland Shore covered with snow looking but little better—Nothing of note transpiring untill we came
oposite Alexandria—when we were hailed by—a Gov. Vessel that
Sent—an officer on board to Examine the papers to see that they
were all right—we were soon allowed to pass on having no difficulty
in showing that we were in Uncle Sams Employ—and that were
goeing to try and do something for the good of our country—if
possible—we Started on our way down the River passing the Spot
nearly where the ashes of Washington Repose[25]—though at this
time presenting nothing of special interest to the Eye—of the
beholder the Snow covering the ground and a thick mist or Fog
continueing through out the day—

made the trip not one of pleasure and observation as it would
have been had the weather been clear And the Sun Shining out

Brightly—the Broad Expanse of water would then have been beautiful with the Many thousands of Ducks Floating and feeding upon
the water it would certainly have been a beautiful Sight—to feast the
Eye upon—After passing down the Potomac untill we came to the
Potomac Creek we passed up the inlet formed by the tide making up
that Small Stream untill we came to what is called Prales [Pratt's?]
Landing where we came to a Halt[26]—

/Bele Plain/

We laid at the landing all night—The next morning we took up
the line of march that we might occupy the position held by the
old Penn[a] Reserve our object being to relieve them—they goeing
[to] Alexandria to do guard Duty—upon Landing we found the
mud almost with out terminous it was actually running down the
hill so much had it been stirred up and so thus had become I had
often heard of corduroy roads and pole Bridges but had never seen
them in perfection untill this time. The many teams that came to
this place put on not more than the fourth of the Load that they
would if the roads were good and thus many of them would Stall
and have to be pulled out—the mules would flounder in the mud
get discouraged Lie down and refuse to get up with kind treatment
or the contrary And many of them would be killed So that it was no
uncommon thing to see dead horses and mules—In Some places
could be seen [as] many as a dozen horses and mules Laying within
a narrow Space—Showing plainly Enough [t]he great Source of
Expense to the [page torn]—Some places you would see a Sutlers
team that had stuck in the mud—And had been left to its fate—the
next team that passed would likely overturn the wagon and leave
it to its fate so that the whole thing would be a dead loss to its
owners—

/February 19, 1863—/

The men plunged through [t]he mud up to their knees up the corderoy road untill they reached the top of the hill—there taking an

Easterly Direction for about two Miles came to the camp of the old Penn[a] Reserve—but for Some Reason it was not thought best for us to pitch camp in this place—but we were taken further to the South and camped near the 149th and 150th Reg.[s] Penna V[ols] with which Regts we were Brigaded about this time—we went into a thick growth of pine—the Men immediately began to chop down the trees and build themselves houses in a manner quite interesting they first built up a peer [pier] of logs Some 4 or 5 feet

Feb 19th 1863. [continued]

high then putting their shelter tents on these for a roof had quite good houses as the timber was cut away the Direction of the streets soon began to be Manifest and it soon began to have quite the appearance of a vilage—And An appearance of neatness and comfort that would astonish persons not accustomed to such things—[A]fter getting into camp and [rain?] coming down these men being much Exposed had considerable Sickness—beside having a number of cases of Measles—this being the most troublesome to treat of all— the catarrhal symptoms in all were severe but those cases that had Pneumonia of which there were several all Sunk into the low form or in other words had Typhoid Pneumonia.

/Typhoid Pneumonia Bele plain/

And in Spite of Every Effort And Remedy us[ed] by us the consequence was that they Sunk and Died—We used the stimulant And Supporting form of treatment—But it appeared to me that the Erruption of the Measles was not only upon the External Surfa[ce] of the Body but that the mucus And Serous membranes[27] of [the] lungs and bowels were Equal[ly] Effected—And owing to the Extreme delicacy of these parts they took on a high state of inflammation So Much So that the vitality of these parts were destroyed—in the manner that gangrene acts we first have congestion then inflammation by which the vessels become so full and Engorged that they are unable to relieve themselves And the result is that they die And the parts

Slough off—but in the case of the Lungs And Mucus Membrane of the bowels—the parts being so Extensive instead of the Sloughing we have a loss of that power by which the blood is oxygenated in the lungs hence the General poisoning of the whole system by impure blood—the Brain [w]orking as usual under such [c]ircumstances— the Bowels of [c]ourse being unable to take up those principles that go to build up the System of course being preoccupied with trying to relieve themselves—remedies used—were External irritation with mustard croton oil Blisters with the administration of copaiba a. turpentine carb Ammonia—Pot. chlor. [potassium chloride] camphor[ae] Liquor[28]—

/Camp Dana Bele plain/

But all the means resorted to by us were unavailing the patients without an Exception Sinking and Dying—by the reasons that those parts by which the functions of life were to be carried on were unable to act hence inducing inaction—And death—

The remainder of ~~April~~ February And And [sic] the Month of April was Extremely Storm[y] there being a great many Sto[rms?] of Snow so that it was very trying on the men doeing Picket Duty[29]—And All this too after having good times in Washington in the Beginning of Winter but the men had no complaint to make doeing their duty cheerfully and without complaint—March I think was the most uncomfortable Month that I have Ever passed in Any part of the country it is in fact the Most Severe Winter they have in Virginia—

The country upon which we Encamped known by the name of Bele plain is a region of Sand with hills and vallies having the appearance of having been [cov]ered with water And taking its [f]orm by the motion of the water in many places there being large deposits of Shells And other indications of marine inhabitants having at one time floated over the surface—the surface of the country is poor—though I think with proper Management I think [sic] the country would be Easily cultivated And in My opinion would make a beautiful country—but one thing is certain there must be a great change not only in the country but in the people—

/Camp Dana Bele Plain/

the class that now occupy the country are not only poor but ignorant in the Extreme the Men wealthy and intelligent living along the rivers and having large plantations—the poor whites being not only very poor none of them being Land holders but at the same time very ignorant being below the Negro Slave in point of Gentili[ty] of course can never raise as long as that institution exists

NOTES

1. In southern Chester County.
2. Possibly Assistant Surgeon Joseph F. Wilson, Emergency Militia.
3. Kirk mustered in on August 20, 1862, and mustered out with his regiment on May 23, 1863.
4. Unidentified.
5. Col. Langhorne Wister, commanding officer of the 150th PA.
6. Possibly Pvt. Thomas Mackey, 121st PA, later wounded at Gettysburg on July 1, 1863.
7. All officers of the 150th PA.
8. Unidentified.
9. Possibly Corcoran, unidentified.
10. Both detailed to the Soldiers' Home to guard President Lincoln.
11. Episodes of typhoid fever among Companies D and K, which provided security for the president, are not mentioned in the regimental history of the 150th PV.
12. Col. J. H. Puleston, Military Agent of Pennsylvania.
13. One of the city's defensive forts, northeast of downtown Washington.
14. Dr. Reamer mustered into service on September 16, 1862; Dr. Scott mustered on September 18, 1862; and Hospital Steward Lewis mustered on September 6, 1862 as a private, Company E, and was promoted to hospital steward on October 1, 1863. Evidently, Lewis performed his new duty in an acting capacity before his promotion.
15. Battle of Stone's River or Murfreesboro, Tennessee, December 31, 1862–January 2, 1863. Maj. Gen. William S. Rosecrans, who commanded the Army of the Cumberland, achieved victory.
16. Harewood General Hospital opened in September 1862, and closed in May 1866. Located in northwest Washington, D.C., the hospital was a short walk north from Glenwood Cemetery. Harewood featured around 2000 beds and was famously visited repeatedly by Walt Whitman.
17. Today, an iron door to a brick-built tomb bears the name "Douglas and Diggs" and contains several interments.

18. James Fulton's younger brother, William T. Fulton, was at this time a major in Maryland's Purnell Legion.

19. Commanding Company F, 143rd PA.

20. Probably 1st Lt. H. M. Gordon.

21. Possibly Pvt. Chas. F. Cook, who served with Company D.

22. Union soldiers termed "contraband" the thousands of enslaved African Americans who fled to Union occupied areas and created makeshift temporary settlements near forts. Contraband camps functioned as a transitional zone for refugees seeking freedom in the North.

23. Ohio Congressman Clement L. Vallandigham. See chapter 7 for a discussion of his significance.

24. The wording is awkward but Fulton appears to say that Vallandigham's treasonous remarks are reckless and cause injury beyond his apparent intent.

25. Mount Vernon.

26. The regiment came to Belle Plain, now called Belle Plains, located along Potomac Creek a few miles east-northeast of Fredericksburg and south of Aquia Creek.

27. Mucous membranes are moist tissues lining the surfaces of openings to the body. Serous membranes line interior cavities and reduce motion-induced muscular friction around some internal organs.

28. See chapter 9.

29. Soldiers on picket duty manned outer guardposts to give warning to the main encampment of incoming threats.

TWO

Chancellorsville and "a Spiteful Morose Scamp"

Diary, February 22, 1863, to June 28, 1863

THE BRIGADE'S MORALE WAS NOT DAMPENED BY A PUNISHING SNOWSTORM: *the soldiers were now ensconced within a theater of war in a part of Virginia where the front line was less a line than a curtain fluttering sinuously over the countryside. When in camp, the soldiers drilled and improved their own lodgings despite the snow, while their officers attended to administrative tasks and improved their own knowledge of tactics during impromptu evening classes. All regiments rotated picket duty, which necessitated equipping soldiers for rations and ammunition for two or three days before posting them along the Rappahannock River.*

—⁓—

February 22ond

This morning [illegible word] commenced Snowing Early And continued throughout the day. It is I think one of the severest Storms that I have Ever seen—the Snow fell to the depth of 14 inches— the Men Are called upon to go on Picket duty which is indeed just leaving good [q]uarters to go into the woods in a terrible Snow Storm without any Shelter Except as they cut the Boughs from the trees and in this way Slightly protects themselves from the Storm—not Under-standing the business it being Entirely new to them they did not take their axes with them and of course had not the chance of Making Much fire—

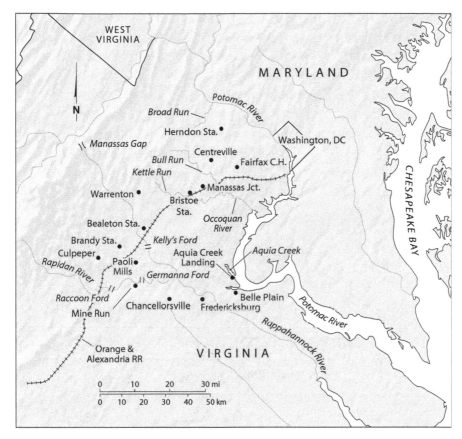

Map 2.1. Central and Northern Virginia

/Camp Dana Bele plain/

for My part I was not called upon to go on Picket but Joe [Private Josiah L. Lewis][1] And Myself Sojourned in camp in our Sibley tent [a conical tent that could accommodate 10 to 12 soldiers invented before the war by Henry Hopkins Sibley] with a Small Sheet Iron Stove—we went about half a mile and gathered up some rails and dragged them through the snow. th[ey] helped us Some but the[n] we could not keep warm—I suffered More in the Night having to get up three times during the night and visit sick Men in camp—After Each visit it was Still More difficult to get warm untill I finally

determined to go to a Small house that was near by and See if it was
Not possible to get warm—upon goeing to the house and knock-
ing I found that old Pap. St Clair[2] And [Vandersort?] had taken up
Lodging there and that they had a good fire in the fire place I went in
And Sat By the fire untill Morning Keeping compar[a]bly comfortable—this I think was the Severest Storm that I have Ever been
called to pass through or at Least I think there was more real suffering from the cold than I Ever Experienced in my life before—The
month of February continued Storming throughout having storms
of snow Every day or two—And they being quite Severe—So much
Moisture And such a feeling of chilliness—

/Camp Dana Bell Plain/

about this my picket duty commenced it being my place to go on
picket about once a week it being sometimes quite pleasant at others
very disagreeable not having any other protection from the storms
than the Bough houses built by the Men—they would keep the
Snow from getting upon a person but when the snow would melt the
~~wather~~ water would run through and be more unpleasant than it was
out of Doors—The picket line presented but little of interest Except
the Burial place of the wife and child of Cap[t]. Taliaferro[3]—Now
General in the Rebel Army—the burial place has at one time been
quite neat and tastily [sic; perhaps Fulton meant tidy] but now the
fence is all down and the ground grown up with undergrowth that
Makes it look rather hard—this region of country is rather better
than about our camp it getting nearer the river but then it is not good
much of it being grown up with pine Showing that is land that has
been worn out—And then thrown out And allowed to grow up with
pine—there is an occasional Strip of good timber though Such is not
at all plentiful—being rather the Exception than the rule—The only
great advantage the country seems to possess is the great number
of good Springs and fine little Streams running down the valies in a
high degree qualifying it as a grazing country for which I think it is
better suited than for every other purpose—

About this time My horse and one of the Majors [horses] got away and after considerable Search we found them tied up among the horses of the 11th Illinois Cavalry[4]—we were Lucky in finding them when we did or the Scamps would have had them sold and then—the chance for getting any more good out off old Bones would been a bad one—Old Bones is fast improving so that he is getting to be quite a good horse he can jump a ditch with any horse in the Regiment he is so large and strong that he is valuable to Me as I can put my three days rations on him with my bed and cooking utensils and go to the picket line without any trouble—

March month 1863—

throughout this month but little of interest the regular routine of Picket Duty—and inspections and reviews—apparently preparing for field operations   things having but little of interest. When our Regts. went to Camp Slocum this day.[5] Being quite Stormy—it was ordered to Encamp on the farm of Mr. Ray[6] the men suffering from the cold attacked the old gentlemans hay and Straw Stacks to make them selves beds that they might the better keep out of the wet and mud. they also took some of his fence to make fire with the old gent was pretty wrathy and put in a Bill of $125.00 but the field officers thinking it too much refused to pay and the matter run along untill in July we were goeing to be paid when we found that there was a claim of $400.00 Doles [dollars] had been filed at the pay department against the Reg. And that we could not be paid untill it was settled the Colonel went to Washington but could do nothing a Col Gibson[7] had joined in with Ray and made such an impression upon the Authorities there that they could not be disabused—and we consequently had to foot the whole Bill—

April 1863.

The Beginning of this Month had been little of interest to the Soldier with the Exception that on the 20th we had orders to take up the

line of march we started about noon taking a direction toward the
Picket line not knowing to what part we were goeing—about 3
oclock in the afternoon it commenced to rain the roads Soon began
to be quite muddy we Marched on untill about 12 o-clock when
we stopped in the wood to have something to Eat—after which
we again took up the line of march plunging through mud many
places being up to the Mens knees in one place we went through
the wood for half a mile the distance being almost impassible—it
was my duty to try and keep up the Hospital teams and a terrible
job it was—Stalling and breaking their Harness and Sometimes
upsetting it was the heaviest task that Ever I had and many times
would have gladly been relieved of the undertaking—but we worked
along through the long dark night—Stopping again at daylight
again to take Some breakfast—about this time we came up with
the Pontoon train they had an awful time to get up a long clay hill
but by doubling their teams and with much swearing and whipping
finally got to the top—I often thought [sic] when at home and the
papers kept saying that the army could not move because the roads
were so bad[8]—but at this time I was fully able to appreciate what it
was to move an army—though we had no Artillery—After taking
Some coffee and hard tack we again took up the line of march untill
dinner time when we came to port Conway that being the point of
destination for the division. there being only one Division under
the Command of General [Abner] Doubleday the object being to
make a feint to draw the attention from Fredericksburg not having any Artillery the Gen ordered the beds to be taken from the
wagons and in the place of [these] logs to be mounted in the place of
them [sic]—

The Pontoons were then taken down to the village at the Edge of the
river. the Pontoons were then taken from the wagons and put on the
ground as though preparing to put in the water the wooden guns
were then put into position to cover the Laying of the pontoons all
this was done about dusk as though the idea was to cross under cover
of the night—but when night set in rightly and it was quite dark we

quietly withdrew and left the Rebs to their reflections—they soon saw however what the object of the move was and the strong force they had then was sent up the river—to meet any other move we might make higher up the stream—

[Major] Gen[eral Joseph] Hooker finding the Effect this move had upon the Rebs immediately Sent the 2ond Division down to cross the river—they did so capturing Some Men And quite a number of mules—though that night when we quit the Bank of the river we retired about two miles into the wood and there camped for the night—the next morning taking up the line of march for our old camp which we reached about 3 o clock of the 22ond of April after one of the most tiresome marches that men have been called to pass through of the Same length—the time being only three days—at Port Conway the Rapahanock is quite a fine Stream here there is some fine farms along the river at this place there was a large field of corn here that had not been husked they were busy fishing and they caught some fine Shad And Sold them quite reasonable to what they did at Potomac Creek—this country would be beautiful if it was only properly cultivated—but all this is left to the negroes—on our way home in the morning Dr. Henderson[9] and myself stoped at King Georges Court House and got our Breakfast—we had quite a good meal for 50 cts warm Biscuit hoe cake Shad and coffee—So that we could go on our way rejoicing. the Lady of the house told us her tale of Sorrow which was in the usual Strain She had been the owner of twenty nigs and she greatly complained of the yankees for coaxing her Nigs to run away from her—among the others She Said that she had a young girl that was nearly white and she hinted though she did not say that they wanted her for their own use—She represented her as being very good looking—if so I must confess it is more than can be said of her mistress—as for the town of King Georges what it was in its Palmy days of greatness and Glory. I am not able to say but at this time the court House is but a quite an ordinary looking building. There not being many other buildings in fact it being but a small vilage to say nothing of it as a county seat—after finish[ing]

our Breakfast we took up the line of march but the troops had turned
of[f] and gone another way—and the Dr. and myself had to [find]
the way back by ourselves—

/Pollocks Mills Virginia/

getting into camp a short time before the troops—after getting
back we again settled down to the old routine of camp duty for a
short time but it was not long untill we were again under marching
orders—And Nothing of importance transpiring between this and
the 28th day of April when we again with our whole Corps took up
the line of March from Pollocks Mills on the Rappahanock[10]—we
came within a mile of the place And then Encamped in the wood
for the Night this time there was Pontoons along but they had quite
a diff[ere]nt look from those at Port Conway and in the place of the
wooden guns we had the genuine dogs of war that not only looked
cross but could bark and bite in the morning the Pontoon train with
the Sharp Shooters went down to the river taking the Rebs Entirely
by Surprise—the Pontoons were down by noon and the 1st Division
of our Corps crossed over and posted themselves on the hill on the
other side—about this time the Rebs began to pass up the River
finding that they had work higher up Stream did not Stop to molest
those that had crossed at this point but went on up to the United
States Ford where Hooker had crossed Several Corps and taken the
Plank road—The Rebs not being disposed to distant[11] [sic] at all the
rest of our Corps laid quietly behind the hills there being nothing to
Break the monotony Excep occasionally a little Shelling—from the
Rebs which was promptly returned from our Batteries on this Side of
the river—

/Chancellorsville or the Wilderness/

I had been detailed by Dr. Hottenstein for Hospital duty at the time
of action—And of course I had to go and help put up the tents and
prepare for recovering the wounded but as good luck would have
it we had no men wounded in our Division—the first Division had
about 12 men hu[rt] in crossing—Col[onel Edmund L.] Dana[12] had
the idea that it was not quite right that all the medical officers should

be taken from the Regiment [and] Petitioned to Dr. Hottenstein that I should go back to the Reg. as he did not feel Satisfied without having one medical officer—I was quite well satisfied as I could then see all that was goeing on—the last days of april and the first day of May were passed without anything of note transpiring—but on May 2nd our Corps had marching orders in the morning at 8 o clock we took up the line of march for Chancellorsville the distance being about 25 miles the day being very warm the men threw away their Blankets— and many of their Shelter tents that they could the better get along— [w]e reached the battlefield at 2 o clock on the morning of May the 3d And fell in ready for action things had been goeing rather badly. the 11th Corps had been driven back and lost much of the advantage that had been gained in the Beginning—but after being kept in line for about an hour we were allowed to lie down on our Arms for the night.

/Chancellorsville May/

On getting up in the morning the Men were assigned a position in the line and immediately commenced throwing up Breast work to protect themselves against the Enemys attack they soon had quite a formidable work with an abbatis[13] in front of trees with the Ends of the limbs toward the Enemy. our Men soon began to Bring in prisoners they were mostly wounded Rebs that were goeing to the Hospital and our men intercepted them on their way and brought them in.

I here took the Ball out of the back of the neck of a wounded Reb who had been shot in the Eye the Ball passing apparently through the Brain—but not killing him—he was taken to the Hospital his Brother had been killed that Morning—he manifested a great Anxiety to get well that he might see his Mother again poor fellow I think his chance of Ever getting to see her is a bad one indeed the poor fellow but hard is their lot many of them forced into the army against their will to be killed and leave their widowed Mothers [to] suffer want and the cold charities of the Confederacy to depend upon for food and raiment which is indeed but a forlorn hope for the future—how sad the tales of Sorrow that many a poor woman has to relate more pitiful far than those related by the negro drivers before

the rebellion broke out about the running away of their negroes and
the taking away of their rights by the northern abolitionists.

/Chancellorsville May/

How much of pain and Remorse must those that did so much
toward Bringing about this unhappy strife have if any conscience
they have to be goaded into remorse—A question that admits some
discussion—

This being the Holy Sabath day did not seem much like that day as
it used to be spent at home with its holy calm and reverential awe.
but in the place of that we had the Booming of canon the rattle
of Musketry the Rebs seemed determined to turn our left and to
that End made about 18 charges upon that part of the line Each
time resulting disastrously to them and with but little gain to us
with the Exception of holding our position. But the Rebs finding
that our Corps had left the positions below Fredericksburg—after
which [Major] Gen[eral John] Sedgwick who had been left there
with the 6th Corps advanced and took possession of the Heights at
Fredericksburg but thinking to form a junction with the Main Army
advanced on up the River toward Chancellorsville—the Rebs finding the shape that things were taking turned their whole force from
Chancellorsville upon Sedgwick and compelled him to recross the
Rappahanock thereby losing all the ground that he had taken—after
which nothing was to be gained by us holding the positions at
Chancellorsville where we thought it best to recross the River—

/Chancellorsville May/

May 7th at two o clock we took up the line of retreat toward the
River which we reached about 5 o clock in the Morning—when we
immediately began to cross before Starting one of the boys belonging to C Co. on taking his gun from his tent drawing the muzzle End
first the gun was discharged and the contents Entering the abdominal cavity just above Pouparts Ligament[14] the Pompion[15] Entering
was taken out but no ball could be found, the poor fellow was carried

to the River about three or 4 miles and then left in the Hospital his
fate has not been learned though it is highly probable that he died
as the Peritoneal inflammation[16] must have set in right away—after
getting Safely across the River and a mile or two on the other side we
partook of some refreshment—but owing to my loosing my haversack. goeing I had nothing to Eat Except such as I could beg from the
boys that being little more than a little hard tack—meat being out of
the question—After we had recrossed the river I never felt so hungry
for meat in my life feeling that I could Eat anything in the shape of
meat—I finally got hold of some raw pork and it was the best meat
that I Ever tasted having the appetite that made it taste good—

After Crossing the River we Marched back toward our old camp as
far as White Oak Church[17] reaching that point at Sun Down in the
Evening but then Col[onel Roy] Stone[18] think[ing] to go back to our
old camp[19] struck out for that point but it soon began to rain very
heavy with thunder and lightning and after wandering about untill
10 o clock at night we had made A circuit of Some four or five Miles
and Landed at white Oak Church the point from which we had
Started about Sundown—by the [sic; Fulton probably meant "that"]
time we were Satisfied to Stop in any place that we Might Escape the
plunge of the Storm And get relieved from wading through the water
in Many places two and three feet deep—

/Chancellorsvile Va./

in the Church the floor had been taken up and the boys had a
fire built on the ground—the house was crowded the Men trying to Make themselves as comfortable as possible under the
Circumstances which was but a poor Show for comfort the house being so much Crowded that but few could get to the fire—the house
being full of smoke Cap.[tain C.M.] Conyngham[20] And myself finally Made up their [sic; Fulton probably meant "our"] mind that we
would hunt another Lodging place if not More Comfortable at least
not So Much crowded—we consequently went back of the Church
to a place that had been used as head qrs [quarters] for one of the
Divisions And there we found a good fire and Some of the 149th had

take[n] up this position for the night—there had been Some poles that were laid down on the ground to Serve as a walk upon these we Spread as [sic; Fulton probably meant "our"] Blankets which were wet and Stretched our Shelter tent over us as well as we possibly could it however affording but little protection against the Storm— we were wet And And [sic] Laid down in we[t] Blankets with the rain Coming down upon us and Slept finely until morning—and felt refreshed by it a[nd] something that I did not think that I could do but we did it and felt nothing the worse for it—

/Retreat from Chancellorsville/
Wednesday May 7th 1863

after getting a little of something to Eat we took up the line of march for our old camp at which place we arrived about noon and immediately set about fixing up but soon learned, that we had made a mistake in coming to Bele[21] as it was designed that we would go into camp near White Oak Church so we made ourselves as comfortable as possible during the night—and in the Morning started for the church where we landed.

May the 8th 1863—

thus having finished up the Chancelorsville Campaign it was not long it is true but then it was made up in severity it being attended with much hard marching and Storms—After getting into to camp we imediately set to work to fix up our hospital as there were many Sick [with] Typh[oid]. Malarial Fever being the prevailing disease with Diarrhea having myself quite a severe time of this uncomfortable disease Lasting about two weeks—those attacked with the Fever were taken down similar to what a person would Expect with Bilious Remittent[22] but then it would keep that form but a short time—soon assumeing a low or Typhoid form with delirium and great prostration—the Main and Most Effectual treatment was turpentine Ar. Spt. Am. Brandy. Qn Sul[23] with the External application of turpentine it was while Laying here that [Private] Lewis Constine[24] had the Misfortune to let his gun discharge the contents into his leg the ball passing between the tibia and fibula—Severing both the Main arteries as we afterward Learned but no hemorrhage taking place and the bones not being injured I thought best in conjunction with the opinions of others that the leg could be saved but about the third day. Symptoms of mortification Manifested themselves—I immediately called on Dr. Hottenstein he thought it best not to operate untill the line of Demarcation[25] would form—Dr. [C. E.] Humphrey[26] being at the time absent at Chancelorsville—attending to our wounded that had been left behind—

But comeing home the 4th day I had him to see the Boy we soon concluded to operate thinking perhaps he might have a chance though it was a slim one—we immediately operated he however lived but three days after though not in so much pain as he had before the operation—had his leg only been amputated at first he would without doubt have recovered—but in trying to save the leg we lost they [sic] Boy—but it was done for the best—about this time [First Lieutenant Charles B.] Stout of Co II[27] was shot accidentally by a pistol in the hand of Serg[eant Jarius] Kauff[28]—the Ball Entering the thigh Just Above the Knee cutting the Femoral artery and splitting the Condyles from the Femur—

/White Oak Church/

in his case the action was plain there was Nothing left but to operate we Amputated at the lower third of the thigh he did well but there being so many, cases of Fever he was taken to the Fitzhugh Hospital and there he was left.—It was about this time that Lieut[enant] Col[onel George E.] Hoyt[29] was taken sick with the Fever. he soon began to sink and desire to go to his home. I made out his certificate and upon making his application he got permission to go home. Where he laid about two weeks when he died[30]—

it was a sad day for us as he was an officer that was much Respected in the Regt and though no resolutions of Respect have been passed by the officers of the Reg to his memory it only a coldness and apathy[31] [*sic*] that is certainly very unbecoming toward an officer so manly honorable and in Every Respect qualified to fill the position he occupied—it was an Event that made me feel sad for the future of our Regiment—well knowing that it would be hard to fill his place—Major [John D.] Musser being in the line of Promotion is made Lieut Colonel Cap Conyngham Being Sr. Captain was made Major—About this time the 150th Reg—was blessed with the addition to their Regt. of Dr. [Philip A.] Quinan[32]—as Surgeon he being the only Surgeon in the Brigade not on detached duty was immediately made acting Brigade Surgeon—in which position he he [*sic*] continued to serve as Long as we staid at this camp—

/White Oak Church/
~~April~~ May. 1863

about this time I made a Requisition for Medicine and in the place of Sending those things wanted he packed up a lot of old trash that he wished to get [illegible word] of and sent to me—whereupon I sent them back stating that they were of no use to me and that we could not—haul them—he got mad as the saying is and said that I should have kept them and if I could not haul them I should throw them away and State that they had been lost in the Service—I came to the conclusion that he might do his own dirty work and not get me to do it and then Lie out of it—he made the threat that he would pay me for it he no doubt will as he Looks like a spiteful morose Scamp—that will hold a grudge for a long time and resort to any means to Gratify his feelings of spleen—And hate such men are seldom good but mostly making up for their want of knowledge and honorable dealing by their acts of Tyrany and oppression toward those that are subject to their Sway. Such men however as a general thing soon run their course as a general thing [*sic*] it is not long untill people get to know them and their race is soon run—

/White Oak Church/

About May 31st we had orders to be in readiness for marching as the Rebs were supposed to be making their way to Penna. The order came to be ready to go by 7 o clock in the morning—and understanding that we were goeing to Falmouth[33] and having quite a number of men that had just recovered from the Fever but were ~~sill~~still quite weak and not having a way to Carry them and their Knapsacks I Started them Early in the Morning toward Falmouth that they might get well on the way before the sun would become too hot for them—there was about a Dozen Such Started on they went until they finally got to Falmouth Station there Stoping to wait for the rest of the army—but the rest did not come that day—and they were Scattered all around and not having Any place to Stop

Gen. Patrie[34] telegraphed to head qrs that a number of Sick Men from our Corps were there without proper Accommodations And that they Must be looked to and provided for—the Matter was soon looked into By Dr. Herd[35] the Surg. in Chief of our Corps And traced down to Me and of course the Blame all all [sic] belonged to me as I had acted Entirely without authority in the case—Dr Herd ordered Dr. Humphrey who was at this time Div Surgeon to put me under ~~arres~~ arrest—Dr. Humphrey came to Me And told [me] what had been done and Stated that he would do all in his power to get me relieved—he went to Dr Herd And Stated that What I had done was done with proper Motive and with[out] having any idea of the result that Might follow—Herd finally agreed to let me off but Said that he wanted Me to come to his office in the Morning—in the Morning I went up to corps head qrs and Saw him he seemed to be in a good humor—And talked to Me in a reasonable gentlemanly Manner of the Consequences that would follow if all would be allowed to send of their sick without proper authority. I finally left him having a high opinion of his Bearing as a soldier and a gentleman having a much higher opinion than I formerly had—I felt quite well pleased to get of[f] so safely—

/White Oak Church/

To Sum up our stay at this camp we had quite a fine Location for our Hospital though the men had not so good a place for camp—the weather being very dry and so much going too and fro the dust was almost intolerable flying in clouds continually—The 10th of June we again got orders to get ready to move in the morning—Every thing was in motion preparing for the Expected move we had quite a number of sick to be sent to Division Hospital at Windmill Point [mouth of the Rappahannock River] near Aqia [Aquia] Creek Landing[36]—where it had been Established in the spring about the 1st of April—Dr [Francis C.] Reamer[37] and [Assistant Surgeon David L.] Scott[38] being Detailed from the Reg. for the purpose of running the machine—In the morning of June 11th we were all up in time to get the men their Break-fast before starting for the Hospital the ambulances coming we got the men aboard and started them and soon our Brigade was in Motion taking the direction toward Falmouth we kept well back from the River out of sight of the Enemy making the move as quietly as possible we marched all day pretty hard getting about half way to Bealton Station[39] that night and Encamping near to a stream about dark—here we had a good nights rest—and nothing of interest transpiring with the Exception that the Men were very tired when they came into Camp. But the night being pleasant all rested well and were in the morning ready to resume the march

/March to Penn[a]/
June 1[2?]th

June 13th.[40] [sic] to day we made a hard march getting to Bealton Station about dark again the country through which we passed to day was better than we have been in for some time the farms having a better appearance that such as we have been in many of them would be good had they only the care and cultivation requisition for good farming—the country through here has a little [of] the appearance of some parts of Penna, that are not much improved there being great many chinquapin Bushes[41] and there being many of those Large nigger head Stones[42] as seen in some parts of Chester County—the country round Bealton is level and apparently good it is certainly a fine country for grass—the pasture is fine and would certainly be a great place to feed cattle and no doubt has been used for that purpose—we moved into the wood and camped for the night about two miles from the Rappahanock—there was a cavalry fight just across the river yesterday—in which we had a large force Engaged and the Rebs got pretty badly whipped and Gen Steward lost his papers in which we learned the whole plan of the invasion of Penn^a. the rail road in this part looks as though there had been no business done for some time—it was greatly used at the Beginning of the Rebelion to cary troops to Manassas junction but now is of no use to the Confederacy as that point is not held by them—

Sunday, June 13th 1863

This was a day that will long be remembered by the portion of the Army that was on this March we left Bealton about 6 o clock in the morning and took up our line of March along the railroad in the direction of Manassas junction we did not halt for dinner untill about two o clock—we started as soon as we were done Eating and went on untill about 9 o clock when we again stoped for Supper—after which we again started for the Junction getting in there about 3 o clock in the morning the object appearing to be to cut of[f] the Rebs and get into the Fortifications at Centreville before they could get there.

By this time it was pretty wel–understood that the programe of the Rebs was to go into Penn^a to make it an invasion on their part and Carry the Strife into the Northern States thinking that Old Virginia had suffered her share and in order to do this properly our officers [thought] it would be of immense advantage to them to cut off our communication by holding the Fortifications at Centreville[43] and thereby compelling us to make the longer march before we could meet them at Manassas there is but little of interest Except that you may see the wreck of many [train] cars that were were destroyed by stone–wall Jackson last Summer—the old wheels and other Iron work Laying round in the profusion goeing to show that the destruction had been great.

/March to Pennsylvania/

There were two or three Earth—works round they did not Look
very formidable but with large guns mounted in them would have
given the Contending force some trouble to have taken the country
through which we passed on this march was of the poorer character
and not so valuable as that near Bealton though in crossing a Stream
in the night Said to Be goose creek.[44] we found the Stream Scirted
[skirted] with fine pasture or at least Timothy[45] the Seemed to be a
good Size so that the horses did fine so long as they had an opportunity to Eat—which of course was not Long I was sorry that we did
not pass this country in daylight so that we could have a chance to
see it better

June 1[3?]th 1863[46]

the Stream Seemed to be quite large in this place—This morning
left the junction about 8 o clock and took up the line of March
for Centreville the distance being about [eight?] miles the first
object of interest being a large Brick house—that had been used by
[Confederate] Gen. [Pierre G. T.] Beuregard [Beauregard] as his
head qrs at the time of the first Bull run fight. The House was quite
a good one—after passing this a short distance we soon got into the
pines where the old Shell's were to be found in great abundance—
Showing that the conflict there had been long and Sharp. Keeping
on about two miles we came to the famous Stream of Bull run a
Stream About the Size of the Elk[47] at Katy Dizards[48] and somewhat
of its appearance—

/March to Penn[a] /
June 17th 1863—Tuesday,

To day we Still Remained in the vicinity of Centreville and rested
we all began to feel pretty good—The Boys took a general Swim
in Bull Run the old Battlefield presents but little of curiosity to
the visitor no graves being visible the careless manner in which
the dead had been buried causing all Signs of the departed to pass

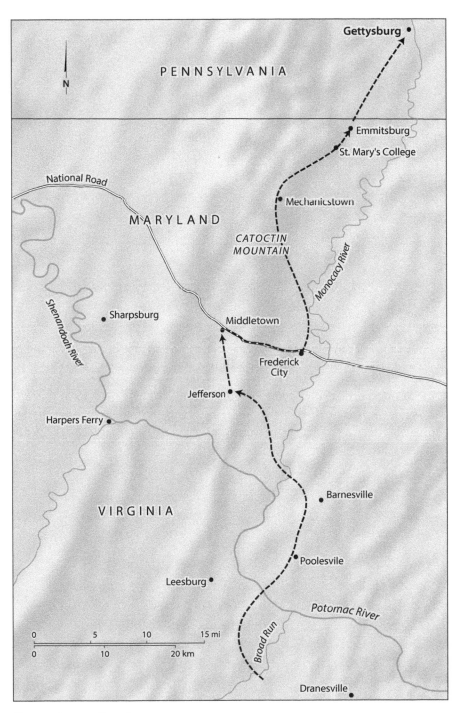

Map 2.2. Route to Gettysburg

away. [ere] long Even of the many, hundreds of Rebs that died with
[space] disease no visible sign now remains of the ravage that the
Climate Severe made upon them from the far South their Lungs not
being able to withstand the rigors of this North Virginia climate the
consequence was that hundreds died many, with the measles—And
many, more with Pneumonia—And Typhoid Fever so that in this
way, the Southern Confederacy lost many of her best men—but
only adding to the Long list of Widows left helpless and hop[e]
less by this unjust war—how must those men feel that used their
influence toward bringing about this State of affairs if they have any
consciences—

/March to Penn[a] /

this ground though presenting but little of importance to the Eye
is yet of great interest to the visitor it being the place where the
forces Loyal to the US met in force the Enemies of their country
and make a desperate Effort to save the country our long train of
Evils—but in that awful conflict in the Providence of God it was
so ordered that our Army was not to be victorious but that of the
Enemy was to triumph And we were to be driven a routed And
Vanquished rabble before the Exulting foe to the very gates of the
Capitol of the nation—after this it was of course a long time before
the Army could again be prepared for Aggressive operations And
put under the Command of [Major] General [George B.] McClelan
[McClellan]—

the people round are generally poor for the reason that they can
do nothing in the way of Farming—And if they could they would
be liable at any time to have their crops destroyed by one army or
the other—As for the Village of Centreville it is An old looking
place with but few houses and those having the appearance of
being very old So that the place is not very Atractive none of the
neatness And beauty that is usually Seen in Country Vilages—the
Situation is a fine one And the Vilage could be Made beautiful—but
then in this As with All Else belonging to Virginia there is no

taste no Enterprise—The Fortification being guarded by the 22[49]ond
Corps under the command of Gen. [Major General Samuel P.]
Heintzelman And having quite a fine position there being but little
to do And good quarters—the duty though Nice is Not the Kind to
be Sought by Good Soldiers that wish to do their duty for their duty
for [sic] their Country—We Soon began to find that the Rebs had no
Notion of disturbing us here and the Cavalry bringing information
that they had had [sic] been Making demonstration in force between
us And the Potomac there was no Need of our longer remaining
~~longer~~ in this position—

/H. Rosenberg March to Penn[a]/
June 26th 1863 –

To Day, we got word of the death of Hiram Rosenberg[50]—who had
been our Hospital Steward—he was a good boy he had two attacks
of Fever and was quite weak and unable to march but would not
ride in an Ambulance. he Laid down at night between two of his
comrades And they did not know of his death until Morning—it
was Near Adamstown Maryland—the Boys buried him as best they
could—it is Said that his wife is a bad woman and was the cause no
doubt of his death[51]—

/March to Penn[a]/
June 17th 1863

This Morning we Struck tents And took up the line of March passing
through I think the first farming Country in Virginia it being in
Loudon [Loudoun] County—Some of the farms Seemed to have
been Kept in a good Condition And the land looked as though it was
good the Most of it being Covered with rich grass with fine Springs
of water Showing that it is a country well Calculated for Grazeing
And in fact would Sent [sic; Fulton probably meant "suit"] me well to
live in having much the appearance of Chester County Being quite
hilly And in some places quite Stony; the houses being built of Stone
And Some of them having Stone Spring houses Made this part of the

Country have quite a good appearance And looking like as if it was inhabited by a Civilized people—

I think the Most of them have Emigrated from the Northern States there is one settlement near this composed of Emigrants from New Jersey, And they have things in good order And live in a degree of comfort And happiness unknown to the old settlers—this days march was a very pleasant one indeed because the country being hilly afforded much of interest we would meet here a running stream And Anon a woody dell affording a variety—that did away with the feeling of weariness so common to marches through a Country where there is so much Sameness and that presents no objects that are new as it is in many parts of Virginia—particularly in the Bele [Belle] Plain Region—

To day we travelled to near Drainsville[52] where the old Bucktails had their first fight in which they gained their first reputation as good fighting men [Major] Gen[eral John F.] Reynolds took up his head qrs at a large Farm house close by our camp—at the house there was a good Spring of water the Major went out to another farm house and got Some fresh butter he sold us a pound this being the first good butter that I had Eaten Since I had been in Penn[a] which was in october 1862. it tasted good After Eating Nothing but hard tack and meat for so long, we put up our tents in an open field it being quite a pleasant place for camp

Near this is a village called Herndon there was an old steam mill that was goeing to ruin there being nothing Else of note it is Situated in the line of the Leesburg Railroad, the road being [in] a ruined condition this part of it not being used at all by Either the Rebs or ourselves—the rails being in many places taken up—we Enjoyed the rest here very much indeed as the weather was very hot and dusty tiring the men greatly the water in some places being Scarce and bad and the men not having a chance to leave the road to go any distance to get water—Suffered at times greatly for that of all things [is most] important to the weary, heated soldier on the March—

/March to Pennᵃ/
June 18ᵗʰ 1863—

This morning before Stoping to get Breakfast we Struck tents And took up the line of march for Broad run[53] the distance being about 4 miles—the most of the distance being along the railroad—the country being poor and most of it overgrown with Scrubpine—And the land that was clear looking as though it was too poor to keep a Whiporwile [whipporwill] from starving Broad run is quite a fine stream with fine timber along the banks I went as soon as I came to it and found a nice place and took[54]—shortly after getting a good place Col Wister [Lieutenant Colonel Henry S.] Hydikooper [Huidekoper] and Major [Thomas] Chamberlain with Adj[utant R. L.] Ashurst[55] also came and we had a splendid bath the water being clean the Bottom being covered with with gravel. after Batheing we went Back to camp—or rather to look for a good place to camp.

I concluded to put up my horse by the side of the stream under some oak trees that were there the ground was covered with a good Sod the grass being Short and and no bushes it was a beautiful place for the purpose—but word soon came for us to lay out a camp and to organize Regularly, as though we were goeing to stay for Sometime we did So and it was not long untill we were fixed up quite comfortably—here was the first place that I had Seen foraging carried on—after getting their tents fixed up it was not Long untill the crack of the rifle could be heard in all directions there being Some fine flocks of Sheep in the neighborhood—the Boys improved their time by getting Some mutton And the way. Sheep and calves had to Suffer was a caution it was not long until [there] might be seen a quarter of Mutton—or veal hanging up by almost Every tent indicating that fresh meat was at least abundant one Evening being aroused from bed by considerable noise. I went out to see what the trouble was and found that the Boys had brought in a Scap [skep] of Bees And that the Bees had not been killed—but in attempting to take out the honey the Bees got out and were crawling all about the ground so that Some with the Sweet were getting Stung to give variety to the Scenes—the Boys also had a good time gathering up horses This Section not having been visited before by Either party had a good many horses in it though Most of them being colts—or very old—they also brought in one good yoke of oxen—they found a Box of Tobacco that had been hid in a hay Stack to keep it from being found but in Staying Several days the hay was used And the tobacco was used—the lucky boy makeing quite a Speck by finding it—he Sold it out making quite a Speck by the operation—the tobacco was as good chewing tobacco as Ever

/March to Penn[a]/

I had the pleasure of chewing—it being the national leaf— Dr. Quinan had been Brigade Surgeon since he came to the Reg. but about this time Dr. Reamer having to skedaddle from Windmill point[56] came back to the Reg[t] and claimed the position of Brigade Surgeon: Quinan being of course unwilling to give up the position and go Back to the Reg.

Stood Somewhat upon his dignity = that being greatly developed in his character—claimed that he merited the position from the fact that he had been an asst Surgeon for Eleven yrs in the Regular Army.—But then the authorities were not able to see the point as Reamer was the Senior Surgeon—So Quinan had to pack his duds and take [sic; Fulton perhaps meant "make"] his way back to his Reg. feeling that the deserving do not at all times get the position and that the great are not at all times appreciated— how Strange that all persons cannot See things as they Should—this Should learn a person wisdom for I Sometimes think that I deserve a better position than I have but when I Reflect that my actions do not appear to others as they do to my self, I Should be contented to wait untill they merit the aproval of those who are my Superiors And then I shall be advanced—if there is in the world one thing more disgusting than another it is a man puffed up in his own conceit to such an Extent that he thinks that no one knows anything but himself and that he is the only one capable of doeing a certain kind of business—

/March to Penn^a/

Now Dr. Quinan felt that he was better Qualified for Brigade Surgeon than any one Else there was And that any one could do the business of the Reg. And further that he was a man of too much importance to be tagging along at the Rear of a Regiment And deciding who are able to march and those that are not—his usual morose disposition and harshness toward the privates was only increased by this sudden turn in his position—

About the time he came to the Reg[imental]. Major Chamberlain made the Remark to me that he was a good [doctor] having been in the Regular Army,—being at that time Brigade Surgeon [and] would Bring Some of the Drs up to the work—the remark though making little ɨp impression on me at the time was nevertheless remembered by me and of course called up when he himself was weighed in the Balance and found wanting—It was on Sunday. June 22. that there was quite a severe cavalry fight between us and the Potomac it Begun Early in the Morning and continued throughout the day—the direction being in the morning Northeast and gradually changing passing to the West untill about 4 o clock in the afternoon. the sound passed away, Entirely our forces having driven the mountain at Snickers Gap it being a pretty warmly contested action and the Enemy getting considerably the worst of the bargain—it cleaned the country of the Enemy's cavalry, and left us a clear course to the Potomac—

/March to Penn^a/

It was while laying at this camp that Js [Josiah] L Lewis joined us[57] he had been acting as hospital Steward at Windmill point—And at the Breaking up of the hospital had been Started with a number of others had been Started [sic] to join the Reg. they went up the Potomac on a canal Boat And there marched across the country by way of Leesburg to join us he—had a Sad tale of distress to tell of his hard marches—And his Suffering from hunger—they had been compelled to march about thirty miles And And [sic] to live on hard tack and pork for two or three days and Even to Stay out a whole night in the rain with[out] any covering but an old blanket—poor Boys.

I guess time will Show that there is more work of a Severe nature in reserve for them—I trust that none of [them] may See any thing worse—if not we may consider ourselves fortunate—It was at this camp that [Private] George Muehler[58] Shot the End of his Big toe this was the first time that I Ever Amputated the great toe— I succeed[ed] in getting good flaps[59]—And I think he will have a fine Stump—he was doeing well when sent away to the Hospital—

/March to Penn[a]/

~~The Boys hada~~ the Boys had quite a time fishing the Creek for clams they hunted it closely and I think cleaned it out pretty well—the shells could be seen laying about in all directions—

On the Night of June 23[d] we were all called out [and] put into line with the Expectation of marching but after Standing in the rain until we got completely wet through we were ordered into camp

and again Standing in as heavy a rain as I have had the misfortune to be Exposed to for a long time—we had a very unpleasant night of it being completely [wet] to the skin—

June 25th 1863—

This Morning we Broke camp this Morning [*sic*] and took up the line of march for the Potomac which we reached about noon. the country through which we passed presenting but little of interest to any, one we Stoped And took dinner after which we again Started crossing the Potomac at the Mouth of goose Creek there being two Pontoons one across the mouth of the creek the [other] across the River we had no trouble in crossing the Streams the Potomac here is a beautiful Stream Goose Creek being also quite a large Stream– it was indeed a beautiful Sight to See the troops crossing the long unbroken column Extending on Each side of the Stream made it a beautiful Sight indeed to Witness

/March to Penn^a/

on the Virginia side there was a large house looking as though it had been a farmhouse though at this time Entirely deserted by its former owners, no one being there Except a few negroes they being the only remnant of once departed fortune the house was a perfect wreck the fences were all down and things in General looked as though some devastating Pestilence had Swept through the place Leaving nothing in its wake that had been good or nice = When we crossed the river and got into Maryland[60] how different the look of things it seemed as though we had got into another country Entirely—the fences were generally good and we soon began to see fields having crops of grass and grain growing—something that we had not Seen since we had been in the State of Virginia—a Some thing that made us feel as though we had left the land of Barbarians and got into one of civilization—

after getting into Maryland we took the road to Poolsville [Poolesville] here we Saw a Sight that did us good and made us feel as though we were getting home—the first School House that I had Seen since I left Washington having School in it. the children were at the doors and windows taking a good look thinking perhaps that they Saw the whole Union Army, And wondering where So many men came from thinking that there was men Enough to whip all the Rebs in Creation when in reality they only Saw one Division of our Corps the Village of Poolsville has the look of having been quite a nice place before the war disturbed it and destroyed the fences round the vilage yard [we] could See that a large force of cavalry had been camped near the town accounting in part for the disappearance of much of the fence that was not visible—the houses of the vilage were Substantial there were not many flags to be seen the people thinking no doubt that in a few days the rebs would be through and that it might only be the worse for them—they however looked on with much apparent interest won-dering to themselves in all probability what thoughts were passing through the minds of the men knowing that many were going to Penn^a to find a final resting place from their long and toilsome

Marches—through hot Sun and rain and Mud—the Men though
tired were all cheerful well Showing that they were good Soldiers
and had the good of their country at heart And were willing to
do anything in their power for that country. Even give up their
lives—for her good,

/March to Penn^a/

after passing Poolsville we marched on untill we came to the
Village of Barnesville where we Stoped for the night. just before
getting to this place however a heavy rain Set in makeing it very
unpleasant about putting up our tents wetting us completely
through before we had Shelter for the night—we however Soon
got freed up and getting Some Supper we Laid down for the night
And were soon locked in the arms of Morpheus—[the] village
was not much of a place though nice beside anything we had seen
in Virginia Some of the officers went into the town and Staid all
night thereby avoiding a good ducking as those who staid out got
for their want of trying for better Lodging the country through
which we passed had quite a good look being somewhat similar in
appearance to Penn^a in their Mode of farming—oxen you would
see the fences good [you would see oxen and good fences], and
things generally looking thrifty as though the people had Some
life and Energy.—About 12 o clock at night the wagon train began
to come into camp and continued to come untill about daylight—
when they were all in this was owing to the tedious process of
crossing the Pontoons at the Ferry. they all crossed safely which
is Something to be wondered at considering the great number of
them that had to cross—

June 26th 1863.—

This morning we Broke camp at an Early hour And took up our line of
march for the Village or near the Vilage of Jeffersonville in Middleton
Manner or Valley[61]— the day being wet the men had a pretty trying

time the roads were very muddy the country soon became hilly and stoney as we approached the mountain—the country did [not] present Anything Striking untill we came to Carl Manor[62]—which could be Seen Stretching out in the distance before us and the mountains on the north—It being such a contrast when compared with what we had been so long accustomed to look upon it seemed as though we had got into the garden of Eden itself Fields of grain of the very best quality covering the Broad Expanse varigated [variegated] here and there with fields of corn and grass all being well fenced

/March to Penn[a] /

the wheat I think I never saw Excelled for beauty and Luxuriance the whole face of the country looking as though about the three fourths of it was in wheat—I had been rather prejudiced against Maryland but this part of it at Least was Equal to any land that I had Ever seen in Chester or Lancaster Counties of Penn[a]—the farms had the appearance that they have in Penn[a]. the building outhouses and every thing about them giving an air of comfort and plenty seen only in Northern States—After crossing the Manor we soon came to the foot of the Katankton [Catoctin] Mountain the ascent of these mountains was long and tiresome we had to stop and wait for the artillery the road being So Mu[d]dy And Steep—

while Stopping [at] one place on this mountain the Boy's learned that a little log house by the wayside had Something for Sale that would Stimulate and the result was that a great running was kept up for a time with caution—however the Artillery Soon got up the hill And then we followed after upon getting to the top of the mountain we Saw Such a Sight as had never greeted my Eyes before. it had been cloudy And Wet all day And now it was Evening the clouds had given way the Sun Shone out in all the beauty of Evening Clear And Mellow here we were at a great hight—the Beautiful Valey of Carl Manor Stretched out at our feet looking More Beautiful than when we crossed the declineing rays of

the sun giving it a richness and beauty that were indescribable
but which could I have seen paintings of Sunset views and of
Landscapes but in all that I have never did my Eye rest upon the
Equal of this beautiful Spot—

/Carl Manor March to Penn^a/

but we did not get long to look for the column Soon began to move
and goeing about two miles we called a halt for the night on the top
of a hill overlooking the Middleton Valley and in sight of the village of Jeffersonville here we had another fine sight—the beautiful
valley Stretched out at our feet clothed in the richest verdure. And
[had] we not so lately looked on the beautiful Manor—this perhaps
would have been the finest valley that we had Ever Seen—though
not Exceeding the other in beauty I think it is fully Equal to it
in richness of soil—having the appearance of being more of a
grazeing country than the other—After getting our tents up And
comfortably fixed for the night I took a Stroll over to the village
of Jeffersonville—the Town has but one Main Street with paved
Side walks there are several good Churches [one] is not in use for
Services As it was in use for Hospital purposes after the battle of
Antietam And Since has not been fixed up for Service—the other
churches are good comfortable buildings—and well suited for
the design after looking through the vilage and comeing to the
Extreme End—

/Carl Manor March to Penn^a/

I met a gentleman that Showed me the place where the Battle of
South Mountain had been fought[63]—as it was in full view of the
End of the village—the Spot though in itself presenting nothing of
interest was in connexion with the Battle of Antietam[64] of Some
consideration—on this days march we crossed the Monaquacy
[Monocacy] River a beautiful Stream indeed Some of the Largest
trees growing upon its Bank's that I have seen—we crossed it on a

beautiful Bridge after crossing we passed along the Stream for some distance and had not the road been so bad And the march so much forced we would have had a fine trip but then being hurried along on a forced march it was all the men could do to Keep along And doeing their best many fell out.

South Mountain

In Summing up this days march I do not think that I have Ever travelled a day that there has been presented to the Sight more of beauty and interest than was in this it Seemed as though the Author of nature had been more than lavish in his dispensation of beauty— and with which this this [sic] part of creation had been adorned. the love[r]—of nature could here feast his Eyes upon the rough and rugged Mountain, crowned with forest, brought in direct contrast with the richest and Lovliest of vallies Spread out beneath like a carpet of richest hues with its Serpentine rivulet meander—through [though] we Americans go to the Alps to see beauty—And yet Know nothing of the rich beauty of our own country—.

/Near Emettsburg/
June 27th 1863—Saturday

This morning we took up the line of march for Middletown passing through Jeffersonville the county being of the finest quality—all the way comeing to Middletown the County Seat of [Frederick] County—it is a very pretty place the Reb Cavalry had been in the town a day or two before we got there they were just Scouting round Seeing what was to be seen—some of our men got after them and made them Skedadle for Frederick City ut from which place they had to go shortly after—the court house in Middletown was quite a good building And Made quite a good appearance comparing favorably with other buildings of the kind in other parts of the county—the churches were good Substantial—Structures And worthy—a people of as much wealth as the county Seemed to posess—

Middletown Maryland
Middletown Valey

After getting into camp and getting fixed up we tried to get
Some butter and other Eatables but Every thing of the kind
had been hunted up by the Many Soldiers that preceeded us the
people had baked up Every pound of flour they [had] Many sending
away all they could possibly for fear the Rebs would come in and
capture it—finding the Search for provisions fruitless I thought
I would go to Middletown And try to get a Nights Lodging—And
Something good to Eat. Upon goeing there and hunting for a time
I finally Succeeded in finding Such a place the gent—of the house
doeing all in his power to make me comfortable—in fact the Bed
was so soft sinking down so much in the feathers that instead of
having such a good nights rest as I had anticipated I could get
but little turning and rolling all the night through to be comfortable. I would get heated up and Sweat So that when Morning
came I found myself but little rested from the fatigues of the
preceeding Day,

/Middleton March to Penn[a] /

In the morning I had quite a good Break fast—My bill being but 50
cts for bed and Breakfast—In the night I was awaked by the noise
of cavalry passing through the town—but on going to the window I
found that it did not open toward the street and of course could get
no Sight of them—they had been out on a Scouting Expedition And
were just returning to camp—

Middletown Maryland
Sunday, June 28th 1863

This morning after getting Breakfast I left the village of Middletown
for camp intending to go back to church but after getting there it was
Said that we would move soon and of course I was afraid to go away,
for fear that I might be left—the 11th Corps had reached the village

before we did and had Encamped just outside of the village—to day about noon the 3ᵈ Corps passed through the 11ᵗʰ Corps followed after they got well passed we took up the line of march for Frederick City we Started about 3 oclock reaching or nearly reaching that place Shortly after dark. The 3 Corps being under the Command of Gen Reynolds he being our Corp's Commander it being the 1ˢᵗ. the orders issued being very strict not allowing any commissioned officer to visit the town—

/Frederick City Maryland March to Pennᵃ/
Frederick City

Many of course of were greatly disappointed in not getting to Spend the Evening in Frederick City but it was Entirely proper—as the command would have been greatly Scattered—And in the Morning when the time came to Start but few would have been on hand to start with—the march though not long was a pleasant one. the men were in fine Spirits And Seemed to Enjoy themselves greatly. the day though warm had a cool Breeze. and it being Even[ing] made it quite pleasant, And beside all had got well rested and consequently the better prepared for the march we passed up the mountain getting a good view of the Surrounding country. but it not being so fine as the other views on account of the valley

Frederic City Md

in this place being contracted and not so fertile As other portions—it tending to roughness—And being stoney though there was Some fine farms in view—but after getting to the top of the Mountain and passing down the long descent we soon began to see good country again—as we came near to Frederick City—the land was rich the farms beautiful being finely farmed—the land being quite Level was well calculated for a farming country and by the appearance of the county the Husbandmen was well repaid for his labor for the crops looked as though they could not be better [and the] fences good—Every thing in a flourishing condition

And looking as though the country was one of happiness and plenty—for the possessors—I would Like to Live in this part of the state myself—

NOTES

1. Promoted to hospital steward on October 1, 1863.

2. Unidentified.

3. Possibly Brig. Gen. William Booth Taliaferro of Gloucester County, Virginia, at this time posted to the Georgia coast.

4. Fulton appears mistaken, because at this time, the 11th Illinois was in Tennessee.

5. More than one Union Army camp was named for Col. John Slocum, 2nd Rhode Island Infantry, killed at the first Battle of Bull Run/Manassas in 1861.

6. Unidentified.

7. Unidentified.

8. Although awkwardly phrased, Fulton appears to say that when he was a civilian and read in the newspaper that the army could not move because of the weather, he did not appreciate the meaning of that statement until he himself experienced it.

9. Assistant Surgeon M. A. Henderson, 150th PA.

10. On the north bank, south of Fredericksburg.

11. Although awkwardly worded, Fulton appears to say that rebel troops were not far away.

12. Commanding the 143rd PA.

13. A structure of cut timber designed to delay and confound the attack of an enemy on foot.

14. Now called the inguinal ligament, which "connects the anterior superior iliac spine with the pubic tubercle." See University of Michigan Medical School, *Anatomy Tables—Inquinal Region,* online at http://www.med.umich.edu/lrc/coursepages/m1/anatomy2010/html/gastrointestinal_system/inguinal_tables.html, accessed October 22, 2018.

15. Tampion, or a plug at the end of the muzzle.

16. Likely peritonitis, an inflammation of the peritoneum, or thin tissue lining the abdominal wall, covering most organs there.

17. About two miles north of Pollock's Mill.

18. Second Brigade commander.

19. At Belle Plain.

20. Commanding Company A, 143rd PA.

21. Belle Plain, according to the memoir of the 150th PA.

22. "Remittent" concerns the periodicity of symptoms; an archaic term denoting a cluster of symptoms, particularly fever and diarrhea, that accompanied malaria and other infections with similar symptoms, sometimes denoted "camp fever."

23. Probably quinine sulfate. See chapter 9.

24. 143rd PA, who accidentally wounded himself on May 11 and died of his wounds on May 18.

25. Zone separating living from dead tissues.

26. Surgeon, 143rd PA.

27. Company C, 143rd PA, discharged for disability on November 7, 1864.

28. 143rd PA.

29. Co. D, 143rd PA.

30. Died on June 1, 1863, in Kingston, PA.

31. Fulton appears to be saying that the lack of any memorial to Colonel Hoyt's service among the officers struck him as particularly cold and apathetic. The lack may have owed to the rising number of casualties, too many for individual memorialization.

32. Mustered as surgeon on May 28, 1863. For more on Quinan, see chapters 7 and 9.

33. About a mile west of Fredericksburg along the Rappahannock.

34. Possibly Brig. Gen. Marsena Patrick, provost marshal, Army of the Potomac, staff to General Hooker.

35. J. Theodore Heard of Boston, US Volunteers, attached to the Medical Director, I Corps.

36. Tributary of the Potomac River.

37. Surgeon, 143rd PA.

38. 143rd PA.

39. A small town on the Orange and Alexandria Railroad, Fauquier County, Virginia.

40. Fulton wrote "June 12th, apparently, at the top of the diary page, but began the diary page with the 13th.

41. Common name for a variety of trees and shrubs in the genii *Castanopsis, Chrysolepis,* and *Castanea.*

42. A common nineteenth-century term in in Maryland, Delaware, and Pennsylvania for Delaware black rock, syenitic granite, or syenite.

43. Next to the Bull Run/Manassas battlefields of 1861 and 1862.

44. Goose Creek crosses the Potomac east of Leesburg.

45. A type of grass.

46. Fulton apparently continues his diary for June 13th.

47. Possibly Big Elk Creek or Little Elk Creek in southwest Chester County.

48. Unidentified.

49. Which had general responsibility for the defense of the capital.

50. Not listed in official records of the regiment.

51. The march north exacted a death toll. The 149th PA lost at least two men to diarrhea.

52. Dranesville, Fairfax County,Virginia.

53. Broad Run was a very small railroad community in Fairfax County, Virginia, named for a stream that passed through it.

54. Fulton did not complete his thought but perhaps would have said, "took off my clothes."

55. Huidekoper, Chamberlain, and Ashurst served with the 150th PA.

56. Mouth of the Rappahannock River.

57. On October 1, 1863, he was promoted from private, Company E to hospital steward.

58. Company E, 143rd PA, transferred to the Veterans Reserve Corps on January 15, 1864.

59. Fulton refers here to the "flap method" of amputation that allowed for extensions of skin above the amputation site to be folded down over the cut to ensure a cushion of skin around severed bone.

60. The 149th PA recorded that the brigade crossed the river at Edward's Ferry, Maryland, directly opposite Goose Creek.

61. The brigade crossed Catoctin Mountain at Jefferson, west into the valley with the South Mountains to the west, continued north to Middleton, and then marched east across Catoctin Mountain toward Frederick.

62. Unidentified. This may be a reference to a building as part of the small community of Catoctin Furnace, an early iron production site.

63. The Battle of South Mountain occurred on September 14, 1862, in which Union forces prevailed over the rebels in three battles at three mountain passes.

64. The Battle of Antietam took place nearby on September 17, 1862.

THREE

Searching for Flour at Gettysburg

Diary, June 29, 1863, to July 4, 1863

FOLLOWING A RESPITE OF SEVERAL WEEKS AFTER THE CHANCELLORSVILLE battle, the three Bucktail regiments—the 143rd, 149th, and 150th Pennsylvania, collectively Stone's Brigade (named for Col. Roy Stone)—dusted themselves off, tightened discipline, and marched north. The June heat created a dust cloud that enveloped the soldiers as they marched over dry dirt roads. Their northward march between the South and Catoctin mountains took them into Maryland's intermittent rain, which produced mud and hard marching, but the soldiers were buoyed by cheers of support as they passed through the small towns of Adamstown, Jefferson, and Middletown. Inchoate news, rumors, and fear of rebel forces nearby kept the soldiers and their commanders alert. By June 28, they learned that Hooker had been removed from command and the Army of the Potomac placed under the direction of Maj. Gen. George Gordon Meade, a dependable, loyal, and meticulous officer but one largely unknown to the brigade. A change of leadership meant a change of strategy, and the brigade was ordered east to Frederick City.

—〰—

/March to Penn^a Frederick City—M^d/
Monday June 29th 1863—

This morning we Broke camp at an Early hour. And took up the Line of march for Emettsburg [Emmitsburg]—It was here when we were about starting that we first heard that Gen Mead [Meade] had taken command of the Army of the Potomac and that Gen. Hooker had been removed we were all thunderstruck not knowing what to think of the intelligence and of course not knowing what the result would be but all supposed that it would be highly injurious to the cause as to Gen Mead we knew but little of him—Hooker all had confidence in as he had done so much for the Army, And had put it into a shape to do good work the Cavalry in particular all had the utmost confidence in him—but there was but little complaint all feeling that they would do their duty when called upon, Contrary to Expectation we did not pass through Frederick City [now Frederick, Maryland] and of course I know nothing of [it] Except by seeing the tops of the steeples in the distance

Judging from the numbers of them it is a place of some size—we did not take the turnpike direct for Emettsburg but kept to the left across fields and through woods—there having been so much rain the roads were very deep and heavy, making it pretty hard marching—we Saw Saw [*sic*] some beautiful farms along the way—we passed Several vilages on our way, the people generally manifesting much Patriotism the Ladies more Particularly by the waving of Flags And singing of Patriotic Songs these demonstrations Seemed to do the Boys much good the cheering of the Ladies in particular here they began to get apple butter and good Bread And thing[s] of this character that Strengthened up the Boys And Kept their Spirits good And made them think that they were getting among friends again

/March to Penna /

the village of Mechanicsville is quite a flourishing place—And doeing quite a business—after passing it a short distance we halted to take dinner—After which we again resumed our March Gen Rawly [Rowley] being in command of our ~~Br~~ Division Gen Doubleday our ~~Division~~ Corp's Commander in Command of the Corps—the country here was generaly rough and Stoney all the way untill within a Short distance of Emettsburg but when within about 3 Miles of Emettsburg we came in view of that old and well known institution

St. ~~Josephs~~ Mary's College for the purpose of Education of Catholic youth for the ministry—the building is Situated in a natural grove on high ground to the left of the road—the building is White and presents quite an imposing appearance being remarkable for its Seclusion and retiredness from all the bustle and din of Society that would naturally take the attention of youth from their Studies—And Lure them Away from the holy calm of their religious Exercises—

here are made many priests that officiate in the churches of Penn[a] and Maryland—the Scholars [of] this institution ranking with those of any other in the depth of Learning and Erudition—After passing this place and goeing about 3 Miles we Came to the celebrated town of Emettsburg here the main item of consideration being the Female School St. Joseph's College in which they have from one to three hundred pupils under instruction all the time the building is rather a Large one though not ostentatious in its appearance, being a plain white Structure of good dimensions—after passing this we passed on untill we Came into the town—the Seminary being out and to the south of the town—about half a mile near a fine Stream

/March to Penn[a]/

the SIsters have quite a fine farm upon which to support those under their care they being mostly orphan children and of course having nothing upon which to live have to depend upon charity—

The town of Emettisburg has the appearance of being rather an old place it had been Somewhat injured by a fire Extensive for a place of its Size—that had destroyed a whole Square of buildings making a rather an unseemly gap in a Small town—after getting to the Centre of the town we turned to the left passing through the Main Street leading in that direction it Seemed to be well supplied with drug Stores and other Stores Showing that it was a place of considerable business

/March to Penn^a/

while passing through here I saw [Major General] Carl Schurz for
the first time—I must confess that his appearance did not come up
to my Expectations for what I had read about him being a midling
large Man with Sandy Whiskers wearing glasses—not having the appearance of being a Man of Superior Mental Capacity however much
of mind he may be possessed one thing must be acknowledged—
that he has managed to get himself into a good position that of Maj
Gen in the army, a place I think that might be occupied by men more
deserving of American birth—though he has the position and has
command of a Division in the 11ᵗʰ Corps And I trust that he will
do his duty as he has a chance to help the reputation of his Corps
very much indeed—as it has a rather a bad odor since the Battle of
Chancellorsville—at which place they lost for us the fortunes of that
Campaign—

After passing through the town and going to the west of it about half
a mile we then learned that we must go on Picket Duty—taking a By
road and going about a mile further we Established a picket line just
on the Penna and Maryland line being fixed up we took camp for
the night—Just about a the Beginning of our Picket Line an old lady
lived that seemed to be very poor and protested again[st] the soldiers
getting any thing that she had Saying that all She had [was] for her
own living—but notwithstanding the Serg[t] Major [Alonso] Holdon
took nearly all her onions—thus proving his cowardly disposition
when the poor woman would come to look for her onions—

/March to Penn^a/

She would find that they had disappeared in the night We Laid
in this place all night in the Morning we went to the neighboring
farm house in the morning myself with Cap [Captain Chester]
Hughes and a few others and got a good breakfast a Something that
we had but Seldom met with on our march. the people Seemed Kind
and wished us well—the country here was quite poor and Stoney
and looked poor the people—being quite poor and having the

appearance of being quite poor and making a bare living—though they seemed to be contented and happy.—

/June 30th 1863—

This morning we took up the line of march in the Penna there being nothing of Special interest Except that at a halt made in the fore-noon the Quartermaster gave out shoes to all those men that needed them Many of the men being Barefooted the Shoes came good to them—about noon we came into camp in the wood and rested the remainder of the day,—Joe[1] and I took a wash in a nice Brook—a short distance from here there was a church that had been visited by the Rebs during the service on the ~~following~~ preceeding Sunday, and all the horses taken from the carriages—goeing to show us that the Report of their being in Penn[a] was only true Enough—

/March to Penn[a]/
July 1st 1863—

This Morning Morning [sic] at an Early hour we Broke camp and took up the line of March for the town of Gettysburg being distant about 4 ~~8~~ Miles [between four and eight miles]—the Morning was very warm with a heavy mist or gentle rain prevailing Keeping us damp all the time nearly wetting us to the Skin until we had our gum blankets on this Morning I packet [packed] Every thing on John and concluded that I would march with the men thinking to Keep their Spirits up and give them the more encouragement by so doing and thereby having the less Straggling—the roads were very muddy—and the march was consequently a very hard [one] the ground being So Slippery that made it hard work for the men to march—the command had not proceeded far untill the Sound of Artillery became audible a Sound that Sounded Strange to the Ears of Pennsylvanians—the State in which Many of us were born And one above all. the others accustomed to the peaceful pursuits of life and it would be no Easy thing to describe the feelings of those that heard the Canon of an invading foe upon the soil of our nativity—the Men did not Say much but that did not indicate a want of interest—there was a deep indescribable feeling of determination to for the country all that feeble Man could do—from the time of Starting in the Morning we had Marched fast not Stopping much to rest—but after getting half Col. [Roy] Stone came back and told us that we were needed to the front And to get along as fast as possible.

/Gettysburg Battle/

the pace was immediately quickened to a double quick—the ground being very Soft and Stoney made it very hard work Sometimes I thought that I would fall but Still I Kept along. we left the Emetsburg Turnpike road a Short distance from Gettysburg goeing to the west of the town through fields of Wheat corn grass and through wood over fences nothing Stopping us untill we had come to the [Lutheran] Theological Seminary Situated to the north of the town in a Beautiful grove. here the Men were halted and formed in line passed across one field when they threw of[f] their Knapsacks—after which they were Marched across a level and then up a rising piece of ground then down a Slight declivity into another hollow piece of ground with a Small Stream or Spring Drain passing through it. this ridge that has just been passed Lays just to the left of the turnpike to the north of the town the field taking or occupying this ridge was covered with corn and to the right of where we passed between us and the road or pike we had a battery planted—but I noticed in passing that all the horses had been killed or wounded and that the Battery was Entirely Silenced[2]—Just across the pike from this Battery was a clove[r] field in which to the left which Gen Reynolds was killed about this time he was making a reconaisance with his Staff And one of the Reb Sharp Shooters picked him of thereby inflicting a heavy Loss upon ou[r] Corps—

/Gettysburg Battle/

it is Said that when Gen Hooker was relieved and Gen Mead given the command of the Army of the Potomac—it was offered to Reynolds how true this is I know not but one thing is certain he had the confidence of all Military Men who knew him—Gen Reynolds

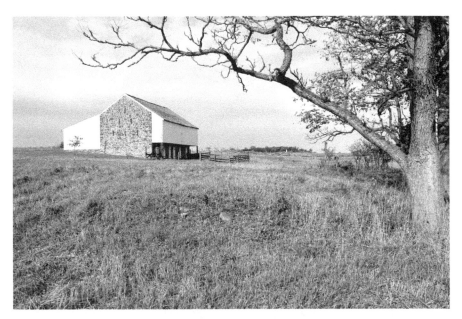

Figure 3.1. Reconstruction of the McPherson farm, Gettysburg. Fulton's brigade positioned itself along the northern and eastern perimeters of the farm for several hours on July 1, 1863, until forced to retreat over Seminary Ridge to the east. Credit: Robert D. Hicks.

being killed Gen Doubleday our Division Commander took command of the Corps—after passing the ravine in front of the Battery the Men passed part way up a moderate Ascent and there Laid down under cover of the ridge in a peach orchard and and [*sic*] there laid down in line of Battle Skirmishers were sent out to reconoitre the Enemy, and feel their position to see whether they were in force.

I followed my Regiment into the field to where they formed the line of Battle in the orchard—to the right of the orchard and between it and the turnpike there was a stone house And barn[3] it was not long after getting here that I was called into the house. upon goeing in I found quite a no. of wounded [soldiers] from our Battery—but upon looking round neither the Steward Jos L Lewis nor My Hospital orderly Ge° Sheldon had ventured to follow the Regt across the field thinking it probably the be Safer part of valor to remain in the

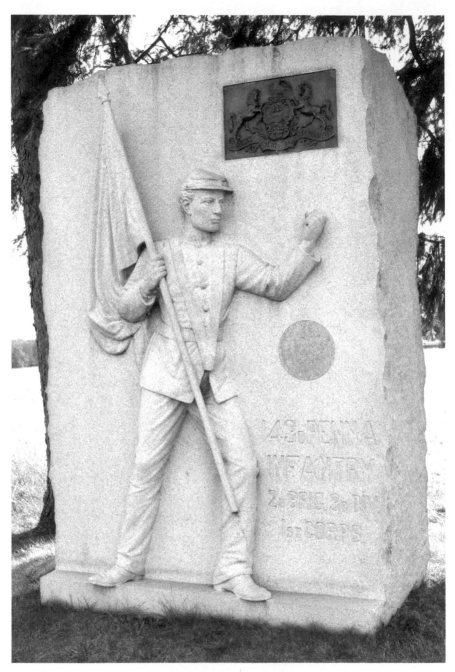

Figure 3.2. Photograph of the monument to Fulton's regiment, the 143rd Pennsylvania Volunteers. This monument is visible to the east of McPherson's farm, Gettysburg, and depicts Sgt. Ben Crippen, the bearer of the colors, shaking his fist at the advancing Confederates, who shot and killed him as he did so. Credit: Robert D. Hicks.

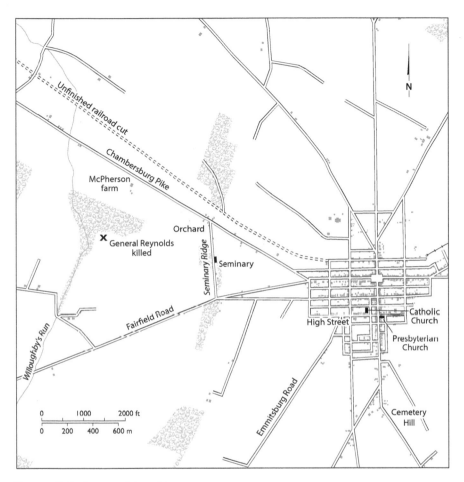

Map 3.1. Gettysburg on July 1, 1863.

wood out of the way of the Shells So when I was ready to go to work
I had nothing to work with So I could not do anything Else than
go back to the wood by the Seminary to See if I could find them
rather Expecting to meet them coming out but on and Still on I went
while I got to the wood but before getting here I met Dr. [White G.]
Hunter[4] comeing to the field to order me to the Hospital for Special
Duty—

/Gettysburg Battle July 1st 1863/

But having left my coat and Sword at the house on the field I had to go back and get them—I did so And in crossing the field that we had crossed in the morning though the Shells and balls flew pretty thick we did not think of any one being hurt. I could now See that quite a number had been Struck Some wounded others Killed one poor fellow Laying on his back though he had not been killed more than an hour his face was already black and Swelled up as though it would burst—on our march in the morning I got George to go to a farm house and get me some apple Butter in a tin can—there was about a pint of it and not having time to Eat it on the way.

I carried it along, to the house on the right of our Regt and put it on the table there Keeping it untill I was ordered to Hospital taking back with me to the Seminary where Dr. [William T.] Humphreys Said our Hospital would be but on goeing there we found that the first Division had already taken possesion of that building and that it was already crowded with their wounded the time being about Eleven oclock [*sic*] in the forenoon—on looking around and making inquiry I found that the Catholic and Presbyterian churches on high Street had been selected as hospitals for the third Division—upon starting to go there Jo and I took what tea we had with the Sugar— we had not been in Town long untill the wounded Began to come in Jos And Myself Began to look round for a place in which we might make tea and Soup.

Two pages of maps appear at this point in the diary, sketched by Colonel Dana, 143rd.

/Gettysburg Battle/

we finally got to Mr. Meyers—And were Soon closely Engaged in Meeting the wants of the poor fellows who had been Brought in wounded and were greatly in need of Something to support and

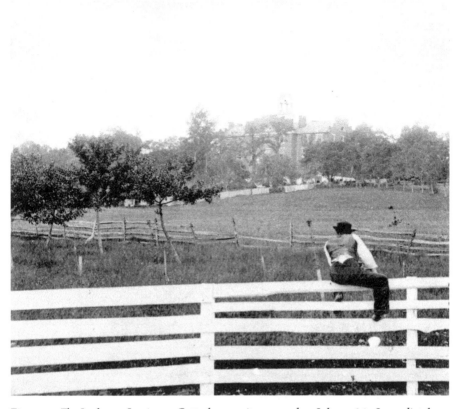

Figure 3.3. The Lutheran Seminary, Gettysburg, as it appeared on July 15, 1863. Immediately following the battle, Fulton worked at this makeshift hospital for several days, where hundreds of Confederate and federal soldiers were treated. The hill was also a battleground on July 1. Credit: MOLLUS Collection, US Army Heritage and Education Center, Carlisle, PA.

nourish them we made up Soup as fast as possible begging Bread And apple Butter for those that could Eat it until we had them pretty well Supplied we had been closely, Engaged in this manner for an hour or two when the canonading began to get nearer and nearer the town while it Seemed to be in it—the Ladies all became very much frightened and fled to the cellar—after a short time they called to me stating that the men were crowding in upon them and that they were afraid. that they would be crushed to death—

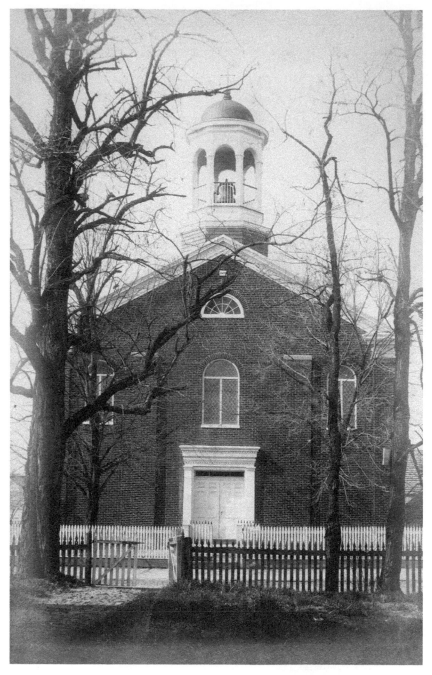

Figure 3.4. Fulton was ordered to assume command of makeshift hospitals in Gettysburg on July 1. Both hospitals were within sight of each other, a half-block apart. One, a Catholic church now known as St. Xavier's Catholic Church, appears here as it did during the battle. This building was replaced by a new church in the twentieth century. Credit: Adams County Historical Society.

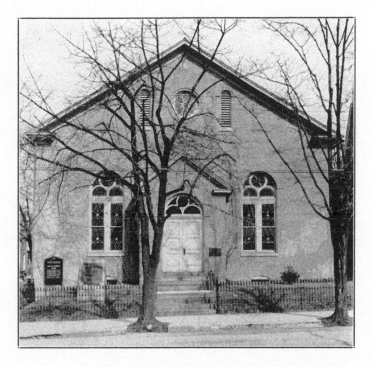

THE PRESBYTERIAN CHURCH
GETTYSBURG, PENNSYLVANIA

Figure 3.5. The second of two churches that Fulton commandeered for a hospital, a Presbyterian church, is shown here as it appeared in 1863. It, too, was rebuilt in the twentieth century. Credit: Presbyterian Historical Society.

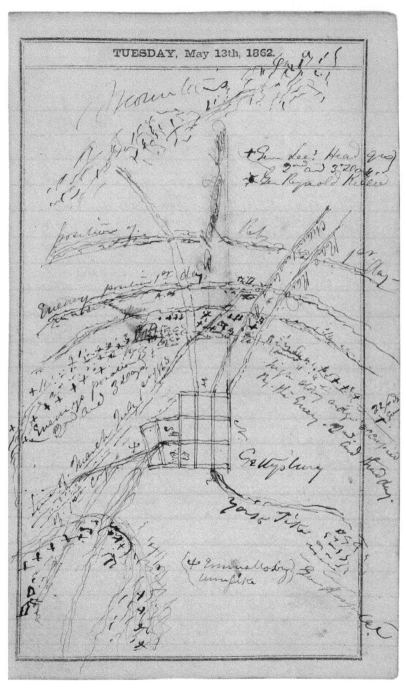

Map 3.2. A sketch drawn by Col. Edmund Dana in Fulton's diary showing the disposition of troops on July 1, 1863, Gettysburg.

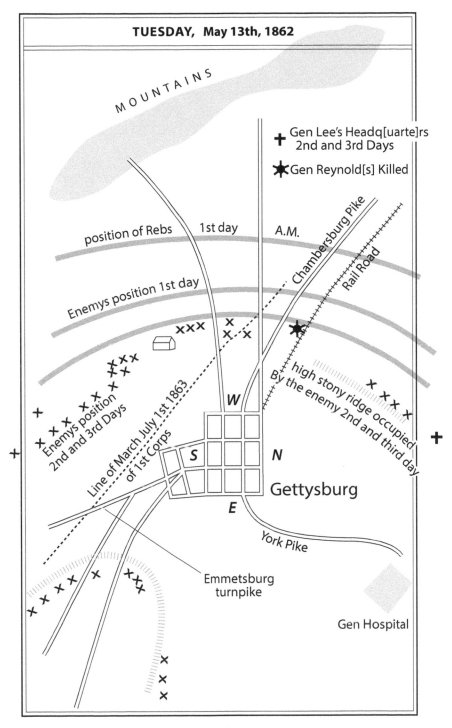

TUESDAY, May 13th, 1862

MOUNTAINS

✚ Gen Lee's Headq[uarte]rs
2nd and 3rd Days

✷ Gen Reynold[s] Killed

position of Rebs   1st day   A.M.

Chambersburg Pike

Rail Road

Enemys position 1st day

position of Rebs

high stony ridge occupied
By the enemy 2nd and third day

Enemys position
2nd and 3rd Days

Line of March July 1st 1863
of 1st Corps

W

S   N

E

Gettysburg

York Pike

Emmetsburg
turnpike

Gen Hospital

Map 3.3. Transcription of Col. Dana's map of July 1, 1863.

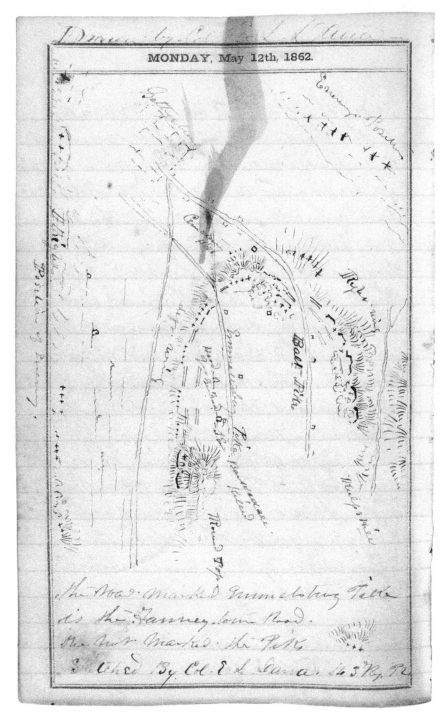

Map 3.4. Col. Dana's sketch in Fulton's diary of the disposition of soldiers on July 2–3, 1863, Gettysburg.

Drawn by Col. E. L. Dana

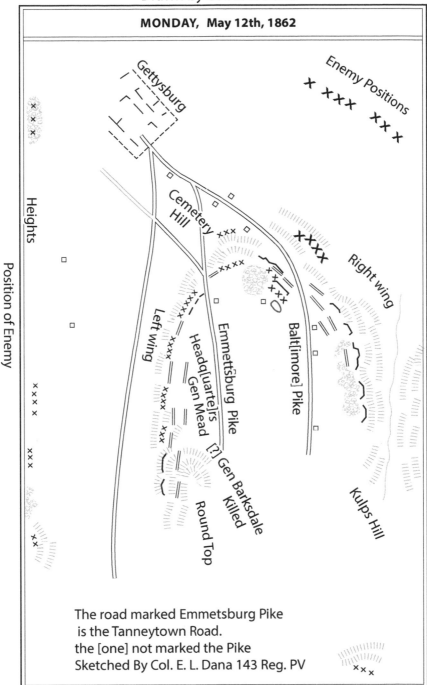

MONDAY, May 12th, 1862

Enemy Positions

x x x x   x x
                x

Gettysburg

Heights

Position of Enemy

Cemetery
Hill

Right wing

Left wing

Head[quarte]rs
Gen Mead

Emmettsburg Pike

[?] Gen Barksdale
Killed

Balt[imore] Pike

Round Top

Kulps Hill

The road marked Emmetsburg Pike
is the Tanneytown Road.
the [one] not marked the Pike
Sketched By Col. E. L. Dana 143 Reg. PV

Map 3.5. Transcription of Col. Dana's map of July 2–3, 1863.

I went down and found that they were all duch [German] and from
the 11th Corps. I asked them what they were Surrounded[6] I told them
to get out but they said that there was no use in it So in a Short time
a few Rebs came in and took them all prisoners without any trouble
they be[ing] very willing to give themselves up as they made no
resistance whatever—Showing that they were a couwardly Set Such
men as are a nuisance to any Army—one Man could take a hundred
prisoners—finding that there was no use in My Staying in the House
I went into the street and the first man I Saw after goeing into the
Street was a Reb he said that he would take My Sword, I handed it
over to him. he told me to go with him to the rear—I did so but on
getting back to [Confederate Lieutenant] Gen. [Richard S.] Ewell[7]
was told that if we had Many wounded I had better go back and assist
in providing for them.

/Gettysburg Battle/

it did not require a Second invitation to cause me to go—on goeing
back to the church I found the door locked and all the Surgeons
Safely E[n]sconced inside Supposing that they were Safe if they only
had the door locked, but after a time the Rebs came along, and made
them unlock the door—I do not know what of one of the Gentleman
has the honor of Suggesting the original idea of Locking a church
door to Save themselves from the assaults of war—the gentlemen
promised to give the Rebs a correct list of all that were about the
Hospital attendants and Surgeons—which seemed to Satisfy
them—when [we] Established ourselves at the Hospital we had all
hitched our horses round the Hospital—

After being released and coming back to the church I found that
My horse with all the others had been taken—before being taken
to the rear I saw George he told Me that he had found a Splendid
place in the Basement of the church perfectly Safe and wanted me
to go in—but I did not see the point nor himself long—as he was
soon marched to the rear but he did not have the privilege of coming
back as he was kept as a prisoner of war and taken along—. had he
been watching the progress of the battle instead of dodging Shells he

might have Saved my horse as well as himself—the Rebs got not only the horse but my Blankets Buffalo Saddle and Bridle Shelter tent one coat And Every thing that belonged to me almost leaving me very poor indeed in case. I Should have to march again—

/Gettysburg Battle/

In the course of the day there were Some things that were quite Amusing that happened—for example about the time I was taken they got Joe but instead of goeing along he dodged up a chimney thinking there to Escape detection but the Rebs were not so Easily fooled—They looked round and finally Brought the boy from his hideing place—looking foolish Enough—he explained to them the dignity of his position and demanded a guard to conduct him to the Hospital—curious to Say that he procured one and was taken Safely through well Showing that the More face a man has the better he gets along—I Save[d] quite a number of our Regiment that had been taken and were being conducted to the rear—

About this time things had a curious and rather alarming appearance our men had been overpowered—there being no troops Engaged on our Side Except the 1st Corps and one Division of the 11th Corps these had to Contend against the Corps of Ewell—being about 30,000 Strong. our Corps numbered about 8000—the Div of the 11th Corps having only two Brigades—So the force pitted against [us] had greatly the advantage in point of numbers they being nearly three times As Strong as we—in falling back through the town they raked the Streets with grape and canister—Many a poor fellow getting Killed and wounded in passing through—the town—our Men passing through the town took position to the south and East of it as Shown in the [Dana] Map in the form of a horse Shoe—

/Gettysburg Battle July 1st 1863/
July 1st 1863

it Seemed to those of us that had been taken as though they had anihilated our little Corps of Brave Boys for all day, had they contended with this powerful force And fell back only when completely flanked on both side[s] and had an Enfilading fire from both quarters when the Rebs got posession of the town they seemed much pleased And thinking that they had things all their own way made many Brags and and [*sic*] Boasts Saying that they would drive us before them to Baltimore And after taking that City would go on to Washington and there dictate terms of peace—

July 1st 1863

but fortunately for us when they got possession of the town they Seemed to be Satisfied for that time and ceased their aggressive operations for that day—giving our forces a chance to get up their reinforcements And to Examine the ground upon which they were to fight the future two days battle—I had not Seen much fighting but one thing [is] certain that when the Rebs were Shelling the Streets after our retreating forces Men falling on Every Side—it presented a Spectacle sad indeed to look upon—you would see a man fall here a horse there and often the carnage ceased, the Sight presented was a Sad one the men that had been Killed and that Still Lay upon the Streets were Stripped of their Shoes and Some of them had their pants taken off—and left there to undergo decomposition in the hot Sun—

/Gettysburg Battle/
July 1st 1863

Old Bobby Carey[8] was driving the Medical Ambulance of our Brigade—It is Somewhat curious to hear him tell his Experiences And how he Made his Escape from the Rebs. He Said that he had four as good horses as a man Ever cracked a whip over—when the Rebs began to crowd round pretty thickly and about the time they felt pretty Sure of their prey he Spoke to his horses and away they went at full flight and as the Rebs would catch at the horses the [illegible word] killed them—others ~~they~~ would be Knocked down by the wheels And crushed beneath them he Says that he does not know how many he Killed but they were ~~very many~~ hundreds—Some think that perhaps the old gut may be a little lively in imagination—he however made his Escape with the Wagon and drugs—

July 1st 1863

Among those that made themselves the most useful of the citizens was M[r] Meyers and family, Mr [Solomon] Powers and his family, Miss Harriet Schilling—Mrs. R Eyster with Whom I had the pleasure of being for Some time—she certainly is one of the finest Ladies of My acquaintance being I think a true and consistant christian not only in walk but in all the Essentials that are to be Expected of person making a profession—9

One other little incident occurred during the ~~first~~ 2nd day that is worthy of note—Dr. Herd | Bache were Stopping with a family being in the corner of high Street and the Street running out to the college10 in [the] morning about 10 minutes after they had arisen from bed and gone down Stairs. a Shell penetrated the wall [of] their room being at the End of the house Exploded in the chimney destroying that part of it the pieces of Shell and Brick flying all over the room knocking the pillows from the bed upon which they had been Sleeping and leaving Scarcely a Square foot of the wall or ceiling that was not cut Either by a piece of a shell or brick—

/Gettysburg Battle/
July 1st 1863

After goeing to down and takeing their Breakfast they had not left the room more than twenty minutes after finishing their Breakfast a Shell Entereed [sic] the room in which they had been Eating the clock Standing on the Mantle was knocked into a thousand fragments—the dishes had not been removed from the table they were all Broken to fragments the pieces being Scattered in Every

Direction over the floor—it is wonderful what persons Escape at
times and at others what trifles destroy life

July 1st 1863

it is the all wise providence that protects us in all our danger
and brings us Safely through all our trials—and difficulties
notwithstanding two Shells Exploded in the House of Mrs. Foster
neither of the Drs. Nor any of the family were injured in the Slightest
but all Escaped without a scratch—In the Evening of the first
day after the Rebs got possession they devoted their time to the
Robbing and plundering of Such houses as had been deserted by
the owners—Such as had not been too much frightened to Stay at
home and take care of their property were not molested and Escaped
without injury—or much Loss further than of their chickens and
vegetables. Except in cases where they went to the cellars and the
Rebs got possession of the uper part of the House in Such cases
they generally took Everything whether of any use to them or
not.—at M[r]s Eysters they took all of her Son Wms good clothes—
a Silver Knife and fork all the coffee She had with the pepper
and Salt—

July 2nd 1863—Gettyburg—Penna.

This morning I asked the Rebs—what the program for the day was
they stated that they were goeing to take the position occupied
by our men at the South East of the town—our centre being the
Cemetery Hill our right Extending along a stoney [Stony] Hill
covered with timber for the distance of two miles to Kulps [Culp's]
hill—the left wing Extended about the same distance to round
top on the Extreme left the position was a good one—So the Rebs
viewed it but Said that we must be knocked out of it—our men in
the mean time had not been idle the 5th Corps with other Corps
had been brought up to the assistance—the Rebs had not been idle
Either [Confederate Lieutenant General James] Longstreet had got

up with his Corps they had their plans matured Gen Longstreet
advanced with his Corps to the left ^{their right} until Ewell took the
position _{centre} opposite the ^{right} centre [Confederate General] A P Hill
opposite the ^{right} centre Wing—11

/Gettysburg/

those of the Rebs that I talked with generally Seemed to be well
informed in regard to the intended movements of their forces for
as they Stated—So they acted and at about 4 oclock being the time
they Said that Longstreet would get round to the Extreme left the
Signal was fired And the artillery duel commenced Exceeding in
grandeur any thing of the Kind that I have Ever witnessed in my life
there being about 400 guns Engaged in all the Rebs having about
200 with them—the Duel Kept up for an hour when Longstreet advanced his column to the charge on the left wing under cover of the
artillery—but the charge was met and Repelled they were compelled
to fall back with heavy loss in the Evening an attack was made upon
the centre with the Same for their unfortunate termination though
they had their hands on the guns the men beat them off with the but
of their guns—useing their Swabs and ramers [rammers] with a right
good Earnest over the heads of the Rebs compelling them to fall
back without capturing a Single gun—their chagrin is more Easily
imagined than Expressed—

/Gettysburg July/

through the day I had felt quite depressed fearing that we had not
force Enough to resist them not having a chance to Know what force
we had got up but when our men had compelled them to fall back
and kept them from being successful in this day's attack I began to
have great hope that we could prevent the Success of any attack that
they—might make—in the Evening I asked the men how things
were goeing they said that our men had such a good position that it
was impossible for any common men to take it—but that it would

have to yield in the morning—we had by this time great difficulty in
getting provision for the wounded they had given most of their Bread
to our soldiers as they passed in the morning of the 1st of July—that
which was left the Rebs took So that but little was to be found—

in looking round I Saw the Baker Ziegler[12]—and in a quiet way he
told me that he had twelve Barells of crackers that he would Sell
us, The chance was a good one so I Immediately engaged them
about the half of them were Soda crackers—And answered a fine
purpose but in goeing back and forth to the Bakery—I Saw one of
the Reb Colonels and he told me that I had better go to [Confederate
Brigadier] Gen [Harry] Hays[13] And he could tell me how to do that
I might get Flouer and Start the Bakery to goeing—I did So and he
told me to go to Gen Ewell and State that we had many wounded
and that there was no way of providing for them unless we could get
Some flour And Start our Bakery—

/Gettysburg July 1863/

I did So[14] I found him having his head quarters on the poor house
road in a Small Barn—before coming to the Barn a shed that had
been used as a wagon house it Seemed as though there was guns
and accoutrements Enough to fit out an army. they had been busy all
morning in gathering up the guns about town. they made our men
who were prisoners carry them to the rear—the men though they
had Escaped fighting by being captured did not Escape work And it
pleased me to see the 11th Corps duchmen [Germans] tugging away
at the guns and carrying them about a mile to the rear—upon asking
about the flour Ewells' adj–General told me that we Should have it
and that he would send it in as soon as possible—

I went back to camp town after getting there I looked round and
found men to run the Bake Shop getting all things in readiness we
waited for the comeing of the flour but through the long day no flour
made its appearance—Gen Ewell was Sitting upon the Bridge of the
Barn Eating his Breakfast in quite a Soldierly like Style. he is apparently not a tall man with a thin face—And Sharp Eye a bald place

about the Size of a Dollar on the top of his head. the Rebs look upon him as the best officer they have next to Lee. he taking precedence—

they Say that they have not got Stonewall Jackson but that they have the man that gave Stonewall his reputation meaning Ewell he certainly is a good commander Managing his command well and turning the fortunes of the day, frequently against us in the Many Engagements in which the two armies have met in Virginia—though there is no command in their army of which our men have so much dread as they had of Jackson when he was living—

/Gettysburg Battle July 2nd 1863/

he was one of those conscientious men believing firmly in the justness of the cause in which he was Engaged [and] went into the work with his whole Soul thinking of nothing but Success And in fact Seldom meeting with Anything Else So long as he was in Command—

This afternoon Gen Ewell and his Staff came along high Street and Stoped oposite our Hospital. Sending his staff in the church to mount the cupola—that they might get a view of the Battle field this was during the time that the cannonade was in progress .at the time the Rebs made the attack upon our left Wing they made the greatest hurrah and Shout to try and cheer their men on to the charge. They appeared to be in the greatest glee—I went up with– them and took a view of the line of battle—but thing goeing so much against us—I Soon got tired looking and came down into the church leaving the South quite jubilant and happy in the [sic] their prospect for the future—but after Sitting in the Gallery about an hour they came down and I noticed that they did not look so well pleased as they had done when I last Saw them but were looking Somewhat dejected this gave me Encouragement and notwithstanding all the Efforts made by them they failed in their undertakings. And things [sic]they made a desperate attack on the centre about dusk they had to fall back a defeated Enemy—notwithstanding all their Blow and Bragadocio—

/Gettysburg/

Friday I Stoped with M[rs] [Catherine] Powers and was kindly
treated in fact we were glad to get a Little of Something any place we
could find it—as the town was so—Strip[p]ed that no one had any
thing to give away—

To day I went to Judge Zeigler[15] and he refused to let me have a
pound of tea for the wounded Soldiers for fear that he would not get
paid for it. At that time things looked dark and it was not certain
which side was goeing to triumph but the prospect was quite as good
for the Rebs as for us—he perhaps was thinking and hoping that
they would be Successful as he was quite intimate with Some of the
Rebel officers as they were closely interested in the result—

/Gettysburg/

Zeigler is certainly a Tory to his country if there is one living in the
State of Penn[a]—Some argue that we have no Tories but if the Man
that has no Sympathy with the cause of his country And that would
be glad to see the Rebels triumph that his own Wicked purposes
might be fulfilled—and who is willing to do and does do all in
his power to weaken and injure and to help the Enemies of our
country—such is the character of many men calling themselves
Democrats—Yet they will [indecipherable word] and Blow about the
persecution of the Democrats saying this is no longer a free country
that the press is no longer free the freedom of speech has been taken

/Gettysburg/

has been taken [sic] from the American people—the only mistak the
Go[v]. [government] Has made in this respect is that we have not been
Sharp Enough on such men a[s] judge Zeigler and his clan here was
a man that pretended to be a friend of his country that was arm in
arm with the Rebs willing to give them information that might assist
them [in] turning us away without a notice—. But future history will
certainly place such men where they belong—The old revolutionary
[tory] was honorable beside such a man he had something to build his

doubts upon—they Launched from an old Established gov. the best
that then Existed in the world and as it were Launched out upon the
ocean of Experiment but not so with those that are wageing the war
for the mantainance of the Gov. we know what we have and what we
want to Keep perfect and intact—May, the God of Nations protect
and guide us to the stance of peace And repose for which [we] are
Laboring with so much of zeal—

I was told a little anecdote of [Brigadier] Gen [George Dashiell]
Bayard[16]—when he received his death wound and was about to die
the Chaplain of one of the New York Regts went to him and began to
talk with him about his future welfare—the Gen thanked him for his
kindness but Said that he had lived a Soldier and would die one thus
dismissing his allusion—he was killed in the first Fredericksburg
fight—

/Gettysburg/
July 3ᵈ 1863

This morning the fight began about daylight the Enemy, attacking our
right heavily with musketry but failing to accomplish anything were
finally compelled to fall back without the action being decisive—
And in the middle of the day and untill about three o clock there
was but Little done—but about that time in the afternoon the
Artillery on both Sides opened—And of all that I have seen in
war this Exceeded in grandeur And Solemnity—about 300 guns playing the Earth as it seemed to us would tremble Shells bursting in air
As they went Screaming over us, an occasional Striking in town made
it not only, a solemn sight but one of danger the people all fled to their
cellers and there Stayed so Long as the duel continued the women all
the time asking if the town was goeing to be sheled upon being told
that it was not they would be contented for a short time but the next
person passing would have the same interogating put to him—
during the Shelling the Reb advanced their lines to the charge makeing a desperate Effort to Break through our lines[17] and though they
caused [a] portion of our line to give back at times they only made
their pursuit to meet with sure destruction or capture—after many

fruitless trials all failing they again fell back to their lines apparently to rest for the night—

/Gettysburg/

this day was of the three the Sourest they had made up their minds that they were goeing to break our lines there never was I think a set of men more confident of success feeling certain that they could accomplish their purpose with such ideas and the prospect of soon Entering the city of Washington And in the Capital of the Nation and there dictate terms of peace after so long a time of war and privation and hardship as they had gone through it is not to be wondered at that such men with the sure promise of peace would fight hard, but notwithstanding all these promises and prospects held out out [sic] to the Enemy they had to fail and fall back once more a defeated though a brave and in many Respects a noble Enemy.

During the fight they Showed to our men many acts of Kindness and Generosity in Bringing them water and caring for them in many ways true Some of them would rob the dead And wounded but they were the Exception And not the rule such men as there are in all armies men that go into the Army for the Sole object of Robbing those that cannot defend themselves—of all the Southern troop that I have met the Georgians are the most of gentlemen—And the whole Army gives them the credit of being the best Soldiers—as with a horse the one that works well will have it to do so they have the most of the fighting to do there being Many wounded of the first Day, this day nor yesterday failed to Bring us Any, more for the reason that those wounded to day And yesterday were Kept within our lines the Enemy did not get any of them but our men got many of theirs.

/July 3ᵈ 1863 3ᵈ days fight Gettysburg/

It was to day that the Sharp Shooters took possession of Mr. McCreary's House[18]in the part of the town near the tannery our men had possession of the Hotel between that and the Cemetery. Our men hurt the Reb Sharp Shooters very much greatly irritating them. they determined to Stop us if possible and finally, brought up one of their best men with his Telescope rifle thinking that he would make Sure work of the thing but failing to do any Execution the first fire he got a Man to watch when he fired the Second Shot the Man told him that he fired too low and too much to the right he Swore that he would bring the Yankee Scoundrel the next Shot—he put a powerful charge in his gun took aim and fired thinking Certain that he had Killed his Man Stepped back and looked to see that his man was Killed—About this time two Men of ours fired about the Same time both Balls Entering the Reb in the Abdomen Killing him nearly instantly—they dragged him down Stairs ~~Killing him nearly instantly~~—Marking the Stairs And walls as they went with the [sentence not completed]

/Gettysburg Battle July 1863—/

In the Room occupied by, the Reb Sharpshooters—it being the best Bedroom the Rebs used the Pitchers and Basins to Relieve themselves being Either too Lazy or afraid to go out of doors for that purpose—it is not hard to imagine what Kind of a room they left. the vessels being in this condition with great Stains of Blood upon the floor that could not be washed out—. The town of Gettysburg had but one citizen has that ~~had~~ patriotism Enough to take his gun and go to the field of Battle and assist the friends of freedom[19] in fighting the great Battle of freedom. of all the places that I have Ever been in I think that this mean town had more of copperheadism[20] and ~~the~~ less of Patriotism than Any place of the Size that I have Ever been in during the time of the fight no men were to be Seen. they had all left the town or were hid in the cellers. the young men in particular the dead that had been Killed on the first of July, Still Lay upon the streets Swollen black and hideous forms Exposed to the gaze of all not a man daring to Show himself or offer his Services to bury the fallen patriots but all keeping at a Safe distance, the Ladies Showed a commendable disposition many of them manifesting a disregard of danger highly commendable to them while the Men the paltry cowards Sneaked into cellers or other places where the Shells of the Enemy, could not reach them,—21

/Gettysburg Pa/

By this time the wounded that had been brought in from the first days had all been operated upon that required an operation most of them being pretty comfortable or as much so as they could be made under the circumstances—we not being able to get up the Hospital Wagons And neither the Gov nor any of the Sanitary Commissions being able to get through the Enemys lines—the men of course had no beds but then there was Straw Brought in and they were made as comfortable with that as it was possible to make them under the circumstances. Col. Hydekooper [Huidekoper] had his arm taken of[f] And was at Mrs. Myers. He is doeing well.—Lieut. [Lyman R.] Nicholson was also Seriously wounded: the Ball Entering the back of the Shoulder and passing through the left Lung—Lieut. [Charles William Betzenberger] Betsenberger of Co I was Killed in the first day's fight he had a presentiment that he was goeing to be Killed— [Sergeant George] Geo C. Fell of Co. B22 was also Killed he was a fine Boy. he had the idea that he was goeing to be Killed And wRote to his parents—to that Effect while on the March to Getysburg it only proved too true—

Cap. [C. M.] Conyngham Cap. [Chester K. Hughes] Hughs Cap [Asher] Gaylord Cap Fells Cap [George N. Reichard] Rickhand23 Col [Roy] Stone Col. [Langhorne] Wister—all wounded in the first days fight Col E[dmund] L Dana was unhurt and the Command of the Brigade devolved upon him—

of the citizens during the fight there was but one Killed And She was a young Lady or at Least calling herself such.24 She had Strong tendencies to the Copperhead persuasion And when the Rebs were in town She told them where an abolitionist had his horse hid they got the horse and took it away.—on the morning of the third day M[r]s Powers thought She would go out on the field of Battle and See if there was not some poor men there who were Suffering for the want of attention She found two and gave them Some water And Soon had one of them brought in And cared for As she best could her and her girls doeing all in their power for the comfort of the poor fellows—

/Gettysburg Pa/
July 4th 1863.—Gettysburg

The morning Mr. Powers came to My Room Door to call me up Stateing that the Rebs had left I could hardly think it but on coming down and goeing into the Street I found it Even as he had told Me they had withdrawn to their fortifications on the ridge back of the town and there had a Strong line to protect their retreat they had their Sharp Shooters between the town and the Seminary—they Kept up a poping all the forenoon but quit it about noon As Soon As I had my breakfast I took a walk to the Seminary to see what had been goeing on there. the Cemetery Seemed to be one Mass of guns it Seemed to Me as though they could not have placed another gun had they wanted to do so. the position was well calculated for the placeing of Artillery and had been well used—

/Gettysburg Penna/

I found the centre oc[c]upied by the 11th Corps our Corps lying to the right and left of them. upon looking round I could see traces of the Severe work that had been done the preceeding three days—but then not so much as I had Expected to see a few of the monuments were broken and here and there you might See traces where the Balls had Struck the fence And Broken it—but no dead were to be seen Laying upon the field all having been buried—or taken away, the Men Seemed to be takeing it quite cool[l]y resting themselves as best they could after Such hard work as they had had—

On the Night of the first of July, Dr. [Surgeon Francis C.] Reamer[25] dispatched Joe out on the ~~turnpike~~ road from Gettysburg to Millerston [about eight miles southwest of Gettysburg] to help to take care of some of our wounded that were among the Rebs—on this day of the fourth he gathered up some chickens and had a regular fourth of July dinner having the Rebs at the Entertainment they had quite a good time—To day the people out in the country began to Bring in things for the Sick and wounded Some would Bring in Bread Butter and apple Butter—others again preserves Milk And various things good And useful to those unable to go for them.

/Gettysburg Penn^a/

the Christian Commission also brought in a wagon to day And Supplied Some things for the comfort of those they could accomadate until such times as they would be—Supplied through the Regular channels—which will likely be Sometime as the Rebs burned the Bridge at or near the town as well as doeing much damage ~~also~~ at Hanover Junction[26] but it does not take us long to repair Such damages as these as we are a people of progress And thrift. To day the army rested on their laurels not certain as yet that the rebs had gone—the Surgeons being busily Engaged with the Sick—And wounded most of the operations being performed upon those that were in the Hospitals in town—

NOTES

1. Probably Josiah L. Lewis, hospital steward.
2. The battery was likely Capt. James A. Hall's Second Maine Battery.
3. McPherson farm.
4. Assistant surgeon, 149th PA.
5. Surgeon, 149th PA.
6. Fulton must have told them that they were surrounded.
7. Commanding the Second Army Corps, Army of Northern Virginia.
8. Pvt. Robert M. Cary, Co. E, 143rd PA.
9. See chapter 7 for additional discussion of these Gettysburg citizens.
10. Pennsylvania, later Gettysburg College.
11. Fulton inserted the super- and subscript words after he had written his diary entry.
12. Unidentified. The Zeiglers were an extended Gettysburg family.
13. Commander of Hays' Brigade, Maj. Gen. Jubal A. Early's Division, Second Army Corps under Lt. Gen. Richard S. Ewell, Army of Northern Virginia.
14. Fulton found Ewell.
15. It is not clear if Baker Ziegler and Judge Zeigler are related. The steward of the Lutheran Theological Seminar was Emmanuel Ziegler and his family.

16. Killed at the Battle of Fredericksburg, December 13, 1862.

17. Pickett's Charge, the advance across one mile of open field led by Major General George Pickett under Lieutenant General James Longstreet, which failed to break the opposing Union line and led to the Confederates' abandonment of the battle.

18. Probably the house of David McCreary, owner of a harness shop, who resided at Baltimore and High streets; hat maker Smith S. McCreary is also a possibility, who lived with his family on Chambersburg Street. See Gregory A. Coco, *A Vast Sea of Misery: A History and Guide to the Union and Confederate Field Hospitals at Gettysburg July 1–November 20, 1863* (Gettysburg, PA: Thomas Publications, 1988), 46; and Christina Ericson, "'The world will little note nor long remember': Gender analysis of civilian responses to the Battle of Gettysburg," in *Making and Remaking Pennsylvania's Civil War*, eds.William Blair and William Pencak (University Park: Pennsylvania State University Press, 2001), 88.

19. Fulton probably refers to John Burns, a local citizen who approached Fulton's brigade and asked to fight with them. See chapter 7.

20. Southern sympathizers.

21. Many Union Army soldiers and nurses later criticized Gettysburg residents, particularly men, for apparent indifference to the outcome of the battle, profiteering by demanding money for food or drink or other assistance, or other perceived failures to display patriotic ardor. See Jim Weeks, "'A disgrace that can never be washed out': Gettysburg and the lingering stigma of 1863," in *Making and Remaking Pennsylvania's Civil War*, 189–210.

22. Nicholson, Betzenberger, and Fell all served with the 143rd PA.

23. "Cap Fells" is probably 1st Lt. Asher M. Fell, 143rd PA. Conyngham, Hughes, Gaylord, and Reichard served with the 143rd PA.

24. Fulton refers to Gettysburg resident Jenny Wade, the only Gettysburg civilian to be killed during the battle. See chapter 7.

25. 143rd PA.

26. In York County, Pennsylvania, where Confederates fought Union forces for control of the town on June 30, 1863.

FOUR

Return to Virginia and Christmas with Secesh

Diary, July 5, 1863, to December 25, 1863

FOLLOWING THE GETTYSBURG BATTLE, A PECULIAR CALM DESCENDED ON THE *town and the battlefield. Rumors circulated that the Confederate forces were withdrawing and marching south to the Potomac River. The sultry, hot weather of the previous days gave way to rain, and the brigade's exhaustion from the battle persisted, with a looming new terror of a possible re-engagement with Confederate Gen. Robert E. Lee's forces. While Dr. Fulton remained in Gettysburg, the Second Brigade was on the march by July 6. By this time, Maj. Gen. Abner Doubleday, who assumed command of I Corps after the death of Gen. Reynolds, had been relieved. His successor, Brig. Gen. Thomas A. Rowley, commander of the 3rd Division, had been replaced by Gen. John Kenly on July 10. Col. Edmund L. Dana, commander of the 143rd Pennsylvania, assumed command of the brigade because Col. Roy Stone, formerly in command, had been left behind in Gettysburg due to wounds. Lt. Col. Walton Dwight, commander of the 149th Pennsylvania, Col. Langhorne Wister, commander of the 150th Pennsylvania, and his second-in-command, Lt. Col. Henry S. Huidekoper, also remained behind due to wounds. By July 20, the brigade reached Middleburg, Virginia, south of Catoctin Mountain. By July 25, the 150th had been assigned to guard the railroad at Warrenton Junction, its effective strength reduced to about a hundred soldiers. For the next several weeks, the brigade bivouacked at Bealton, Virginia, and regained health and a spit-and-polish appearance, while officers departed to recruit to fill the vacant ranks. Fulton's diary reminds us that the business of war was far from over in Gettysburg, although soldiers well enough to march had already departed in pursuit of Lee. Thousands of casualties remained in care in or around Gettysburg. Fulton remained in Gettysburg until August 10.*

—⁓—

July 5th 1863—

To day it was made Manifest that the Rebs had left the vicinity of Gettysburg and were Making their way as fast as possible for the Potomac or Virginia to make themselves Safe for the reason that they were well nigh out of Amunition And though they had lived well on their Stealings they could not long live in this way So far from their Base of Supplies—our men followed them up with vigor the Rebs getting of[f] as fast as possible but losing much of their train and many of their prisoners in this way they made their way back to the Potomac where they Expected to cross on a Pontoon Bridge but in the meantime the Bridge had been destroyed by [diary page ends and sentence is not completed on the next page] had been destroyed by our cavalry for Some time the River being high they had to cross their wounded in a common Ferry Boat. when the river fell they forded

/Gettysburg Penn[a]/

it is Said that many were drowned in So doeing but then it is not certain it is only Report—this Day Dr. W[illiam] T Humphrey[1] and all the Surgeons that could go were taken from the Hospitals to go with the army Expecting an Engagement before they reached the river Dr. Humphrey placed me in charge of the third Division Hospital—the Catholic and Presbyterian Church. Dr. [Philip A.] Quinan[2] wanted to Stay but was ordered to go with his Regiment—he did not like it much but had to acquiesce In the decision

July 6th 1863.

To day the wounded that had not been brought in from the farm houses round were brought in by the Ambulances we received one hundred and forty—it being difficult to find room in which to place them Many of them had to be placed upon the floor in the doorway And any other place that they could get to lay down- to day Quinan got permission of Dr W T Humphrey, to

come back to town to buy a horse from Col. [Langhorne] Wister[3]
after getting to town he immediately went to Dr Taylor[4] and
made a complaint about the third Div Hospital Stating that I was
not fit to have charge of it and that the men were not properly,
cared for and finally succeeded in getting Dr. Jayne[5] to put
him in charge of it and of course left Me Subordinate to . . . P A
Quinan—the Hospital of course was not in a good condition for
the reason that we had not received Any Stores to do it with—
And that there was So many that had just been [illegible word]
without proper places. for my part I did not care much though I
felt capable of performing the duty that had been assigned to Me
but Still I could find plenty to do And Still make my self as useful
or more so than before

/Gettysburg Penna/

I Remained at Gettysburg from the first of July until the 10/11 of
August, 1863 And during that time had Some three changes from the
Presbyterian Church to the Court House from the Court House to
the Seminary Hospital—Dr. [Robert] Loughran[6] being in charge I
Relieved Dr. [Harris?]—I had quite a pleasant time having the patients on the third floor under my charge being mostly amputations
of the number one belonged to the 143d Reg.

I dressed the men my self Every day useing the chlorinated Soda
pretty freely in the water with which the wounds were cleansed,
it helping to stimulate the granulations[7] as well to Keep the odor
good—we also used alcohol pretty freely as a Stimulant to the
granulations. the stumps all did well under My care and not a single
patient died—a fact that was to me quite Gratifying—

/Home/

Dr. Loughran And my self Roomed together And we had quite
a pleasant time of it—About the first of August Wm[8] came
down to see me in company with Corporal Johnson[9] they had
been out with the Militia and had first been discharged And

came by Gettysburg on their way home we passed over most
of the Battlefield Seeing as much as possible of the curiosities
attached thereto they were quite well pleased with this visit
And in the morning took their Leave for the Relay House—to
see his old Regt the Purnell Legion while at Gettysburg we had
quite a number of visitors from Chester County And it gave
me great pleasure to see them after being absent from them so
long—Being Relieved at Gettysburg the tenth of August I got
transportation for Washington from there to go on and join My
Regt. but after getting to Washington I went to [Major] Gen[eral
Henry W.] Halleck[10] [and] stated that the Rebs had captured all
My Equipment and asked permission to remain until the 18th
of August he soon granted my Request.[11] I then went to the pay
Department And there got four Months pay . . . Something that
was as much needed by me as any thing Else—

/Bealton/

After getting things fixed I took My Leave of Washington leaving
at 6 [p.m.?] in the Evening and getting to Phil[a] About one clock
that Night—I went to the Commercial Hotel And Staid until
morning taking the Eight o clock train went to Penn Station And
thence walked up home finding all well. I had quite a pleasant time
at home until the 18th of August when I again took Leave of home
And friends for the Army of the Potomac when it was Expected
that there would soon be a fight. I found the army at Bealton
[Bealeton] Station [Virginia] on the Evening of the 19th of August.
I found our Regt. quite small there being a great Many Men and
officers absent on account of wounds and sickness—from this
time untill about the middle of September we Stayed at Bealton
Doeing guard Duty the Labors not being very arduous we had
quite a nice time of it and got pretty well rested up for the fall
Campaign which we commenced about the Middle of September
by goeing from Bealton to Stevensburg [Virginia] a distance of
about 12 miles where we found the rest of our Corps in camp—
here we got two months pay. July And August—after Stay—here

a few days we moved camp for a few miles and then camped again for a few days but not getting to stay long Enough in any one place to fix up—

/Rapid Ann/

but in a Short time we Moved again from here to within sight of the Mountains along the Rapid Ann [Rapidan River] the Men here doeing picket Duty Along that Stream they had quite a good time while they Stayed here. the Boys had Rocking chairs to sit on and could find plenty of veal and Pork—they visited the House of Dr Stringfellow Brother of the notorious Kansas Stringfellow—[12]

When our Cavalry had driven the Enemy back from the Rappahanock [Rappahannock River] Many of the Sympathyzers [sympathizers] left Culpepper [Virginia] and crossed the Rapid Ann to be within the Enemys lines but being considerably humid when they got to the River quite a number of families failed to get across and one house there had seventeen women in it Showing that they were willing to live pretty thick rather than give up their treasonable and worthless opinions which I trust they will be compelled Soon to give up by force of surrounding circumstances—they have held and preached their doctrines of treason long Enough for their own good as well as the good of the whole country—they are not at all Backward in Saying that they are Rebs and Showing their proclivities for the cause of the Rebellion—

After leaving Raccoon ford[13] we went to Germania ford[14] Expecting that we were goeing to cross the River and beard the Lion in his den but in the Meantime [Major] Gen[eral George G.] Mead[e] had Learned that the Rebs were passing round by Culpepper and getting round the right Flank of the army, and he was in consequence thereof compelled to fall Back toward the Rappahanock we commenced to fall Back the night we got to Germania Ford

and that night went as far as Stevensburg getting there about two
oclock on Sunday Morning we camped for the rest of the night but
it being very cold I could not Sleep any of any account Laying down
on the ground without ~~fire~~ a tent and wood being Scarce so that we
could not have much fire—but we [worried?] through the rest of the
night in the best Manner possible keeping warm as best we could
thinking to sleep in the future—

in fact it was nothing new to sit by the fire all night and not get any
sleep—Sunday Morning we Left Stephensburg on our way to the
Rappahanock goeing toward Kellys Ford[15] passing through a rough
Country—most of it being poor untill we got to the River where
as is usual to see the Land is again pretty good—at Kellyville[16] on
the south side of the River there are several pretty good houses and
a good Mile though some of the buildings have been destroyed the
places Look as though it might have been Respectable at one time
though—Now Looking the worse for the war.

October 11th 1863

when we got to the River we found Some little fortifications thrown
up to protect our crossing we waited untill our wagon trains And
Artillery had all crossed and then crossed ourselves without any
accident or trouble whatever—though all day long we heard the
Sound of Artillery and Musketry. Shortly after leaving Stevensburg
the Reb cavalry came in and captured one of of [sic] our men that
had been lef[t] behind Sick—they followed us up pretty close and
near Brandy Station there was quite a heavy fight quite as heavy a
fight of the character as has taken place during the war.

/Oc 14th 1863 Oc 12th Battle of Bristow Station/

After crossing the River we Stoped in the wood that night and all
day Monday Oc. 12th and part of the night leaving at two o clock
on the Morning of Tuesday Oc 13th we took up the line of march
toward Bealton Station—after getting on the Railroad passing on to
Warrenton Junction when we found the army drawn up in line—and

a large quantity of artillery planted on the Eminence and controlling the country upon which the Enemy could be likely to approach— after taking dinner we passed on to Bristow Station where we Stoped for the night—

/Battle of Bristow Oc 14th 1863/

Oc 14th to day we left Bristow Station And took the line of march for Centreville getting there in good time—and putting up for the night behind the fortifications this day there was quite a Brisk little fight the Rebs though[t] to attack and take the wagon train of the 2nd Corps but they were Mistaken in the work they had to accomplish the Rebs made the attack with a Battery and one Brigade of A P Hills Corps the third Division of the 2nd Corps Lay behind the Railroad Bank the Reb Cavalry made a charge upon our line but were immediately Driven back with heavy Loss—they then made a charge with a Brigade of infantry but they too were doomed to the Same or a worse fate for they were not only Driven back with great Loss in Killed and wounded but with the Loss of four hundred and fifty prisoners and failed to get any wagons and provisions that they Seemed to be so much in need of. but they are no worse of[f] for food than they are for Shoes as many of them are Barefooted.

/Haymarket/
October 1863—Thursday 15 Friday 16 Saturday 17 Sunday 18th

to day Thursday we went on Picket on the road toward Edwards Ferry[17], And Staid out all night coming back the next morning we again went into the Fortifications and there we Start all the time hearing the sound of Artillery—hopeing and Expecting that the Enemy would make an attack upon us while in the fortification at Centreville we having there a good position indeed—the rebs being as [sic; probably "a"] little to[o] Sharp to attack us in such a position it being their policy to get the best position at all times or they are not willing to give battle on Monday the 19th of October we

were again ordered to take up the line of march for Haymarket to
make a reconoisance—and See what the Rebs were doeing in that
Direction when we got to there we soon found that the Jonnies were
doeing their best as they had met our Cavalry and at least frightened
some of them considerably and they came flying in some without
hats Showing that [they] had at Least come away from the scene of
conflict in quite a hurry—

Tuesday Oc 20th Haymarket

our Regt was drawn up in Line to Support the Cavalry Expecting
that they would immediately make a charge of a formidable nature
and that a good force of infantry would [be] necessary to Repel it
but they made no charge And we Soon went Back and put up our
quarters for the night—the next morning we went from there back
and Laid there untill toward Evening when we again took the line of
march for Thoroughfare Gap[18] Reaching that place about Dark we
passed through the Gap a short Distance and stoped for the night
the night being dark we could not see much

/Thoroughfare Gap./
Thoroughfare Gap.
Wednesday Oc. 21st 1863—

This Morning we Broke Camp and moved a Short Distance round
the Hill and there found quite a good camping ground for the
country here is good being the best that I have seen in Virginia in
fact the Army has not been through this part of Virginia and of
course the fences had not been disturbed and there had been pretty
good Crops—though the country has been more used for grazing
than for growing grain—it Looks much like Chester And Lancaster
Counties though I think that the Country is naturally Better than
it is there if we did not use lime and Manure as Extensively as we
do—I often thought that I would Like to Live in this Beautiful
Country Known by the name of Louden [Loudoun] Valley—it is

comprised between the Bull River Mountains and the Blue Ridge and is quite Extensive—it indeed could be made Beautiful if it only had the Enterprise—

the Farms in which we were Encamped contained about 250 acres and a gentleman told me that it cost 10.000 [10,000] Dollars and it was considered a very high price it had a good house and the land was certainly of the finest quality for grazeing and raising wheat—but Something Keeps them Back—a Man Living here said that E McClenaghan[19] lived about fifteen miles from him And that his son had been to his mill he Stated that the old gent. had died in the Summer—The poor man Ended his days with those he was in Sympathy with his heart no doubt being in unison with the Rebels and their cause—

/March to Bristow Station/

it is hoped that he got forgiveness for his Sin And died happy though his poor wife must feel Lonely And Sad Leaving her friends in Penn[a]. the spring the Rebellion broke out And Seeing three of her family buried in Virginia with her only Remaining son in the Rebel Army, what a picture of Sadness is here presented—I had a notion to write a letter for her and Leave it with this gentleman for him to Send to her but then we had to Move again Sooner than I Expected And I did not get it done—[Joe] Staid here over the 22[ond] and 23[d]. on [in] the morning we Broke camp and took up the line of march for Bristow Station Being detailed as wagon guard we got to gainsville [Gainesville] about noon from which we took up the line of march again after getting dinner getting to Broad run about dark. when the teamsters were takeing their Supper they soon harnessed their teams and again took up the March all having to wade the Stream it being quite deep and the night very cold

Oc 23[d]—

how the poor fellows did Suffer—it was late when we got to the Station And wood being scarce we had a hard time to get up any

fire the Men did the Best they could to keep warm for My part
I did not Sleep an hour the whole night it was very cold—as
we came through the no[t]ch we had a fine view of the rugged
character of the Mountain there is a Large Stream [that] passes
through with a large mill Situated in the gap—the Mill is owned
by a gentleman in Newyork. but at this time all is Ruin and water
the houses being in a State of Delapidation—And decay for the
want of care and use—the property has been a fine one at one time
though the time has passed And the consequence is that farmers
have to go a long distance to Mill Some of them as much as fifteen
miles which is quite a consideration to the pleasure of Living in
the country. after dawn.

/Manassas Junction—/
October

the Railroad passes through this gap from Manassas Junction to
Manassas Gap it certainly has a very Serpentine course through the
mountain but at one time I suppose did quite an Extensive business
though now it is not doing any thing Except to Gainsville to which
place all the supplies come for the army of the Potomac while the
Road is being Repaired to the Rappahanock—

October
Bristow Station 24th to 25

Nothing of importance occurring to note in the morning of
the 26th we had orders about two o clock to take up the line of
March [to] Manassas Junction at which place we got [to] about
Daylight—here we Staid for Some time doeing guard Duty—at the
Junction there being [a] Large number of Cars stopping here all
the time the duty was quite a pleasant one—we could find plenty
of Wares and other materials to make fire places and chimneys so
that we soon began to be quite comfortable and were quite sorry
to Leave as the Season is getting so far advanced that it is of great
importance that we should have plenty of fire—we had another

advantage here we could trade Sugar and Coffee for butter And Eggs, Poultry And in fact almost anything that a soldier might want in the way of Eating

/Manassas Junction Nov. 1ᵗ to 6th—/

we got acquainted with quite a number of citizens round And they were disposed to be quite Sociable And Said that they Knew nothing of guerillas A Miss Conrad[20] came for me to go and attend her brother who was sick with the Fever—they lived on the old Bull Run Battle field—She made me a present of a Basket made from the Burs—She gathered from the Battle field—She gave it to Me as a Relic She had given away quite a number of them—and they are certainly quite a nice little memento by which to Remember the two Bloody Fields—

Nov 6 1863

the country around Manassas I think Exceeds anything for persimons that I have Ever seen in my travels people there Say that they make An Elegant Beer they first crush them then Bake them And then put them in cold water when they undergo Fermentation And it is Said to be Equal to hard Cider—it is Said that Distillers will give as much for them as for corn to make whiskey—there is certainly plenty of them—We Staid at Manassas until Nov 6 th we took up the line of March for Warrenton Junction Reaching there on the morning of Nov 7 th where we found the rest of the Brigade—After Stoping about An hour with the Regt we turned across the Railroad—

/Warrenton Junction Nov 1863—/

To day we had quite a heavy fight at the the Rappahanock the 6th Corps being the force mostly Engaged they Stormed the Enemy's works takeing about Eighteen hundred prisoners with Eleven pieces of artillery—taken all together it was a Brilliant af- [line break] affair—it is not often that a whole force is captured—they were putting up winter qrs [quarters] And Were goeing to make them Selves

comfortable thinking they were goeing to get to rest the remainder
of the season—but the poor fellows were Sadly Mistaken for about
they [sic] time they began to feel secure in their new habitation Gen.
Sedgwick pounced upon them and they will now have a chance of
Spending the winter in Washington where they will Likely get as
much to Eat as they did in the Confederacy—

Sunday Nov 8th 1863

this Morning after Sick Call I took a walk over to the Depot to See
the Jonnies come in that had been Captured—And Shortly after
they began to file in the poor fellows looked Ragged and dirty as
usual Some were in their Bare feet—there was a pile of Broken hard
Bread that had been thrown out and they soon began to put it in
their haversacks—I helped them to put them in as they had but little
time And Seemed quite hungry—those that Stoped got quite a good
Supply And seemed to be well pleased with what they had found—it
did me good to be able to help them.

/Seven Men Captured by one—Warrenton Junction/

Notwithstanding they are the sworn Enemys of our country they
were Loaded on the Cars and Sent to Washington a portion of our
Brigade was to go as guard but owing to them being 5 Minutes too
late they Missed the job and had to March back to camp a disappointed Set of Men. So much for not being prompt—Cap[tain
Oliver K.] Moore[21] was considerably provoked by the way things
turned out as he would like to have had the trip to Washington with
Nearly two thousand Rebs—It was to day that a guerilla came to our
picket Line—he rode between Seven of our Men and their guns he
ordered them to Surrender. they did So without a word he marched
them of[f] at a double quick about two Miles to a farm house where
he got a woman to hold his pistol to them while a young Lady Kissed
him Several times and he wrote them paroles—

Since the Regt has been organized never has so disgraceful a thing
happened to it the Men Belonged to Company K—And Cap[tain

Issac S.] Little[22] Says that if he had been called upon to furnish
Seven for a dangerous and difficult task there was no Seven in his
company that he would have picked sooner than those Captured
why it was that they Suffered themselves to be taken ignominiously
is one of the Mysterys of war that cannot be accounted for. Men
Sometimes get panic Stricken when no Reason can be assigned or
imagined and they will fly as though pursued by some Demon incarnate which did they not Escape their destruction would be inevitable
and terrible when possibly it May be as at Bull Run the second when
they had ~~whp~~ whipped the Enemy from Every position that could
take and Even from their fortifications at Centreville on the third
day, when the work was well nigh done—they became panic stricken
and fled from the field and passed the fortifications at Centreville—
pele mele [pell-mell] on to Washington where only they felt Safe—

/Prisoners Sent from Warrenton Junction/
Sunday Nov 8th 1863—

when we look at the ground and weigh Every consideration it is as
difficult to See a reason for Gen Popes Retreat as it is to account for
Seven Men being Captured by one—but Such is Man at times particularly when Congregated together The rustling of a leaf the Ripple
of a Stream will Strike terror to their hearts And Send them flying as
a flock of sheep that is pursued by wolves—to certain destruction.
the Railroad as yet is not finished to Bealton so that the Cars only
run as far as the Junction with rations and forage So that it Makes
this place one of great importance—there being a Large Amount of
Stores we have thrown up in front of our three Regts. Quite a good
Breast work so that if Mosby or White[23] should pay us a visit we will
Be pretty well prepared to Meet him—though I think they all find
plenty to do in other places without troubling us—

/Warrenton Junction Virginia/
November 14th 1863

This is certainly a beautiful day And the true type of Indian
Summer. the Air Smoky and Warm—the Dead and Lean Leaf Still

clinging to the Oaks, the Hickory with other trees with their deep crimson foliage giving variety and beauty to [all] arround—And Enticing the Lover of nature to the woody haunts And there holding him Entranced with natures variety And beauties in all its manifold forms—how pleasant to get away from the turmoils and troubles of camp and walk—out and commune with Nature with all its Lovliness—And there for a time at Least be in communion with something natural And that is in accordance with the will and wish of the Creator—war in all its Bearing And in all Connexion being foreign to the will of him who wishes th all things pure And good— instead of wounds And Sickness health And happiness Might be the happy Lot of thousands that are now Suffering from these causes in a climate hostile to them while confronting a hostile foe—But God in his own good time will cause the wrath of Man to praise him And the remainder of wrath will he restrain—these things when called to mind affords at Least one fealing of Satisfaction And that is that At Some time not far distant all will yet be well with our once happy country And that we will have The happy privilege of again joining our families in happiness And there remain the remainder of our days Secure from the new alarm of war—

/Warrenton Junction Nov 14th 1863—/

No More has the Ear pained with the groans And Shrieks of the Wounded and dying—but that the course of us An[d] our Country May be onward from prosperity to prosperity until the Sun Shall Shine upon a people no more free no No [sic] More happy in his wide domain—

the indian Summer has already lasted quite a week And the prospect is that it will Continue quite a length of time Longer— Everything now is favorable Military operations And the only thing that prevents [them] is the railroad to Carry Supplies to the front which is in progress as as [sic] fast as possible And will Likely soon be Completed—it is to be hoped that the work will Soon be accomplished And that the Army will be able to Strike a Speedy and Effective Blow—that will be felt by the Enemy with Crushing

Effect And that will cool their Audacity And Lead them to feal that it is futile in them to Still persist in their Efforts to build up an Aristocracy within the United States that it is time for them to humble themselves And Submit to the fact that they are Nothing more than Men And that it is useless to Strive against God, who in his all wise providence has determined to humble them And bring them with ourselves to Confess our great sin that we have committed in his sight—

/Warrenton Junction Nov 14th 1863—/

Yesterday I am told fifty More prisoners were sent to Washington this make[s] About two thousand that have been sent on within a week. I trust the tide will Continue in our favor as [Private] John McRoy of Co H24 of Co H has returned from Richmond and his haggard countenance bears testimony that the treatment there received is anything but well calculated to favor the growth And development of the human Body—the Cavalry had a reconoisance to the front the day before yesterday but with what result we are not Able to Say at the present writing as we as yet have had no intelligence the fireing was heavy And Continuous. this Evening we are having quite a brisk thunder Shower with Considerable lighting and thunder

Rebel Prisoners—

As I passed the junction to day I saw quite a number of Rebel Prisoners upon inquiry I was told that there were Eighty five of them they presented their usual ragged and dirty appearance doubtless Many of them glad to be taken as they will now get plenty to Eat and have nothing to do—to day I was out to the Picket line and there saw a family that before the Rebellion had commenced were in good Circumstances—but are now begging us to furnish them with flour they have two cases of Typhoid fever in the house with a sick child. the Lady seemed to be quite intelligent. they are by the name of Smith—and have a good house quite Equal to the average in Virginia

/General Med's Official Report of the Battle of Gettysburg July [2–5?]/

We have waited untill Now for Gen Meads official Report of
the Battle of Gettysburg—he he States our Loss in Killed 2334
wounded—13.709. Missing 6643 total 23186 we captured from the
Enemy, 13.000 prisoners their guns forty one Standards or colors—
picket up on the field 24.978. Small Arms—this he gives as the direct
result of the Battle with the driving the Enemy from Penn[a] and
Maryland which is not the least result produced in the three day's
fight at Gettysburg—the Report is concise and pertinent devoid of
Bombast—the records are under rather than overdrawn altogether it
argues well for the Author

Nov 18th.

we are Still at the Junction doeing guard Duty and the Men Seem
quite willing to Stay here So Long as they have the privilege of doeing so as they are fixed up in as Comfortable Manner—More so than
they could be if we should have to Move Every day or two—Most
of them having fire places in their tents—the powers of acquisition
possessed by the yankee Soldier are truely wonderful—Should he
be placed in Juxtaposition with a camp that has just been deserted
you will see their goeing And Coming in crowds some carrying old
clothes others Boards—Stoves and all Kinds of trumpery they they
[*sic*] May be Expecting to Man at any time yet they take as Much
pain to fix up and Make themselves comfortable as though they
Expected to Stay a year—

/Warrenton Junction Nov 18th 1863—/

one will have a neat Stone fireplace—Another a Subterranean
Stove—And So on untill it would Seem that the whole branch
of the Science and philosophy of caloric[25] had been studied
And brought to bear in the preparation of these humble though
comfortable tenements—that possibly are to be deserted a few

Short hours After Completion yet when the order comes all Move of[f] with a good will probably to undergo a few Miles distant the Same course of construction and gathering together—the Soldier's life is Said to be An idle one though if he is watched it will be found that he usually finds plenty to do to Keep his mind Engaged And Enough to Keep him free from diversion And one peculiarity of character is truely Strikeing it is that which Enables the Soldier No Matter how Much Labor he has bestowed upon his house to Leave it or rebuild another And all without a complaint but takeing all as a matter of course in his Every day business of Life—

the Army cannot be Said to be religious though all Seem to have a profound Respect for religion—And talk of death as a something not [Do] unlikely to cross their path and stop their Earthly cares but with little fear—there is a calusness [callousness] and resignation manifested that is truely to be admired—And well worthy of imitation—As it is Expected the true and humble Christian dies so due they with a feeling of honorable pride that in their death much has been done for the future freedom and happiness of Millions

/Rebs [illegible word] to Cross the Rapid Ann— Nov 16th 1863/

Last Sunday Nov 16th we heard considerably Artillery fireing And have since Learned that a Large Rebel force attempted to Cross the Rapid Ann but were repulsed with heavy Loss by our forces on this—side[26]—though the particulars have not been stated as—yet—there is some talk of our Brigade goeing to Brandy Station to do guard Duty as it is Said that Supplies will be Sent forward to that place—the weather Still Continues [to be] beautiful And it would seem that if we are goeing to Make an advance upon the Enemy it is high time that it was done as wounded Men Suffer Enough in warm weather without haveing to undergo Exposure from cold—

Thursday
Warrenton Junction Nov 19th 1863

This is the day for the Meeting at Gettysburg to Dedicate the National Cemetery on the old Battlefield—it is a step highly to be commended as a testimonial of Respect to the Many departed heroes that fell upon that Blood Stained [field] the Many of our rank And file that had their Blood Swallowed up by the Mother Earth to whose Bosom will Now be Entrusted the Ashes of the departed Heroes—It is to be hoped that our Country will make No human thing of it but that in appearance it will be Something to attract visitors from Every Nation Every clime to the great Battlefield of America—And there do homage to the heroism of her Departed great—[27]

/Warrenton Junction Inspection By Cap Osborn[28]—/
Nov 19th 1863

to day at two o Clock we had inspection. Dr. [David L.] Scott[29] And Myself were—the Col would not Excuse us I guess he wanted to have some fun at our Expense for when we advanced then he ordered us to right Dress And we were So green that we did not Know how it should be done—For My part I care but little as Military outside of our particular Duties And of Course get but little attention—this has been a beautiful one a continuation of Indian Summer—the Air Smoky And Calm—beautiful indeed—

Warrenton Junction Nov 21st

To Day we got our pay for the Months August and September—I paid quarter Master $110.00 for the gray horse John Market US—and for which he gives me a warrant—that the horse was his own private property—

/Warrenton Junction to Manassas Junction/
Sunday Nov 22^{ond} 1863

Last Night I got a letter from W^m[30] Stating that Father is quite Sick with dropsy[31] and that he wanted to see Me thinking that I could

give him Something that would benefit him. I accordingly went to
Dr. Humphrey and Stated the case upon doeing So was told that there
was no use in Making application untill the [March?] of the Army
was over as no Leaves of Absence would be granted on Any pretext
whatever though he Said that I Might go up and See Dr. Herd[32] and
Know for certain whether or not I could get home—but on goeing to
the Picket line—I found [Colonel Langhorne] Wister there and was
told that the Guerillas were very numerous in the Vicinity of Bealton
Station And that it would not be safe for for [*sic*] Me to venture that
distance from camp unless I wanted to be captured

/Warrenton To Manassas Nov 22nd 1863/

this I did not want—and accordingly went back to camp there
to await the orders for Moveing which came about dark when we
took the line of March for Manassas Junction at which place we
arrived about 3 o.clock in the Morning after Marching Seventeen
Miles—the men were quite tired indeed and were glad to stop and
rest. the 150th Stoped in camp at Warrenton Junction—the 149th
Stoped at Bristow we came on to the Junction to guard this part of
the road—it was a nice Night for Marching had it not been we would
have had More Straglers than there was—there was plenty as it
was—Cap[tain] Rickhard[33] with his Company was left ~~back with~~ at
the Bridge nearest Manassas

/The [illegible word]—Arrive this year/

When we came to Catlett Station[34] we found the whole road Blocked
up with cars the reason being a Locomotive had ran of[f] the track
And they had Considerable trouble to get it on the track. There was
the Most Cars that I had Seen together in one place for a long time—
we Staid here about two hours untill they got the Engine on the track
when we again Moved on—at Kettle run[35] the Men Crossed the
railroad Bridge—this Makes the fourth time that we have crossed
this Stream and travelled this road—And I am indeed quite well
Satisfied with the travelling for this year and hope that it will not be
required of us to travel it again this year—

Nov 23ᵈ 24ᵗʰ 25ᵗʰ 1863—

These three days we have been busily Engaged in fixing up our quarters And Most of us have Succeeded in Making ourselves comfortable And if we only got to stay here we will have a place quite Comfortable to Live in—the people are bringing in things for us to Eat and if we only get to stay here we can Live pretty well on the 23ᵈ the Army of the Potomac was to make a forward Move and the Rail Road was to be Abandoned and a new Base of Supplies to be taken by Fredericksburg—Via Aquia Creek but owing to the rain the Army does not move—there is a great many cattle and horses goeing down to the Army but not much food for Men Mostly ~~ration~~ forage—there being an immense quantity of that apparently being acquired probably for the Cavalry—

/Army of the Potomac Crosses the Rapid Ann—/
Monday Nov 27th 1863—

to day the army of the Potomac Began to Move toward the Rapid Ann and crossing it at three different fords that they might attack the Rebel Strong holds on the opposite Banks—at Raccoon ford the cavalry[36] of [Brigadier General Hugh J.] Kilpatric[k] Met with Some opposition but finally Succeeded in crossing. there was some fighting throughout the day but no Decisive engagement was brought on. we could hear artillery fireing throughout the day Here at the junction And were led to think that a general Engagement was goeing on but have since Learned that such was not the case—the Enemy began Soon to fall back toward Gordonsville thinking probably to Make a Stand there and if possible cope with our forces—our Corps the 1ˢᵗ crossed the Rapid Ann opposite Culpepper the name I do not Remember the the [sic] two Fords were Germania and Raccoon

Nov 29th

there being Some fighting to day on our Right wing being the position held by the 2ᵒⁿᵈ Corps they took about nine hundred prisoners

the Loss in Killed and wounded being about three hundred—One
Lieut[enant] Colonel being among the Killed—the cars now run
only to the Rappahanock so that we get but Little News from the
front—And have to depend upon the papers we get for what Little
of information we have of the Movements of the Army—We have
succeeded in getting fixed up pretty well we have a good fire place
and chimney and can Live pretty comfortably this cold weather as
we are getting it pretty Sharp for old Virginia—but we only have two
or three cold days at a time

/Army of the Potomac—Fighting Near [illegible word] Court House/
Monday Nov 30

this a Bitter cold day for this country the wind blew a gale the
weather having been so warm and pleasant it sets hard on us as for
Myself I Soon get chilled not having my winter clothes they being
in a box at the Express office at Washington—I have Sent for it two
or three times but of no avail as they Still Refuse to Send it on My
order—the roast pig in the Box I think is getting a little Stale by
this time And I am a little afraid that My clothes will Be Spoiled by
the time I get them as they have been lightly cared for the Last four
weeks—And is Likely to stay there untill the army is done Moving
which I trust will Soon be Successfully done. as the Men wounded
on the field of Battle in addition to their wounds will suffer with cold
which is as Much as the other—

/Army of the Cumberland Victory of Chatanooga/

Sunday—the past week has Made Much of History for America
during the time Gen Grant And Thomas and Hooker have attacked
the Enemy at Chatanooga [Chattanooga, Tennessee] and have
routed them with a Loss of sixty pieces of artillery and Several
thousand prisoners And Sent them howling back to their dens in
Macon Georgia—where they are attemting to Make a Stand we trust
to be only the worse whipped when they Should be attacked which

we think will not be Long—[Union Major] Gen[eral] [Ambrose] Burnside has been Keeping [Confederate Lieutenant General James] Longstreet at Bay untill he has been ordered by [Confederate Lieutenant General Braxton] Bragg to join the Main Army, which he is at this time trying to do by taking circuitous [a circuitous route] south—But it is thought that he will Meet with difficulties before he gets there as Grant will Make use of all the Means in his power to crush him and use up his army before he can concentrate with Bragg—

December 1863—
1st 2ond 3d 4th

We have Still been Enjoying our selves for these four days we have a good fire place and Chimneys and we are Capable of Keeping ourselves as comfortable as though we were at home in good houses the women round the country Keep Bringing us in plenty of pies roast turkeys chickens Butter Eggs Milk—So that we have been able to live quite well indeed—as our Army has crossed the Rapid Ann And driven the Enemy from their first line of works there is but little or no transportation upon the road and of course but few trains running it is quite dull to what it was when there were about twenty trains goeing Every day—

Saturday Dec 5th 1863—

To day we were relieved about Noon by the 3d Brigade of the Penna Reserves and were ordered to Report at Rappahanock Station we accordingly packed up our [illegible word] And started getting under weigh about two O Clock in the Afternoon. we passed along the line of the Rail Road untill we got to Catlett Station when it was fully dark. there we camped for the Night—in course of the Night it Blowed up bitter cold So that with the scarcity of wood it was a pretty trying night to Lay upon the ground without Shelter any other than the Blue As the one Vault of heaven—But we were called up at one o clock and took up the line of March about two we still Kept

the [page break] the line of the Rail Road passed Bealton about
Sun Rise—After passing on from there about a Mile we Stoped for
Breakfast—

/The Fight at Mill Run/
Dec 6th 1863—

We had quite an interesting account of the advance to Mill run
from the Rapid Ann. they drove the Enemy Steadily back untill
they found the Enemy Strongly Entrenched upon this Stream—the
Roads were Exceedingly heavy, Making it difficult for the Artillery
to get along the weather was Extremely cold the Men Say that they
have never Suffered Since they have been in the service—it Being
So Cold that Several of the Men froze to death while on Picket
they not being allowed to have any fire—They were about to storm
the works by makeing a night attack but when they came to Mill run
they found that the Enemy had made a Succession of dams upon
the Stream Making it about 5 feet deep and fourteen wide so that
the Men if they had crossed would [have] been wet from head to
foot And Many of them would have undoubtedly have [sic] perished
with the cold—upon Mature deliberation by officers it was decided
to be impractible they accordingly withdrew the Army from the
Enemy's front and recrossed the Rapid Ann—without Serious
Loss—

/The Advance to Mill Run—Dec 1st 1863—/

The Rebs having performed one of their Sharp tricks the 5th
Corps in taking their position had passed too far to the Left and
were ordered back—their ammunition trains in the Rear as they
were following the Men—an officer Rode up to the Lieutenant in
charge of the train And told him that the General desired him to
take Another Road at the time pointing [to] it the train of the 1st
Division accordingly took his advice the others Refusing thinking
that there was Something wrong in the Arrangement—but after
the trains that went as directed had gone about a Mile they found

that they were in the hands of the Rebs who immediately took the
guard prisoners with the train drivers—then took the Mules and
horses from the wagons—applied the Match and Blowed up the
whole Business—had the whole train followed the Reb [advance?]
a whole Corps would have been without Ammunition Except
Such as they Carried with them—they have the particular faculty
of deceiving our Men—a person would think that we had been
cheated often Enough to Know them but it appears that it Can Still
be done—

Dec 6th 1863—

After takeing Breakfast near Bealton we continued our March untill
we came to Rappahanock Station there we Stoped for Dinner the
Men drew two day's Rations of hard Bread here we could See the
Effects of the fight—there being Many Newly Made graves where
our poor fellows had been buried after their Successful [attack]
upon the Fort and the Capturing two Brigades of Rebs—we here
crossed the River on a Pontoon Bridge we have left the Rail Road
taking the direction of Paoli Mills which place we Reached about
four o clock we then put up for the Night—this is the place that had
been Selected as Winter quarters for [Confederate Major General
Edward] Johnsons Division of [Lieutenant General Richard S.]
Ewells Corps (Reb) they had up Log houses with fire places and
chimneys and Roofs Made of Shingles that they had Split out of the
Surrounding timber—

they in fact were fixed So that they could have lived quite comfortable through the winter—but our Boys coming upon them
Caused them to Leave in a hurry they build if anything better
quarters than our Men. Not having Shelter tents are compelled
to put on Roofs of Shingles or Boards or Some other Material
that will turn rain—they had their Streets Laid out quite nicely
the houses are quite Large and Roomy for the number of men
that have to live in them And if they only have plenty to Eat most
Certainly [can] Live quite comfortably through the winter—the

Night being cold And the Maryland and the 1st Brigade takeing all the quarters that had been Left after the 1st and 2ond Divisions of our Corps had taken up their quarters we were compelled to take up our quarters on the ground under a tree—the night being cold. the night was not a very pleasant one to Ma[n]y of our poor Soldier Boys we had a good fire and plenty of Blankets and Made out to Sleep pretty well—

/Camp at Paoli Mills Va/
Monday Dec 7th 1863—

This Morning our camp was Laid out And Soon the Boys began the work of building houses Cutting trees Carrying logs and Mud and Stones goeing all over the Country looking for Boards and other Lumber. the Bucktails attacked a house and other buildings at the Mill with great Rigor tearing the Roof from the Porch of the house in which the people were Living—they Laid in a complaint to [Major] Gen[eral John] Newton[37] he ordered Col[onel Langhorne] Wister to be put under arrest And Col[onel Edmund L.] Dana then Commanded the Brigade he Stoped the Bad business in a very Short time the Men then had to depend on the timber in the Wood for their houses which they find will answer Every purpose—if Rightly used. they Soon Learn to make themselves Handy—

8 + 9 December.

Nothing particular happening these two days the Men Still working at their quarters and Every Effort to procure Soft Bread failing—No Potatoes to be had—Joe [Josiah L. Lewis] our Hospital Steward put in for a furlough for fifteen days—he is certainly Much Exercised thereby And I hope he will be Successful if not it will certainly Make him sick as I have never seen any one so Much set on getting home as he is he goes to the Col Several times daily to Make inquiries about his papers to Know whether they are goeing right or not—

/Go to Brandy Station for Supplies/
Dec 10th 1863.

To day I was detailed by Dr Mitchell[38] to go to Brandy Station to
get Medicine for the Division—I Reported to Dr. Mitchell in the
Shortest possible Notice. he gave me the Requisitions to Be Signed
by Dr. Herd. I then Started the team that I had been ordered to take
from Division Hospital on toward the Station telling him to follow
the telegraph line after getting the Requisitions fixed up I Started
after him and when coming to or in Sight of a Small Stream that was
at the Edge of a great wood I Saw a wagon ahead and it looked as
though it was Set upon its [far?] End. upon coming I found that three
of the Mules were down in the Mud. I told the teamster to unharness
those—that he could get out and then the others could get up he did
So but found that one of them could Not get out So he had to hitch
his two Leaders to him and pull him out of the Mud—

the Mule could not Stand after he was up—he concluded to tie the
well one to the tree and Leave him there untill we came back with
[medicines]—we then went on to the Station without Meeting with
any other Misfortunes on the way. getting there about two o clock
upon getting there I found Dr. [John H.] Brinton to be Medical
Purveyor for the Army of the Potomac. I had not Seen him Since the
Battle of Gettysburg I was quite glad to Meet some one that I knew—

/Trip to Brandy Station Supplies/

I Set to work to find some place on the ground that I could get
something to Eat but found that it there being No Eating house
[not finding a place that sells food] and no Sutler Except one that
Sold to the Negro Employees on the Railroad and a white Man could
get Nothing Except he got a Negro to buy it for him And then at the
Most Extravagant prices. I tried all the Cars but no one had anything
to Sell So I had to give it up thinking that while a person is in the
Army he Should at all times carry his haversack and Blanket if he
Leaves Camp—After about two hours we got the Requisitions filled
the goods

Loaded and Started on our [way] Back Leaving the Station at four
o clock the Road is certainly a very rough and bad one—they are
putting Corderoy [corduroy] on a good part of the Road but Still it
will be bad Let them do as they will—

when we got back to the place where we left the Mules we found that
they were gone So that we were two Mules out of Pocket coming
back with four Mules instead of six—Dr. [Francis C.] Reamer[39] being at home on Furlough did not have an opportunity to Blow—So
that we had No trouble that night—Not Eating anything Since
Morning before Sunrise and it being Now dark—I felt quite hungry
And I was glad to find Supper in the Shortest possible time—on our
way home we passed the ruins of Several good buildings that had
been burned Showing that the work of destruction still goes on. had
the people only have stayed at home their property would not have
been burned—still if they had not been traitors they would have
seen no danger—

/Mrs. Thom⁵ residence/

The Burned buildings [we] Saw on the way was the private
Residence of Col Thom[40] formerly and Mrs Thom it is not Long
Since She had it refitted and fixed up in fine Style as a Summer
residence—our soldiers burned it at the time that Mead Crossed
the Rapid Ann the Soldiers Say the reason they burned was that
they were told that it Belonged to [Colonel John S.] Moseby[41]—if
it did not belong to him it was the property of those that are No
More Loyal than he is—the Situation is a fine one and the place in
its Palmy Days was one that would compare favorably with those of
our Northern states. The Rebs in this Neighborhood Seem to Mourn
considerably on the vandalism of the Yankees—

December 15th 1863.

To day there was a Med board Met to Examine Cap[tain Oliver K.]
Moore[42] for discharge Lafrance[43] for transfer to Hospital—[Private]

E[benezer] S Fisk[44]—OK Moore[s] papers with ES Fisks were
approved while Lafrance was Rejected—two of the Surgeons
had been in the Purnell Legion of Maryland, And well Knew My
Brother—they Said [they saw] a resemblance between Myself and
him—immediately they wished to be Remembered to him—they
Speak of him highly as an officer—but Say ~~that~~ he was broken down
Not So Much by disease as by trouble of Mind—they went on to
give a rather discouraging account of the Purnell Legion Saying that
Colonel is a Copperhead—

/Dr. Green asst Surg. Gen of Pen. visits us—/
Dec 16th 1863.

To day we had a heavy rain Storm which continued throughout the
day. it having Every appearance that winter with its usual array of
rain Storms has Set in as incident to this climate. Mountain river is
very high the Bridge that we cross in goeing to Brigade Commissary,
is covered with water—there are flying rumors that we will not Stay
here but [go] to the rear More toward Manassas Junction as the Line
by which we get our Supplies is so long that the Expense [is] so great
in Supplying us we have a Long distance also to have them by wagon
and through a country like this is quite an item.

Dec 17th 1863

—to day was quite Stormy—the roads are getting very bad—
Dr Green Asst. Surgeon Gen of Penn[a45] was here yesterday and
made an inspection of the [hospital supplies and beds] it is he
thinks in a good condition the number Excused from duty being
Eleven—the number present for duty being 763 Making the sick
List quite Small in proportion to the number of men present—To
day there was general of the Reg. the men made quite a good appearance—the Men had taken great pains to fix up and be in as
good condition as possible I am glad to see them looking so well
as it is Said that on their appearance to day Much depends their
chance for getting Furloughs this winter And as I would like to

See all the Men who have been in the Service More than one year
have a chance to visit home I trust they will be Successful—Joes[46]
Furlough has been back for correction makeing him feel quite
uneasy indeed but he Says that it is all right it being all the way
through Even up at Corp's head quarters—

/Rain Storm [mountains?] [illegible words] taken away./
December 18th 1863.

This Morning Sun Shone out Brightly—though Last night it rained
hard all Night—And ~~the~~ carried away the Bridge by which we
crossed Mountain river—the roads to day are very heavy And it will
be a long time before it will be possible to haul Much of a Load—
there is Strong talk to day of us goeing back to fairfax station to do
guard duty on the Railroad it is Said that the Rebs made an attack
upon the Road with a force of about 700 Men and burned a train of
cars And doeing considerable damage—And it is said that we go
to guard that part of the Road. To day Cap[tain Asher] Gaylord[47]
Returned to the Reg. from Hospital he left it the day being wounded
[Gaylord left the hospital on this date having been incapacitated
since July 1] in the first day's fight at Gettysburg he was Shot through
both legs—

/Eherehart Zaner sick./

to day Cap[tain] Moore heard that his discharge was not goeing to
go through if he fails he says that he will resign unconditionally—To
day the Col[onel Dana] Came to Me and Said that Eherehart
Zaner[48] a black Duchman of Co A was very sick and Must be sent
to Division Hospital—on Examination I found that he had been
Laying on a trash pile for several days and Nights without any
Shelter from the storm And that in consequence though he is now
quite Sick—he is So dirty and Lousy that no one will take him into
their quarters and the poor fellow has in consequence of his Laziness
made himself sick—

Saturday Dec. 19th 1863—

To day we had a Board of Surgeons again to Examine Eight Men
for Discharge they [are] [First] Lieutenant H[iram] S [H., not S]
Travis Co D[49] [Private] John [R.] Smith [Sr.] Co B[50]—[Private]
Leonard Shaffer Co A[51] [Private George] Ge° Leutz[52] [Private]
Jesse Herrington[53] Co I—[Private Patrick] Patric Hart[54] [Private
Charles] Chas Williams Co D[55]—and [Private] Henry C Matter Co
H.[56] of the number Matter Leutz Herrington And Lieut Travis—
they concluded to discharge the others to be sent to the invalid
Corps—this Evening the Furloughs of our Regiment were returned
approved—and the Col. Quartermaster Lieut [Crepp?] [Thomas]
Davenport[57] with Several Privates and Non-Commissioned
officers—they will be at home just in time to Enjoy Christmas
they have ten day's Leave

/Furloughs approved—Sutlers prices/
Sunday, Dec 20th 1863.

this Morning the Col[onel] with Joe [Lewis] and the others took
their Leave of Camp for their trips home An Ambulance Came
And took them to the Depot they went to Brandy Station—I Made
an inspection of camp this morning and find it in a bad condition
I Reported the facts to Lieut[enant] Col. [John D.] Musser[58] Now
Commanding the Regiment he promises fairly to have the difficulty corrected And I trust that he Will have the thing properly
attended to and remove the odeum [odium] that has so long hung
to the Reg[t]. D. Yesterday a Board was Called to fix a price List for
the Sutler—

Sutlers Price List

the Sutler did not much like the idea of being curtailed in his
prices—Col Dana was much opposed to interfering with him—
those of the officers that are fond of Whiskey—of course are
favorably inclined to him as he Brings them in Liberal Supplies of

of [sic] that article but it is high time Such things were Stoped—the Men or Soldiers have to pay the Expense of the treats given to the officers—they as a general thing having to pay Sixty cents a pound for butter when the officers get it for fifty—this is a gross injustice as the difference should be the other way.—I hope he will have to Stand to the Mark More Closely in the future And do justice by all

Monday. Dec ~~Tuesday 22ond 1863.~~

This Monday, but Little of Interest Except that there is Some Effort to to [sic] get the Camp in a better condition that we have been accustomed to have our Regt.—I hope that it will work out—Last winter Col then Major Musser Said that if he was only in the Position that the Lieut Col then had he would Show a different State of affairs but Since he has got the position he has done Little or Nothing—but Now Says that if he was only Colonel he would Show a different [illegible word] in our favor—so with us we can accomplish something that we have No business better than Our allotted work—Always Looking to the future for something great and Neglecting our present Duties—to Day Dr Janett[59] was ordered By [Brigadier] Gen[eral John Reese] Kenly[60] to Come and Examine John A. Ward of Company A[61]. Who while on detached duty with Col[onel Chapman] Biddle[62] at Noakesville [Nokesville, Virginia] was arested by Col Biddle and had one half of his head Shaved and thrown up in a Blanket twenty times daily For gambling it was said at the time of his arrest that he had about Six thousand Dollars on his person he is a Substitute And says that he came to the Service with the intention of following his profession he being professional gambler—when he was Mustered And was asked his profession or business he said a gentleman—But after his trial and sentence thinking it too Much for his Dignity he immediately wrote to the Secretary of War Stateing the facts in his own way—the Secretary of War immediately ordered his case to be inquired into And if Col Biddle did anything that resulted in the injury of the Said Soldier he would be visited with Severe and condign punishment—for inhuman And improper treatment of a private Soldier—But all seem to think that he has been properly punished

Tuesday Dec 22ond 1863—

to Day I Made a Certificate of Discharge for Lieutenant H S
Travis—Also for Lieut W Lafrance for furlough And one for
Dr D L Scott[63] Sick Leave—the Dr. has been Suffering for a long
time with Dyspepsia which is at this time Much worse in addition
to that he has a Catarrhal affection together with a tendency to
Diarrhea. Travis claims to have been in the United States Service
for twenty years—being fifty-one years of age with bad sight And
general Debility deserves to go home and spend the rest of his days
in peace and quiet being nothing more than he deserves—

/Zaners Death./

Lafrance is Suffering with a Nervous pain in the Shoulder Caused
by by [sic] a gun Shot wound. Received at Gettysburg the first day
of July,—And says that he Cannot Slep at Night, doceing it Mostly in
the Morning—he has chancres on his Penis—And I guess it is them
that Make him feel So uneasy about getting away—And I trust that
he will succeed as I am quite tired of hearing his Complaints To day
we get intelligence of the death of Zaner— of Co A.—he has been
gone to the Hospital about four Day's—

December 24th 1863—

Last Night we had orders to be prepared to March at daylight this
Morning accordingly we Made Every preparation And this Morning
at 3 o clock we got up and began to pack our Medicines And Books
for the March—And after goeing through the usual paraphernalia
of getting our Sick into ambulances we at Nine o clock to took up
the Line of March in the direction of Brandy Station from there to
Culpepper Court House—it being said that there were barracks
built for our Corps there but upon getting to the place we Not only
found that there was No barracks but that the Cavalry we were goeing to relieve had not gone And that they did not intend to go untill
the next day—we therefore camped down on the ground Expecting
the next day to have better [accommodation][64]—

/March to Culpepper Court House/

it Seemed to be rather a cool way of Spending Christmas Eve—it
is certainly the coldest weather of the Season though clear and
frosty—we built a large fire in the front of our tent and Spent
Most of the Night pretty comfortably—or as Much So as could be
Expected under the circumstances—On the March there was but
little of interest the Country between our Camp And Brandy being
very flat and wet but Now being frozen Now we could March over it
without getting Swamped in the Mire—

When we got to Brandy [Station] we took the west side of the
rail Road to Culpepper passing through a portion of country
that before the war had been in a high State of Cultivation the
buildings good though Many of them had been destroyed and
others Much injured—the fences were Entirely gone—Some of
the houses were built in the Latest Style some of them after the
Cottage fashion— one of the prettiest Situations along the way
had been Entirely destroyed the buildings burned the Cedars
that hedged the Lane or avenue to the house Mostly being cut
down And burned for wood by the troops that were Camped in
the vicinity—in fact Every thing bears the Mark the Mark [sic] of
Devastation And ruin—

/Culpepper Court House/

Culpepper is Not a Large town And is Called a Village the court
house is a middling building though not to compare with such
buildings in the North there are two Middling good Churches—
one very good one for a small town—the houses generally good
though Many of them old fashioned And Many of them Small—
there are a few that are built in the Modern Style it Looks as though
the people Lived in Comfort before the war broke out—though
Now Many of them hardly know one day what they will get to Eat
the Next—they of Course as usual Curse the Yankees for all their
trouble And think that their want and the destruction of their

property is all to be blamed upon—them—it is Strange to see with what pertinacity they hang on to their old Notions about the war—the Streets are Narrow and dirty about Equal our Mud Lanes in the Country, but that is the general Characteristic of the towns of Virginia

/Christmas Day 1863/
Friday De^c 25th 1863 Christmas

Well this is Not a Very Merry Christmas. Laying round in the cold upon the ground—and not having Anything to Eat but hard tack and raw pork—at Noon I thought that I would go into town And See if it would afford Anything better—After inquiring all round I was directed to the hotel down by the Depot And was then told that I could get Dinner at two o clock—I accordingly waited with great patience for the time when the Bell would Sound a charge on Turkey's geese Mince pies and all other good things—the Bell finally rang but on getting to the table nary a turkey was to be seen. we had boiled Cabbage and Potatoes And Roast Beef—after which we had Mince pie—

/Reb Grave yard Culpepper Court House/

the only one of the Many good things that I Expected to get after dinner I paid My half Dollar And took My departure for Camp— during the day I took a walk to the Cemetery back of town And found that it had been used to bury Reb Soldiers there was about five hundred burried in the Lot the graves were fixed up quite Nicely with head boards Made of pine plank two inches thick painted white And Nicely Lettered the records Showing that Most of them had been Georgians—they had Mostly died from desease though Some of them had been wounded in Skirmishes And battles in Virginia— Even in the first Bull run fight—these are but a very few of those that repose in the soil of Va—

/Ball at Culpepper By [Carols?]/

To Night the officers of the Cavalry are to have a Ball the Secesh
Ladies of Culpepper are to participate And I Suppose they will go
and dance And flirt with our officers and after they will Make fun of
the green and awkward Yankees as is their Custom—but I Suppose
all our fellows want is a little fun in the way of a dance not Careing
what the Ladies Say about it afterward—

The Cavalry has Not Moved yet And we still have to rough it how
Much Longer this will Last I do Not Know but the way the weather
is we hope it will not be Long—

NOTES

1. Surgeon, 143rd PA.
2. Surgeon, 150th PA.
3. Wounded commander of the 150th PA and temporary brigade commander during the Gettysburg battle.
4. Probably Surgeon John Howard Taylor, commissioned into US Volunteers Medical Staff on October 2, 1861.
5. Probably Surgeon Henry Janes, US Volunteers, surgeon in charge of approximately 60 hospitals in the town of Gettysburg.
6. Surgeon, 80th New York Infantry, placed in charge of Seminary Hospital at this time.
7. New tissue formation in the healing wound.
8. William T. Fulton, James's brother.
9. Possibly Cpl. James Johnson of Co. A.
10. At this time General-in-Chief of the Union Army.
11. See discussion of Halleck in chapter 7.
12. See chapter 7.
13. About eight miles southwest by south of Culpeper.
14. Germanna Ford, about eight miles southeast of Stevensburg.
15. On the Rappahannock River about six miles north from Stevensburg.
16. A small hamlet on the south side of the Rappahannock adjacent to Kelly's Mill and opposite Kelly's Ford on the north side. The village does not exist today. See *Map of the Battle of Kelly's Ford* by Robert Knox Sneden, 1863–65, *Encyclopedia Virginia*, online at http://www .encyclopediavirginia.org/media_player?mets_filename=evm00002375mets.xml, accessed October 22, 2018.
17. On the east side of the Potomac where Goose Creek joins the Potomac River.
18. Located on the border between Fauquier County and Prince William County in the Bull Run Mountains, part of the Blue Ridge Mountains.
19. Unidentified.
20. Unidentified.
21. Commanding Company A, 143rd PA.

22. Commanding Company K, 143rd PA.

23. Probably Lt. Col. Elijah V. White, leader of another partisan unit nicknamed "White's Comanches," formally the 35th Battalion, Virginia Cavalry.

24. Also spelled M'Roy in Pennsylvania records, 143rd PA.

25. A tenet of chemistry at the time, caloric referred to heat as a substance, possibly fluid or gas, that passes from a hot source to a cold one.

26. Neither the histories of the 149th nor 150th Pennsylvania Volunteers record a fight at this time. Fulton may have an incorrect date for this action.

27. Fulton here recounts the dedication of the Gettysburg cemetery by President Lincoln and the occasion of his famous address. See chapter 7.

28. Possibly Capt. Edwin Sylvanus Osborne, Co. F, 149th PA.

29. Assistant surgeon, 143rd PA.

30. James's brother, William T. Fulton.

31. An old term for swelling due to an accumulation of water in the tissues.

32. Surgeon J. Theodore Heard.

33. George N. Reichard of Company C, 143rd PA.

34. About two miles north of Warrenton Junction.

35. Kettle Run extends east to west between Bristoe Station to the north and Warrenton to the south.

36. Cavalry Corps, Army of the Potomac.

37. Commanding V Corps.

38. Unidentified.

39. 143rd PA.

40. Unidentified.

41. 43rd Battalion, Virginia Cavalry.

42. Resigned January 24, 1864.

43. 2nd Lt. William LaFrance, promoted later and discharged on November 16, 1864, Company E.

44. Company K, 143rd PA, discharged on December 24, 1864, on a Surgeon's Certificate.

45. Possibly James Montgomery Greene, MD, one of Fulton's examiners at the University of Pennsylvania in August 1862.

46. Fulton's hospital steward, Josiah L Lewis.

47. Co. D, 143rd PA, killed at Hatcher's Run, Virginia, February 7, 1865.

48. Pvt. Earhart Zanner, Company A, 143rd PA, died on December 8, 1863, and was buried in a temporary cemetery at Paoli Mills on December 23, and later moved to the National Cemetery in Culpeper.

49. 143rd PA, resigned December 29, 1863.

50. 143rd PA, transferred to the Veterans Reserve Corps on January 29, 1864.

51. 143rd PA, discharged for disability on March 22, 1864.

52. Lutz, 143rd PA, discharged for disability on February 29, 1864.

53. Harington, 143rd PA, discharged for disability on February 29, 1864.

54. Heart, 143rd PA, transferred to Veterans Reserve Corps on January 25, 1864.

55. 143rd PA, transferred to Veterans Reserve Corps on January 25, 1864.

56. 143rd PA, discharged for disability on April 20, 1864.

57. Company I, 143rd PA, discharged for disability on October 21, 1864.

58. Promoted from major on June 2, 1863; originally first lieutenant with Company K; killed at the Battle of the Wilderness on May 6, 1864.

59. Unidentified.

60. Commanding the Maryland Brigade.

61. Private, died of wounds received at the Battle of the Wilderness, May 12, 1864.

62. Commanding the 121st Pennsylvania; discharged on December 10, 1863, because of a wound received at Gettysburg.

63. Discharged April 8, 1864.

64. At least three times, the brigade tried to settle down in prolonged winter quarters.

FIVE

"To Bring Man in Communion with His God"

Diary, December 26, 1863, to January 29, 1864

THIS CHAPTER CONCLUDES THE DIARY, BUT IMMEDIATELY FOLLOWING THE *transcription are two other segments that conclude Fulton's use of the pocket diary. The second segment consists of another narrative, written upside down and proceeding page by page from the back of the diary toward the front. Given the detail and the precision of his dates, Fulton must have written the second narrative as a first attempt to edit his diary entries into a finished piece. Although Fulton heads the second (incomplete) narrative as a summary of 1863, the events he recounts all fall within 1862 and the organization of the brigade, which included the 143rd, 149th, and 150th Pennsylvania Volunteer Regiments. The final segment includes several pages of medicinal recipes.*

/Mrs. Graves Farm Camp/
Saturday Dec 26th 1863.

To day the Cavalry Not having Moved we Still Stay in the Same position though there are rumors that we would Move at 4 oClock—to day I—again visited Culpepper though I Saw but Little More of Interest than before the day fine though cold and frosty. Last Night we had a heavy white frost—we got orders toward Night that we would Move in the Morning—to Night it begins to look cloudy and hazy and as though tomorrow Might be a wet day—[Lieutenant] Col[onel] Hydekooper[1] was along And Looked out a camp for the 150th Reg we will Move further on—they have the choice of ground.

Sunday Dec. 27th 1863—

This Morning we broke camp and Moved to the Southwest of CC.
H.[2] And Camped on the farm of Mrs. Graves—She is a widow
Lady, quite young her brother is Surgeon of [Major] Gen[eral James
L.] Kempers Brigade—and they all think that Kemper is about
right—Mrs Graves has Eight hundred acres of Land and has quite a
number of negroes about her. She with all the rest round are Strong
Secesh—though I think they do not talk quite so Savagely, as the
family did—they seem to talk as though they had No doubt but what
the Southern Confederacy would succeed—and they will ultimately
gain their independence—they said that there was No use of any
More fighting and I Said that the South Might Certainly See by this
time that their Cause is hopeless they say that the North Might see
that the South Cannot be Subjugated And So it goes Each thinking
that the other is wrong—but they are Certainly beginning to See the
folly of their course as well as its hopelessness—

/Mrs. Graves Farm Camp/

This has certainly been a fine agricultural country through here
before the war it is rolling with plenty of water Elegant Spring[s] and
little Streams Starting and Coursing Among The hills—though now
it is hard to tell Much about the Country at this time as the fences
are destroyed, with Many of the buildings destroyed.

To day is Exceedingly unpleasant the Morning Set in with a heavy
mist And throughout the day this Continued with occasoonally,
heavy Showers of rain—there being but few Axes in the Reg[t]—there
was a detail Made and they with all the axes were sent into the
woods to chop timber for the whole Regt. that they Might all have
some timber toward building up their quarters—there being but
little timber on the ground upon which we Camped the Cavalry
had been Camped round upon this ground and had used up Most
of the timber though what there is, is good being Mostly black oak
Splits well and the Men Seem Anxious to get at it but [Lieutenant]
Col[onel John D.] Musser[3] Seems Anxious to Keep it as a Kind
of a reserve

/Mrs Graves Farm Camp/
Wet And Cold—

it looks hard indeed to See the poor fellows Sitting and Laying round
in the cold and rain without Shelter waiting for An opportunity
to get themselves up houses to protect them from the Storm—
[Assistant Surgeon] Dr. [David L.] Scott[4] thought they had the time
for the line officers Established And accordingly to work to have his
tent put up, but after a time the Col. got to work and put the Line of
our tents far in the rear of where our tent was Located[5] So that we
were left alone to flounder in the Mud—which got to be about an
inch deep in the bottom of our tent it indeed was the Most gloomy
time that I have seen Change—

Cold And wet.—

Since I have been in the Service—with no fire Except Such as a little
green black oak wood would Make in the front and outside of our
tent the columns of Smoke from which was continually blinding
a person So that it was a punishment almost to come Near the
fire—but we Laid our bed down in the Mud And Laid ourselves
down upon the bed and Made out to get a pretty good Nights
rest, Contrary to Expectations—it rained hard all Night—and
our Camp is getting to be a perfect Swamp—though the ground
does Lay upon the high ground—the 149th Reg. Joins us And Lay
between us and CCH.[6] they have a Nice Situation and are getting
up good houses

/Wet Wet Wet Wet/
Monday Dec– 28th 1863—

To day was Spent Amid the rain And Storm by the Men in trying
to get their houses up they were getting along Slowly—owing
to the want of tools And the Storm—it rains Continually and is
Certainly very cold—to day [Hospital Steward] Geo. Sheldon—
Commenced—to build—us a fire place out of Such Small stones
as he Could gather up round but they being of Such a poor

quality he Could Not cover Much Speed And once it fell down owing to the fact he Said that the Stones were So wet and that the Mud would Not hold them together I ~~wath~~ watched the work with Much interest hopeing that it would succeed for by that Means we would be relieved from the Exposure to which we had ~~so~~ been So Severely Subjected for Some days past—but Night found us with but little done to it—however this Evening the Col found that there was a lot of Bricks in town And he immediately went to see about them and got permission of the Provost Marshal to take them to Camp all the teams were immediately Set to work to haul them to camp—there was quite a large lot of them they were bricks from Cornice being grooved on one side but there they were very good for us he Makes the Quarter Masters Department Step Round quite Lively it is time to wake them up a little.

/Building Chimney/
Tuesday Dec. 29th 1863—

This Morning there was Evident Signs that we would have clear weather before Long again And About Nine o Clock the Sun Shone out beautifully the contrast being Very great between to day And yesterday the rain brought All the frost out of the ground—And to day it is quite Muddy though the ground is beginning to dry, And should the weather Keep So for a few days we will have it quite pleasant under foot—As for the Sky And Air that is as pleasant as Summer, in fact we have just Such weather as I have Seen only in Virginia in December And such I think as they do Not have Any place Else in this Month

/1st and 2ond Brigades Consolidated/

to day we got some brick furnished our fire place and built our Chimney up So that it would Not Smoke then put up our tent And felt at home and Comfortable once More—And it will Not be Many days untill we have forgotten all about the hardships of the past few days in the Comforts of the present—Brigade HdQrs being Still in town I went there to see what had become of Dr. Scotts application for furlough which he Sent in before we Started on the Move. [1st Lieutenant and Adjutant John Emory] Parsons told Me that it had been sent up Several days before—they told Me that the 1st and 2ond Brigade had been Consolidated.[7]

/Camp Near Culpepper C. H./
Wednesday, Dec. 30th 1863

This was a beautiful day, Equal to May or June Except that it was Not So warm—though warm Enough to be pleasant—~~Last~~ to Night about dark I was Called to See a little daughter of Mrs. Green. She has an abscess on her Ear And is Suffering Considerably with [it]—I ordered her Morphia—and a flax Seed poultice to the Ear—And promised to see her Again in the Morning—

Last Day of 1863—
Thursday Dec 31st 1863.

This was a day of Rain And Storm—It is I think one of the Severest Storms that we have Experienced this Season—the Men Are Suffering Much on account of the Storm—Many of them not having their quarters up yet—the work seems to go on slow—timber being scarce And the Men Still having but few Axes to work with—they I hope will have a better Chance Soon to go on with their work We have our fire place And Chimney So that it works well we have a little Smoke at times that we can get along quite [well] if it does Not trouble us More in the future than at the present—

/New Years Day in Camp 1864/
January 1st 1864.

This Morning the Sun rose bright and clear and we were greeted with a beautiful Sight—In the distance Could be Seen the Blue Ridge [Mountains] their tops Capped with Snow Every little Elevation could be traced with And [an] outline clearly market [marked] Reflecting the Suns Rays in all their beauty—the distance is Said to be about thirty Miles—this is the first time that I have Ever seen Mountains Covered with Snow, the impression

Made upon My Mind was one as is rarely felt And only at such times as the Mind is Strongly And Solemnly impressed with the beautiful in Nature And Such a Sight as is well Calculated to bring Man in communion with his God—well calculated to impress Man with Solemnity And Awe in Consideration of the great Superiority of the being that has brought into form And Made to Loom up before Made Work of such Magnitude And beauty—we Can see the Range of Mountains Laying Along the horizon to the west of us—To day the Air is Sensibly impressed by passing over the snow—the air Commenced to get Cold Early in the Morning and Continued to increase through out the day And by the time Night Set in the Cold had attained a degree of Severity far Exceeding that of any previous day this Season—

/New Years Day in Camp/

To day I have been busily [busy] in Makeing out My Reports to day we have had to Make a Morning a weekly a Monthly And a yearly Report Making a good amount of work for one day—though by patience And perseverance And diligence we have Succeeded in accomplishing the work—those of them have been sent in and the third the yearly is in Readiness to send to the Surgeon General—To day Some of the Captains Treated their Men Cap[tain]. [Oliver K.] Moore[8] And Cap. [Isaac S.] Little[9] Bought Each a Barrell of apples for their Men Lieut Pla[o?]tz[10] Bought Seven Canteens of Whiskey the[y] also got one Ration of Whiskey So that Some of them got a pretty good Share of their Corn Juice—there was No Sports in Camp as the Men are generally Closely Engaged in getting up their quarters up they have no time for Sport untill they can have a place where they Can Keep warm and be protected from the Storm—To day Joe[11] Returned from his visit to see his friends and had quite an interesting tale to tell of his adventures among the the [sic] people of Wilkesbarre of his goeing And Returning—there was fifteen home on Furlough—the talk in Camp is that No More Furloughs will be granted on account of So Many Reinlisting in the Veteran Corps—they all get thirty days and the talk is that the army will be too Much weakened by letting fifteen go out of those Regiments that do Not Reinlist—

/New Years day 1864/
1864 1864 [sic]

how Much truth there May be in the Report I do Not Know, but one thing is certain we would all Like to have a chance of getting to see our homes And friends—though all feel that whatever is right they would Like to do—And I do hope that it will be right for all to get Furloughs And go home as they have Most of them been good And faithful Soldiers—And Many of them have Now been from home about fourteen Months and are Certainly Entitled to the privilege of Visiting their families—

Saturday Dec 12 2ond 1864.

To day Dr. Scott had his application for Leave of absence Returned—it went through Correct untill it came to the office of the Medical Director of the Army of the Potomac—where it was disapproved by the Acting Medical Director Dr. [Jonathan] Letterman being absent—it Returned this Evening—This evening Lieut Griffin[13] Came to Me [and] presented Me with a Small Document Stating that he wanted a Surgeon's Certificate of Disability—I told him that I could not give him one but sent him to Dr. Ramsey[14], the Present Brigade Surgeon to see whether a board Could be Called and have him Examined—and then I would give him a Certificate According to instructions

/Lieut Griffin—Resignation 1864./

—but on goeing to the Dr he was told that he Must have a Certificate to Start with And told him to come back to Me And get one—but on coming back I told him that I could Not give him one as I did Not Know that he had been Sick—he then Said that he would send a Statement to Hd Quarters that the Medical Department refused to give him the Required papers—the threat did Not have the [desired] Effect And he cooled down, but I do Not

Know what he Concluded to do—The day has been a very Cold one indeed I think quite as Cold as Any weather we had at Washington Last Winter there Seems to be a Mania in the Rgt. for Resigning Cap[tain Oliver K.] Moore[15] is waiting for his papers to come in Cap[tain Asher] Gaylord[16] Sent his in to day—Lieutenant [Hiram H.]Travis[17] of the same Company got his two or three days ago—it Looks as though all the officers would Resign could they only get away—but fortunately they Cannot Resign Except on Surgeon[s] Certificate And of Course there Are Many of them that will Not be able to procure this—

/Getting up hospital and putting in Flue/
Sunday, January, 3[d] 1864.

This has been a beautiful day—this Morning Dr Ramsey, was here And told Me that we would get a hospital tent And that it would be Sent to us in the Course of the day And that we Must Send And get Some Railroad Iron to Make a flue—to warm it—this Evening our tent came and I immediately had a detail and the tent was put up I think in good Style—I was anxious to get it up the weather Looking as though we were goeing to have Storm—the tops of the Blue Ridge are Still covered with Snow and I think we will have More before Long.

Monday Jan 4th 1864—

To day, we got—a team And Sent out and found three Bars of Railroad Iron—and we immediately went to work to Make a flue through the tent—And then dug a hole at the Mouth in which to Make the fire—after getting the furnace And flue we then Laid down the Iron. the Next thing was to get a chimney this [Private] george Moore[18] Made for us we Made it about four feet high—after which we Made a fire And beyond My Expectation the thing draws well and promises to Answer the purpose admirably—As it is a Matter of great importance to warm a hospital we have accomplished one great object—

/A Case off Smallpox./
Tuesday Jan 5th 1864.

To day, we have been busily Engaged in fixing up our Hospital
we have a detail to go to the woods for forks and poles—to Make
Bunks And Sinks[19]—they Succeeded in Bringing plenty to finish
the job—the ground being So hard it is difficult to get Much done
though we got the tent ditched [pitched] on one side And So Soon
as the frost Comes out we hope to finish the Job—to Day, Day, [sic]
D. L. Scott was called to see H. M. Porter[20] sick in quarters—After
an Examination he pronounced the the [sic] case one of Rheumatism
and prescribed for him accordingly—

Wednesday, Jan 6th 1864—

Still busy at our Hospital tent and Cook House—when the teamster brought our tent he gave us a hospital Fly [a cover or awning],
Extra And we thought that we might as well have a good Cook
house dispensary And place to have sick Call—so we went to work
immediately to put up a house—but Dr Mitchell [unidentified]
Came Along to day And Saw that we had an Extra [tent] Fly And
told Me that there were Several of the tents that had No Flys And
that the one we had was Needed and that it would be Sent for—but
we went on and finished the house thinking that when they did
Send they Might have the one on the Hospital thinking that we
could get along without a fly on it as well as we could without a
dispensary.

/Small Pox H L Porter Co H/

to day, I Saw [Private Henry M.] porter Examined him Carefully,
found his tongue heavily furred with a thick white Fur And deeply
Marked with the impression of his teeth Nausea So great that he
could Retain Nothing in his Stomac great pain in his back—it
Seemed Like a Strange Kind of Rheumatism to Me—he also had
high fever—I gave him Something to control the febrile action his
face was Much Swelled but with No Sign of irruption.[21]

Thursday Jan 7th 1863[22]

Last Night Dr. Scott had his Leave of Absence sent in he has permission to Visit his home for the Space of ten days though he thinks it is but a Short time to be at home when a Man has been from his family fourteen Months—he Started this Morning in the 8th train from Culpeper—And will get to Washington this afternoon About two o. clock—he will Stay there untill tomorrow—And will then go on home by way of Harrisburg—to day, I again Visited [Private Henry M.] Porter And found him very bad indeed with Evident Symptoms of Small Pox. I ordered him Some Liquor And in the Course of the day the irruptions Made its appearance—

/H L Porter Small Pox—/

we had him Sent as Soon as possible to the Small Pox Hospital of the 2ond Division this Evening Dr Ramsey Sent Me a Small portion of Vaccine Matter[23] with which I will first Vaccinate Company H. then as Many of the others as I can—To day, I had a bunk fixed up in My tent And Am Now fixed up in Such a Manner that I Can Live Comfortably—if they will only let us stay—there is Some talk of us Moveing the Cavalry are goeing to the front again—the [Union Army] Sixth Corps have gone into the Valey of Virginia And Are Now Located there it is Said that [Confederate Major General Jubal] Early is trying to get Round in that Region—it is hoped the [VI Corps Commander Major John] Sedgwick[24] will foil him in any attempts that he May Make as he is certainly one of our ablest and Most Energetic officers—

Captain [Chester K.] Hughes[25] and [First] Lieut[enant Thomas] Davenport[26] Succeeded in getting their wives down from Washington yesterday and they have them Now at Culpepper at $7.00 per week though that is Not as high as they had to pay at the Metropolitan Hotel the three were there charged twelve dollars per day—this would seem to be pretty Steep Board for Ladies—Captain Hughes has been suffering with the piles since his wife has come down and will Likely Not be able for duty as Long as she stays

/Case of Small Pox Fatal/
~~Thursday~~ Friday 8th 1864.

This Morning we had intelligence from Hospital that H M Porter
died during the Night—this has been a case of short duration he
has been sick only three days the patient dying the day that the
rash Made its appearance—this Morning I vaccinated the [*sic*]
Most of Company H hopeing if possible to prevent the Spread of
the disease—part of the Company are out on picket And will be in
tomorrow when I Shall try to finish the work—to day, we got a detail
of 3 Men for Nurses for our Hospital— we will get about 3 More And
that I think will be Enough—

This Evening I got a letter from Coff. James[27] Stateing that he had
been paying a visit to Maryland and Delaware and that he had Spent
Some time in talking with Gen [illegible word] and thinks that he is
a good union Man. he also Saw [Major] Gen[eral Irvin] McDowell
And Gen[eral Erasmus Darwin] Keys [Keyes] Key's thinks they
are both Copperheads And that it is No wonder they failed in their
Campaigns [He] thinks that the Service is well rid of them he Says
that the people in that Section of Maryland are Much Exercised
about their negroes. the Colored individuals seem to have quite a
Notion of goeing into the Army And Making Bold Sojer Boyes—it
will weaken the Rebels And strengthen us—Each one that joins our
army—

/[letre?] Letter from C. James—I W Pratt & C/

he also Says that in a conversation with I W Pratt [unidentified] of
Kimbleville[28] that Gentleman told him Among other things that
he was strongly in favor of the prosecution of the War untill the
president Issued his Emancipation Proclamation And that since
he offered some opposition—this is only one of his Copperhead
Subterfuges he Sayed that the proclamation [had] Not influenced
him but that the officers of the Army all tendered their Resignation
on Rece[i]pt of the document and that I Send in Mine it was Not accepted And that I was Kept in the Army Contrary to My wish this I

say here is false I did tender My Resignation but it was because of My wifes Bad health at the time.

After a time She recovered her health Since which time I have felt perfectly Satisfied that I Am here And in fact near Liked Any duty in which I have been Engaged as well—Even better than Practice at home—the only objection being Compelled to be absent from home so long—I[n] conclusion I think that the town of Kimbleville as far Exceeds Any place that I have Seen in Virginia in its fondness for secession as Penn^a—does that State in prosperity And Enterprise and general industry And if they only had their just dues they would be Sent through the lines among their friends—

~~Friday~~ Saturday January 9th 1864

Col. E L Dana is at Brigade Headquarters commanding the Brigade Col. [Langhorne] Wister is at home on Leave of absence—Major [C.M.] Conyngham[29] is in Command of the Regiment—We are busily Engaged in Policeing the Camp—there is Nothing of Particular interest transpiring in the Country Except that old [Confederate Major General Jubal] Early is Making a Raid in Western Virginia. they have Succeeded in Capturing a train of two hundred wagons—with about one hundred Men. It is one of the Most Successful raids they have Made for Some time—though it was not Anything to Brag about—

Sunday Jan 10th 1864.

this Morning Major and Myself Made a tour of the Camp And Examined the Streets And the quarters of the Men from one End of the Camp to the other—And but two Streets presented Any appearance of Neatness. Co. C^s Street And Co G^s. the others were Certainly very Careless And dirty—the Major Said that if I would issue an order to the Commanders of Companies Makeing them Responsible he would Sign it And see that it was Carried out. I wrote out the order Stateing that the Men on getting up in the Morning Must Either put their Blankets out to Air or fold them up Nicely And

Lay them away, then Sweep or Clean the houses wash their hands and faces—

And after Breakfast their utensils used in Cooking And Eating Must be Cleanly washed and put Carefully away—their Sheets Nicely [folded?] [illegible word]—for all of which the commanders of Company's would be Responsible—the Major Seems to be determined that our Camp Shall come up to the Standard of the Regular Army and for My part I will try And do all that is possible in My line toward bringing up the Standard of our Regiment—We have at this time about thirteen Excused from duty Makeing a Very Respectable Sick List indeed for our Regiment—

Monday Jan 11th 1864.

Yesterday Evening Dr. Ramsey, was here to Examine two cases that have the premonitory Symptoms of Small Pox, but as yet there is No irruptions And other Symptoms to Mark Clearly that the disease is Small pox, And he wished Me to Examine the Cases Carefully, this Morning And Report to him at as Early an hour as possible the progress of the Cases after sick call this Morning I visited the Inn of the two Men Sick—one of the Men had an irruption on his arms but on No other part of his body—the febrile Symptoms had abated considerably—the pulse Natural and other general symptoms favorable

/Introduced to the Ladies of Col Hugh[es] + Lieut Davenport/

To day, I Examined the quarters of Company C And I found them in good condition—the Major issued an order that Each hut should have its pole for Each hut [sic]—so that the Men can hang out their Blankets this Evening I had an introduction to the wives of Capt Hughes and Lieutenant [Davenport]—To day, Col Dana visited the Camp's And Hospitals of the Brigade and gave us the credit of having one of the best in the Brigade—Yesterday we took out the Flue—the Bars of Iron for the want of Support at the End had bent down when they became heated—and contracted the flue—it now works well—

/Capt Morris applies for certificate/

this afternoon Capt. Morris Made Me a Visit—being desirous that
I Should give him a Surgeons Certificate on which to ground An
Application for discharge—I agreed to do So As he has been un-
able for duty the whole of the past years Campaign—I think that it
will Not only be a Kindness to him but doeing a good turn for the
Service—Lieutenant [Michael] Keenan[30] will then hold the position
of Captain—And I think will Make a good and Efficient Officer—
Cap Gaylord was also in Applying for a Certificate—on which to
Make An application. he wishes to Make his wound the Basis of his
application—he is quite lame at times—

Tuesday, Jan 12th 1864.

this Morning I Examined Wm Porter And found that the Rash was
More fully developed upon his body Legs and arms so much as to
Satisfy Me that the case was one of Varioloid[31] without any doubt—
And accordingly I have dispatched a note to Dr. Ramsey[32] wishing
him to Come And Examine that case that all May be Satisfied And
that No Mistake Can possibly arise—I feel quite anxious that he
Should do so as he intimated that the case of his Brother was probably one of cerebral Meningitis. for My part I am perfectly Satisfied
the case was one of clearly Marked Small pox though I have No doubt
that the Meningitis of the Brain Might have—been More or Less
implicated as he had involuntary evacuattions the day before he died

January 1864

I think that Wm Porter will have Nothing More than Varioloid as the
Vaccine is beginning to work And I think will Modify the other disease Considerably—Make it a Mild Case of Varioloid— though on
the Limbs And body in Some places they Look as though they were
goeing to be confluent[33]—he is fully Satisfied in his own Mind that
he has the Small pox and is quite Anxious that he Should be sent to
the Hospital that No one Else May get the disease from him—Last
Night there was an order issued for Company Drill—

Wednesday, Jan 13th.

To day, but Little of Interest transpired Except that we Sent Another Man Wm Porter of Co H to Varioloid Hospital. Dr. Ramsey Came And Examined him And was fully Satisfied in his own Mind that he had the disease—Nothing of importance is Now transpiring in the way of Military Every thing Seems to indicate that both Armies have quietly Settled down for the Rest of the winter it is to be hoped that they May Not change their Notion until Spring Comes Again—

Thursday, Jan 14th 1864.

To day, Dr. Ramsey was here And Approved Another order to send away [Private] R[obert] Miller Co H[34] to Varioloid Hospital this Makes the fourth Man that we have sent—And I do honestly hope that we May Not have to Send Any More—I think we have already had to send Enough—Major Conyngham is Still in Command of the Regiment though Mussers time is about out—to day, I looked through the Camp of the 149th Pa it is quite Neat And good—

Jan 15th until Jan. 20th

But little of interest transpired Except that we were busily Engaged in beautifying our hospital grounds and takeing precaution against the Sp[r]ead of Small pox—to day, Dr. Scott—returned—and I immediately Made application for furlough asking for ten day[s]—there has been several [possibly senior medical officers] Visiting the Regt. And all were quite well Satisfied with the general appearance of things all thinking that we have a fine situation and Nicely improved—We have fine springs and the water is generally good coming out of the hills—wood is not very plenty—

Jan 20th untill Jan 29th 1864

during this time I was anxiously awaiting the return of My papers though Most were returned in three days Mine did Not Come for More than a week—Dr. Jarrett[35] thought I think that I could Not be

Spared from the Regt. And for that reason did Not approve it untill hurried up by Some Suggestion from head quarters—During the time the weather has been Exceedingly fine looking More like Spring than winter—the roads are drying up finely—and are Now quite good— the Snow has gone from the Blue Ridge and they Lay Stretched out to the west of us like a great Bank of Cloud—And Certainly present a prospect truely Magnificent to the Lover of the Beauties of Nature—

the condition of our Regt. at this time is truly gratifying there being but two Men that are really sick—there are it is true four Men that had their feet frost bitten but they are getting along finely And will soon be well—[Brigadier] Gen. [John Reese] Kenly[36] was Along on inspection And Said that he had Learned An idea in Regard to the Airing of Blankets—he we have two forks and a pole for Each tent upon which the Men hang their Blankets Every Clear day—and thus drive out all the moisture they Collect during the Night Makeing it at once More healthy and more pleasant for them.

—⁂—

Fulton's diary effectively ends here. The next 44 pages are blank. When Fulton began to adapt his blank pocketbook 1862 daily diary as a journal of his military experience, he began his account at the beginning of the book. Although his last entry dates to the end of January 1864, he remained in the service until April 8, 1864. During February and March, he doubtless had many administrative tasks to conduct to place his regiment and brigade in as healthy a condition as possible. He may have discontinued writing because he felt that his experience had naturally concluded because of his regiment's inactivity in winter quarters.

During his early days in the service, dating to his initial assignment to the 150th Pennsylvania, Fulton may have recorded the medicinal recipes that appear in the final pages of the pocket diary. On the page immediately before the recipes begin (as read from the front of the diary forward), Fulton began a new narrative, written back to front. It is unclear when he wrote the new narrative, but internal evidence points to Fulton's having written it soon after the events narrated. Fulton abruptly leaves off with this narrative, too, and one can only speculate about why he abandoned it.

Both the second narrative and medical recipes that follow have been reordered to preserve readability (reversing the original back-to-front sequence).

Gettysburg July 1st 1863.

On the first day of the fight at Gettysburg [Confederate] Gen A P Hill in giving an Explanation of the ground And the different positions Occupied by the Contending forces to a British Correspondent that was with the Reb Army And As Afterward published by him in the Blackwood Magazine—he took the English officer to the railroad cut where the fight had been bloody And persistent And pointed out where one Regt had made a Stand in the field and where a Color bearer Staid back after his Regt had fallen back. And two or three times flaunted the Stars and Stripes in the face of the advancing foe Gen Hill Said that he was Sorry when he saw the Brave Yankee fall as he did shot through the Body By a Musket Ball—

/Ben Crippen the Brave Color Sergeant And Gen. AP Hill/

the Regt was the 143 Pa And the Brave Color Bearer was Benj Crippen of Co E 143 Pa. Among the Many instances of Bravery that day Manifested no one Stands out in Bolder Relief than that of Ben Crippen—but alas he died in his Glory. his life was Not prolonged to Enjoy his Laurels as with Many Another Brave boy—that went into the action that Morning full of Life And promise—the sun set upon him him a Shattered Lifeless Corp's—

Dr.s Cannot Stand fire

On the third day of July, while the Battle of Gettysburg was rageing Dr. D L Scott was attending to the wounded in the rear of our Line of Battle one Man whose wound he had dressed And had Left but a few Moments when a Shell Struck the man Exploding blew him to fragments—the Dr. Makeing but a Narrow—Escape—the Same day, a Surgeon of one of the Regts who had been Engaged with the wounded in the rear had in the interval of the Shelling Seized the opportunity to Visit his Regt. while there the Shelling Commenced More furious than at any previous time—the Surgeon mounted his horse putting Spurs to his horse set off at full Speed his Sash and Coat tails Streaming in the wind. before he had gone far his hat flew of—but Stopping Not or halting on he flead regardless of cap untill he got to a safe distance—

The 149th Regt. of our Brigade is Situated beside us in Camp at Paoli Mills—Col [Walton] Dwight[37] Made the teams of the Regt turn out And haul Stone and Lumber for the Men to Make their quarters before there was any hauling done for headquarters this Making the Men Comfortable before the officers did anything toward fixing up their quarters—I have Called the attention of our officers to the facts in the case of the 149th but they pay No attention but Still go on in the old way, finding for Each Suggestion a Corresponding Excuse for the filthy and bad condition of the Camp—no [illegible word] will arouse them to Action—

Dr. [Surgeon Philip A.] Quinan[38] through his intrigue displaced Me from the third Div Hospital got the position Himself—then played off got a leave of absence went to Phila there got a position in hospital there he Stayed Week after week and Month after Month Notwithstanding repeated orders for him to Return to his Regiment—untill finally the Department would Endure it No Longer—when he was preemptively dis and dishonorably discharged [from] the Service that by his duplicity And dishonorable Conduct disgracing himself for Life—when at Gettysburg his superiority of rank gave him an advantage over Me his Lying was believed—

I was Rewarded—he was placed in the position I went to another post and performed My Duty faithfully—he kept on with his

intrigue untill he has finally reac[h]ed the End of his Rope—has at
Last Ended his Career in disgrace never More to hold an office of
honor under the government while I though Submitting to the disgrace though feeling it hard at the time did My duty faithfully—and
feel thankful that to day I have an honorable Standing Among those
of My profession And trust that I May be able so to act that Such
May be the case in the future

A number of Quinans, Friends would be pleased to See him as he
owes fifty Dollars to Lieut Da[l?]glish his Mess Bill he forgot to pay
when he went away,—as well as Several other little Bills—The Best
policy in Life is at all times to do honestly And Conscientiously the
duty assigned to one And Should though [one] not hold as high positions as others they will at Least have clear Consciences—and feel at
the Last that they have acted well their part—

Ja³ Fulton

Sumary for the Year 1863.

On the seventeenth of July of this year I was Examined at the
University of Penn^a for position in the Volunteer Service of the
United States As An Assistant Surgeon And by Professor Leidy on
Anatomy Smith on Surgery Dr. Green on Practice and Dr. Stewart
on Materia Medica—And was admited the Surgeon General
H H Smith told us to Report to him on the morning of the following
we then after giving orders for our Military Suits Started for home
Expecting to Meet again on the following Monday Expecting to be
sent to Harrison's Landing at which place the Army of the Potomac
was then Lying—

but when Monday Came [and] I fixed Myself up for goeing I
was told that there was no hurry as the Cars would Not be along
for Some time—but when we got within Sight of the Railroad
Lo and behold along they rushed I whipped And Cut but all of
No use they took on what passengers there was and on went the
Iron horse heeding not how Anxious I was to go And Left Me

to bewail My fate—Not Knowing the Consequences—I felt
pretty sour about it—but Since I [*sic*] as Circumstances have
turned out I have thought differently And in thinking of the
past have as often been thankful that what I considered at that
time a Misfortune Irremidiable has turned out to be a piece of
as good fortune as Ever befell Me—had I been Successful in
getting to the City that day in time I should have been Sent to
the Peninsula and as nearly all the others had an attack of fever I
Should in all [likelihood?] been Sick with it too though I Might
have Escaped it—

But failing to Report on that I day I went back and waited untill the
Seventeenth day of August when I got a Communication from
the Surgeon General ordering Me to Report to Harrisburg in the
Shortest possible time—I got the order at Noon—and that Evening
at 3 o ClocK took the Cars for Phila And found Dr. L R Kirk—on
Board Bound for for the Same destination—we Staid all Night in the
City And the Nex[t] day went to Harrisburg he was assigned to the
131st Reg. which left Harrisburg that Night I was assigned to the
143d which was then Recruiting at Phila And the Next Morning left
Harrisburg to join the Regt. while Dr Kirk went on to Washington
to join his—I felt quite Sad to part with him as we hoped Both to be
in the same Regiment—

after being in the City a Short time I again went to Harrisburg with
the Rgt. And the four Companies of Phila were Consolidated with
four ~~Cot~~ Six companies from the Western part of the State And
the organization took the Name of the 150th. we On the 5th day of
September we Left Harrisburg for Washington And got there the
next Morning about daylight—we were all Night in the Cars And
it was Certainly Very Cold And unpleasant—the Sixth day of Sep
we took up the Line of March for Harpers Ferry. the Army of the
Potomac were all or the Most of them Lying within the defences of
Washington. And as we passed out Seventh Street we Saw [Major
General Ambrose Everett] Burnsides forces Camped in the open
fields Skirting that Street—they Looked pretty well tired out And

Sunburned—this was just the Last Bull run Retreat And the failure of the Peninsular Campaign

And things Looked gloomy in the truest Sense the people at home had Lost Confidence the Army had lost confidence As [Major General George Brinton McClellan] McClelan with the finest Army in the world had failed to accomplish anything And the Rebs appeared Stronger And in a better Condition than Since the Commencement of the Rebellion—[Major General John] Pope as Commander of the Army of Virginia had failed to accomplish anything through a want of Cooperation of his Lower officers they being influenced by Jealousy And a fear that Pope Might Eclipse McClellan—Caused his failure—and almost the ruin of the Entire army—

after this Battle a Short time it was found that the Rebel Army was Making its way into Penna or Mary land—McClellan immediately Set his Army in Motion And the result was that a general Engagement was fought at Antietam about the 15th of September the result being the defeat of the Rebels with the Loss to them of Many prisoners—beside the immense Loss in Killed And wounded—the Enemy recrossed the Potomac—McClelan was ordered to follow them up and give them Battle So Soon as he Could Come up with them And force them into an Engagement—he failed to do So giving as an Excuse that his Army had to be clothed and rested Not being then in a condition to Move he Kept his Army idle Near

Near [sic] the Battlefield untill he had Lost Many by disease untill finally he [preventively?] refused to obey the President's [order] to Move when he was relieved from Command and General Burnside Made Commander in Chief of the Army of the Potomac to the great distaste of Many of the Officers And Men in the Army who at that time thought he was the only Man Capable of Comdg [commanding] So Large An Army—but as they took the Second Sober Look at Matters they Most of them changed their Notions And Settled down to the idea that the administration was wise in

its policy—though a chance one is to be found in the Army Still
who thinks he was correct in his Policy—after Gen Burnside took
Command And Much delay he Moved on the Rebel defences at
[narrative ends]

—⁓—

*The final section of the diary contains medical recipes. Fulton (or others)
wrote them back-to-front, but they are presented here front-to-back for
readability. See chapter 9 for analysis of the recipes. Apothecary units are
expressed by ℥ for ounce, gr for grain, ℨ for dram, ℈ for scruple, O for pint,
f℥ for fluid ounce, and gtt for drop. Quantities appear in lowercased roman
numerals, with j sometimes used in place of i. Other terms include ss (semis,
half), qs (quantum sufficiat, a sufficient quantity), āā (ana, of each), M
(misce, mix), and Fiat (make). Each recipe begins with the symbol ℞.*

—⁓—

~~Men Examined~~ For
the Bucktail Brigade
~~For Cap~~ Pine
~~Charles Fogel~~
~~Samuel Le [Mathews]~~
~~John Scott~~
~~Charles N Ravenov~~
℞
Oleum Cubebs ℥ ss
Oleum Juniperus ℥ ss
Spts Aetheris Nitrici Dulcis ℥ ss
Oleum Terebinthinae ℥ ss
Dose teas spoon three times daily
For Gonorrhoea—
Antimonial Saline Proff. Gross
Antimony Et Pot tartras gr. i ss
Magnes Sulphas ℥ i
Morphia Sulphas gr. ss

Sach Abba [Alba]— ℨ ii
Aqua Distilatta ℥ vi Dose
℥ ss.

[page break]

℞
Zinci Oxidium ℨ i
Morphia Sul. gr. vi
Alcohol ℨ ij
aqua pura ℥ vii ss
To use by syringe—
℞
Pulv. Alumina—℥ ss
Pulv. Cubeba ℨ ij
Antimonii Et Pot Tartras gr. i ss
Morphia Sul. gr. i
Potassa Nit. ℈ ij
Pulv. gum accacia ℨ iij
Aniseed qs for ℥ viii mixture
Orderly Sergeant W. S. Leach

[page break]

~~Cap. Elsegood~~
Red Ointment
Oleum Linii Oi
Camphor ℥ i
Resin ℥ i
Red Lead lbs. ss
Subject to gentle heat stirring
Untill of Proper consistency
           Linament For throat
Cholera Cordial
℞
Spts Lavandula Comp^d O ss.
Tan[n]in ℥ iii

Tinc Zingiber

Aqua Cin[n]amonia O āā ss [Dose indicated for both Zingiber and
    Aqua Cinamonia]

Aqua Camphorae. f℥ iv

Brandy

Alcohol

Water āā O j [Dose indicated for Brandy, Alcohol, and Water]

Morph. Sulph Ə i

Chloroform f℥ iij

Dose f℥ i for an adult. Dissolve the Tannin
In the water by heat, then add the other—

[page break]

[continued from previous page]
ingredients and filter. the Chloroform
must not be added untill the mixture
is filtered.
For for [sic] Pain in the Stomach, Bowels,
Flatulence, Colic &c.
    Neutral Mixture
Acid Citrici— Ʒ ij
Sach Alba— Ʒ ij
Aqua Font—℥ iij
after dissolving—add
Potassa Bicarb Ʒ ij—
Dose table Spoonful
As often as necessary—
~~Dys~~ Dyspepsia Oxaluria
Acid Nitric Acid Muriatic
āā Ʒ ss. Tinᶜ Gentian Co. ℥ j—
Infus. Gentian Co ℥. v—Dose
table Spoonful to be taken
three times daily—
Practice Bennett—

[page break]

~~Captain Janey~~
For Syphilis—Secondary,
℞ Pill Hydg. ʒ i
Ferri Sulph Exxic ʒ ss
Divide into 30 pills one ʒ
times daily—
or
℞
Hydg cum creta ʒ i
Quinia Sulph ʒ ss
Divide into 30 pills one three
times daily—
℞
Hydg Bichloridi gr ii
tinc gentian comp^d. ʒ iv M: a
tea spoonful
℞
Hydg Prot. Iodidi gr x
make 20 pills one after
Each meal—

[page break]

℞
Hydg Bichloridi gr ii
Pot. Iodidi ʒ ij
tinc Gentian Co ʒ ij.
Aqua ʒ ij. Dose
a teaspoonful
℞
Hydg Bichloridi
Ammonia Muriatis āā gr ii
dissolve in a Sufficient
quantity of water and add
powdered cracker qs.
Syrup accacia qs M [W?]
In 36 pills—

[page break]

Capt Gimber
Linament—
Oleum Olivae ℥ ij
Aqua Ammonia ℥ ij
Oleum Terebin ℥ i
Chloroform ℨ ij—
Misc—
P̶l̶ Linament for Sore
Throat. ℞
Oleum Olivae ℥ ij
Aqua Ammoniae ℥ i
Oleum Sassafrass ℥ ss
Oleum terebin ℥ i
Misc—
To Check
Haemorrhage
Plaster of Paris
also Pulv Ergotae
    D L Scott[39]

[page break]

Strychnia—Formulas
℞
Ex Colycinth Comp^d ℨ i
Podophyllin gr. iv
Ex Rhei gr. xxx
Ol Carc[in?] gtt xv
Strychnia gr ij
Fiat Mass. Et Divide in pill xxx
℞
Feni Citrat[e] ℨ i
Sulph quinae gr xxx (30)
Strychniae gr ii
Ex Gentianae ℨ i

Fiat Mass Et Divide in
pill no. xxx (30)

[page break]

P Fred ~~Leld~~
P Fred Lehlback [unidentified]
Applicant for Hospital
    Steward—

NOTES

1. Huidekoper, 150th PA.
2. Culpeper Court House.
3. Promoted to this rank on June 2, 1863, at this time second-in-command of the 143rd PA, later killed at the Wilderness, Virginia, on May 6, 1864.
4. 143rd PA.
5. The line of tents for the 143rd was to the rear of where Fulton's tent was set up.
6. Culpeper Court House.
7. See chapter 7 for details of the consolidation.
8. Co. A, 143rd PA.
9. Co. K.
10. Charles C. Plotze, promoted to captain on February 1, 1864.
11. Josiah L. Lewis, hospital steward.
12. Evidently an error, as Fulton should have entered January.
13. Ezra S. Griffin, commissioned second lieutenant, Co. E, 143rd PA, on September 9, 1862, promoted to captain on January 30, 1863, and died of wounds on July 11, 1864 (nature of wounds and when and where received unknown).
14. Likely Surgeon George W. Ramsay, at Gettysburg the surgeon in charge, 1st Division, 1st Corps, and a member of the 95th New York Infantry.
15. Co. A, 143rd PA, resigned January 24, 1864. See previous chapter.
16. Co. D, 143rd PA, killed at Hatcher's Run, Virginia, February 7, 1865.
17. Co. D, 143rd PA, resigned December 29, 1863.
18. Co. F, 143rd PA, killed May 5, 1864 at the Battle of the Wilderness, Virginia.
19. Latrines.
20. Pvt. Henry M. Porter, Co. H, 143rd PA, died of disease at Culpeper, Virginia, January 8, 1864.
21. Sudden appearance of lesions, pustules, or blisters.
22. Fulton's mistake: 1864.
23. Vaccine matter consisted of lymph, or the liquid that filled raised skin pustules of vaccinia (vaccine disease) sufferers, or pulverized scabs that formed from pustules at a later phase of the disease. These substances were introduced subcutaneously by lancet into healthy arms.
24. Killed on May 9, 1864, at the Battle of Spotsylvania Court House, Virginia.
25. Co. I, 143rd PA.
26. Co. I, discharged for disability October 21, 1864.

27. Unidentified.

28. Kemblesville, Franklin Township, Chester County, Pennsylvania.

29. Promoted from captain, Company A on September 1, 1863, and discharged due to wounds received at the Battle of Spotsylvania Court House, May 12, 1864.

30. Co. H, 143rd PA, promoted to captain on April 19, 1864, wounded at the Wilderness on May 6, 1864, and died of wounds on June 1, 1864.

31. Smallpox.

32. The identity of Dr. Ramsey is uncertain. During the Gettysburg battle, Assistant Surgeon William R. Ramsey worked at the Lutheran Seminary when Fulton was present. Alternatively, Fulton may be referring to Surgeon George W. Ramsey, 95th New York, who was also present at Gettysburg. In January, 1864, the 95th was assigned to the Second Brigade, First Division, I Corps, which participated in the same post-Gettysburg activities as Fulton's brigade.

33. Smallpox or varioloid came in two varieties, distinct and confluent. In the confluent cases, individual raised pustules merged with others to form large masses of inflamed flesh. These cases experienced high mortality.

34. 143rd PA, who recovered from illness and mustered out with the regiment on June 12, 1865.

35. Unidentified.

36. Kenly became commander of the Third Division, I Corps, following Gettysburg.

37. Commanding the 149th Pennsylvania.

38. 150th Pennsylvania, mustered in May 28, 1863, and discharged on November 23, 1863.

39. Assistant surgeon Scott evidently entered the "To Check" recipe as it is not in Fulton's hand and appears to be signed by Scott.

SIX

Dr. Fulton after 1864

RETURNING HOME

From about the time James Fulton submitted his resignation in early 1864 until his final discharge months later, he made no further entries in his diary. Possibly during this time he began a second narrative in the same pocket diary, evidently an attempt to frame his Gettysburg experience into a polished narrative. Special Order No. 193, issued by the Adjutant General's Office, dated June 1, 1864, recognized Fulton's honorable discharge effective April 8, 1864.

Although he had begun a medical practice in Jennersville, where he had met his wife, before the war, Fulton returned to a home in nearby New London that was soon populated with children and occupied by the businesses of farming and medicine. This home he occupied for the rest of his life. It thereafter remained the home of his widow until her death in 1932 at ninety years old. Fulton's farming and medical practice evidently yielded a respectable if not lucrative family life. By 1870, Fulton's real estate was valued at $17,800 and his personal property at $2,400. By 1870, the household included daughters Rebecca (b. 1862) and Mary (b. 1869, also known as Mamie), and son James Jr. (b. 1865). Fulton's wife, Anna, consistently listed in census records as "keeping house," also managed the administrative work of the medical practice.[1]

By 1880, the Fulton household had enlarged by son William (b. 1872) and daughters Carrie (sometimes appearing as Caroline in the census, b. 1876) and Gertrude (also known as Girtie, b. 1880). During his fiftieth year in 1882, Fulton's surprise birthday party was reported in the local news as being attended "by a large number of his friends" at which a "very good time was had by all."[2] Throughout the years, the family remained close. By 1900, son James Jr., had died (1898), but Carrie, Gertrude, and Mary

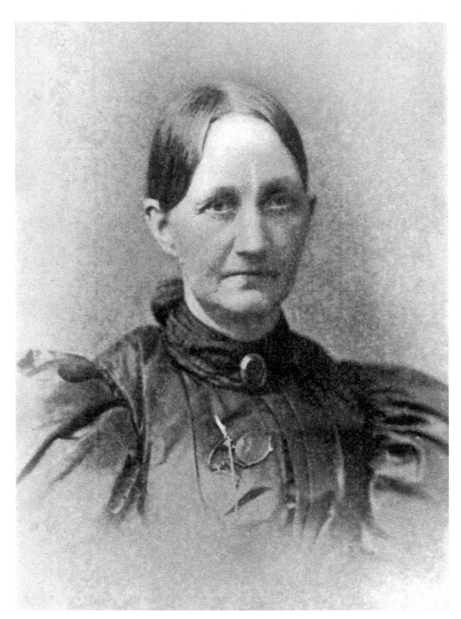

Figure 6.1. James Fulton's wife, Anna Johnson, probably taken during the 1870s. Credit: Hugh R. Fulton, ed., *Genealogy of the Fulton Family*, Lancaster, PA, 1900. Courtesy of David Smith.

remained single and still resided in the house. Son William, also single, lived in the house and managed the farm. Rebecca had married and moved to Pittsburgh.

A few years later, Fulton, now seventy-five, was experiencing a deterioration of health due to heart disease. Nevertheless, the extended family and many friends held a forty-sixth wedding anniversary celebration of James and Anna in 1907, which attracted at least two hundred guests and press attention. The community "rejoiced in the opportunity to pay their respects to the Doctor and his wife, and the affair in a social sense was most enjoyable." Brother Hugh, an indefatigable organizer of family events, recited his own poem of tribute to the couple who had "spent their married life at their comfortable farm home in New London." Daughter Carrie, still single, had moved to Pittsburgh, possibly joining her older sister Rebecca.[3]

Two years later, James Fulton "succumbed to an attack of neuralgia of the heart." His death certificate listed the cause as "organic heart disease." The obituary recounted his lineage, his Civil War experiences, and his work and reputation as a physician. It noted that he had lived his postwar life in New London, "where he spent the rest of his life building up a large practice throughout the entire countryside and taking a prominent part in all the activities of that particular section." In addition to citing Fulton's work as the federal government–designated physician to examine pension claims, the news article highlighted Fulton's commitment to the New London Presbyterian Church, where he served for many years as an elder. At this time, in addition to his wife and five surviving offspring, Fulton's brothers William and Hugh remained alive and working.[4]

After Fulton's death, Anna functioned as head of household in company with unmarried children Mary, Gertrude, and farmer William. By 1920, Anna still reigned as the householder over a diminished household of Gertrude and William, daughter Mary having died in 1915 of cancer. Unfortunately, the long arc of Anna's life can only be constructed circumstantially, as no correspondence or other family record for her exists. She clearly functioned efficiently and resourcefully as James's administrative assistant and office manager, and still ran a household and raised several children. We can speculate on her paramedical role in James's clinic: Did she perform quasi-nursing duties to assist her husband? Did she order, store, and retrieve medicines? Did she prepare some of his professional correspondence? What was her

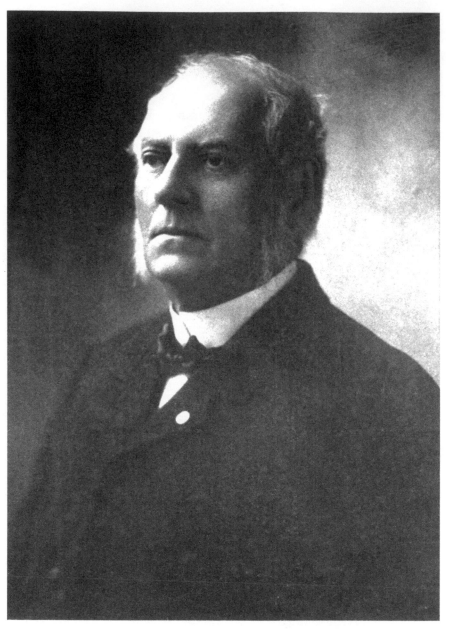

Figure 6.2. James Fulton as he appeared during the 1880s or 1890s. Credit: Hugh R. Fulton, ed., *Genealogy of the Fulton Family*, Lancaster, PA, 1900. Courtesy of David Smith.

education? What were her interests? The best that we can do is to recognize a space for her within the Fulton household within which we register these questions with knowledge that Anna's life merits elucidation.

Gertrude died of tuberculosis in 1916. Carrie had married but still lived nearby. Census records over the years show occasional household servants and farmhands in residence. In the 1930 census, Anna still presided over the house, while William, who married after 1920, ran the farm. By the time of Anna's death in 1932 at the age of ninety, she had outlived daughter Rebecca, who had married in 1889 and lived in Massachusetts at the time of her death. Anna was survived by William, who died in 1954, and Carrie, who died in 1963.

Fulton's three brothers also returned home after army service. The brothers mirrored one another in their commitment to the community, involvement in Presbyterian Church affairs, willingness to serve in civic functions, and ardent Republicanism. They also worked at a variety of artisanal jobs before finding careers. Before the war had ended, William had been elected a justice of the peace (1863) and was subsequently re-elected (1868 and 1878). A lawyer, he became a director of the Oxford National Bank and served as counsel for the Philadelphia and Baltimore Central Railroad. He also got elected as a Republican state legislator. Joseph pursued a career in merchandising, first in Maryland and later in New London. In the family home locality, Joseph ran a drugstore, having graduated from the Philadelphia College of Pharmacy. After teaching school for a short while, Hugh read law under his brother, William, and attended the University of Michigan Law School. He returned to practice law in Lancaster, but then went on a grand tour of western states before returning to legal work in Lancaster, later serving as city and then county solicitor. He helped found Lancaster General Hospital and became the president and director of the local YMCA.

Consistent with their roles as middle-class professional men with deep community roots, the brothers joined fraternal organizations to cement business and personal relationships and retain community standing. James and Joseph were members of the Free and Accepted Freemasons, New London Lodge; James and William were members of the Independent Order of Odd Fellows; brother Hugh was a member of the Ancient York Masons, Oxford Lodge, and the Junior Order of the United American Mechanics. James and William joined the local William S. Thompson Post 132, Grand Army of

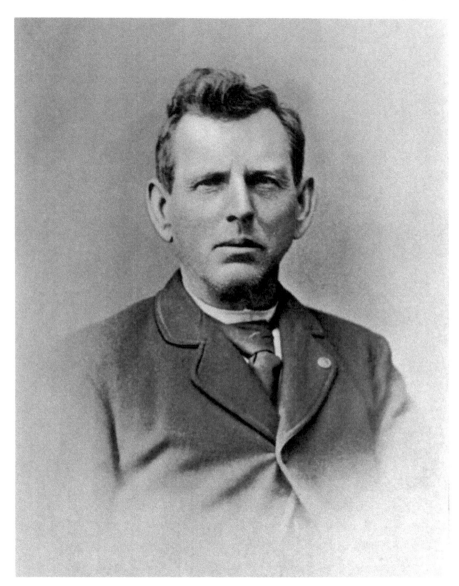

Figure 6.3. William T. Fulton, brother of James, who also served in Maryland and Pennsylvania regiments during the war. He and James occasionally met during the war. The diary recounts a meeting immediately following the Gettysburg battle. Credit: Hugh R. Fulton, ed., *Genealogy of the Fulton Family*, Lancaster, PA, 1900. Courtesy of David Smith.

the Republic (GAR), the veterans' organization, and took an active role in promoting Civil War memory by sponsoring meetings and reunions. James returned to Gettysburg many times. Hugh also promoted memory of the Civil War through GAR Lancaster Post 84.

FOSTERING A MEDICAL COMMUNITY

When James Fulton returned to Chester County in 1864, he established his practice in New London. With Anna keeping the business records, Fulton settled in as a country general practitioner. Son William eventually became the farmer who managed the farm, and life went on in a lively household as children were born and raised. Fulton became active within the Chester County Medical Society, and he was elected president of the society in 1873 and again 1888.[5] In addition to establishing and maintaining standards of practice (including fixing standard rates for various services), the society administered the poorhouse.

When the war was still in progress and through the turbulent years of Reconstruction, Fulton certainly followed events. Perhaps he was able to combine his GAR membership with medical society work. In 1873, the society received a copy of the *Medical and Surgical History of the War of the Rebellion*, the government-published encyclopedia of everything learned by physicians during the war. Possibly the society hosted speakers who reminisced about medical work during the war. During the late nineteenth century, medical societies North and South reciprocally invited former military surgeons to speak about their work, a gesture of reunion that was common at the time. Fulton also maintained contact with the veteran community. In 1875, he received a federal appointment to serve as "examining surgeon for Southern Chester county, to examine invalid pensioners of the United States and applicants for pensions."[6]

Fulton's pension work doubtless placed him in touch with many veterans, including those disabled and in poverty. He may have secured jobs for some or relief for others; we do not know. He may have used his GAR connections to help veterans. His medical work with veterans certainly returned both doctor and patient to their soldier lives, a shared reality increasingly alien to other Americans. Fulton performed pension exams during an era when veterans came to be seen as importuning old men whose pension claims were draining the federal treasury, men who had become "eccentric caricatures." Such public perceptions may have fueled Fulton's participation at GAR events, where he and fellow Union veterans "devised their own rituals, created their own spaces, and even developed their own lexicon and sense of time."[7]

To become sufficiently proficient in medicine to receive appointments to medical school lectureships or hospitals, physicians of the nineteenth century traveled to Europe to study at one of the centers of medical learning, particularly Paris around the time of the war. There is no evidence that Fulton traveled farther than regionally on either medical business (society meetings) or for GAR events. Whatever efforts he expended to remain current in medical practice probably occurred during meetings of physicians. In 1900, the president of the Chester County Medical Society reflected on the half century of its existence. At first, the handful of physicians who created the society met irregularly, but by the early 1850s they had created a formal link to the Medical Society of the State of Pennsylvania, itself founded in 1848, now the Pennsylvania Medical Society. A few years before the war, in 1857, the Chester County Medical Society hosted the annual meeting of the Medical Society of Pennsylvania, a signal event to mark the maturing respectability of the county society.[8] The society president in 1900 reviewed epochal moments in medical history: those moments also marked international achievements, including improvements in medical training and hospital management, the advent of antisepsis and new vaccines, the emerging scientific basis for clinical work, and public health laws and practices to limit the damage of disease outbreaks. As a prominent member of the Chester County Medical Society, Fulton would have integrated medical developments into his practice and contributed to the medical society legacy.

A TALE FOR THE FUTURE

In 1898, *The National Tribune*, a newspaper of the GAR, published Fulton's memoir, "Gettysburg Reminiscences. A Surgeon's Story" (see Appendix B for a transcript). He doubtless referred to his diary as a basis for the essay, but, layered as Fulton's experiences were thirty years on with battlefield visits, celebratory events, and a growth industry in war memoirs, the essay contains tropes common to the genre. Here is the assertion of the resilience of Pennsylvanians to defend hearth and home. Here the behavior of Confederate soldiers receives chastisement for stealing worshippers' horses outside of a church. Unlike the diary, Fulton here presents a fluent, polished narrative. On July 1, 1863, Union soldiers march quickly to the field; fighting becomes intense at the McPherson farm; Fulton and fellow physicians make do without sufficient bandages, medicines, or equipment; Fulton's orderly (who has equipment) cannot be found; Fulton repairs to Seminary Ridge, where he finds the orderly, and both are sent into town to makeshift hospitals at the Catholic and Presbyterian churches.

Fulton quickly determines that the need for food occupies the highest priority, so he goes door to door to beg. He obtains some bread and apple butter, then finds a bakery where the proprietor is willing to bake loaves, but has no flour. The baker nevertheless gives Fulton barrels of crackers that he had had hidden. Neighbor Mr. Meyers fires up his house stove to make beef tea, and several women emerge from cellars to volunteer their help and distribute the crackers. Now a prisoner, Fulton appeals to Confederate leaders for flour. First, he approaches Lt. Gen. A. P. Hill, who directs him to return to the wounded. He then tries Brig. Gen. Harry Hays, who forwards Fulton to Lt. Gen. Richard S. Ewell, who promises flour, but none ever comes. Ewell's haughty behavior did not give Fulton "a very exalted opinion of the man. His bearing toward me was that of great superiority." Throughout Fulton's frantic movements under guard and under fire in Gettysburg to find food, he encounters exhausted soldiers of the Union 11th Corps who had retreated into town when their line collapsed against Ewell's onslaught. While Fulton criticizes them in the diary for their resignation to being captured, in the memoir, he is more generous, crediting them for having delayed the rebel advance.

Fulton cuts a curious figure during the brief rebel occupation of Gettysburg, as he has been assigned a guard but is permitted the liberty of the town. On July 2, Confederate officers enter the Catholic church and ascend to the belfry—accompanied by Fulton—to view the battle as far as distant Big Round Top. This reminiscence affords Fulton a chance to narrate Longstreet's attack on the position occupied by troops of Maj. Gen. Daniel Sickles, which Fulton certainly drew from other accounts. On July 3, Fulton discusses the tactics and strategy of unfolding events with Confederate officers and turns attention to captured Confederate Brig. Gen. James L. Kemper, who was wounded during Pickett's Charge. Kemper receives no mention in the diary, but Fulton develops an acquaintance with him while both are at the temporary hospital at the Lutheran Seminary, a period unaddressed in the diary. In the GAR article, Fulton highlights his conversation with Kemper: "A warm friendship sprung up between Kemper and me. He was a gentleman of whom I learned to think highly before we were separated by the fortunes of war." There is no evidence that this friendship extended beyond the brief time Kemper was a hospital patient. At the time Fulton's essay was published, accounts by veterans on both sides had taken on a character of mutual respect in recognizing that the war was fought by honorable men motivated by equally virtuous ideologies. By this time, then, "the War became a reason for national gratulation rather than a subject for reflective soul-searching."[9] Fulton's essay, like the diary, does not offer any summary statement on the war, argue its inevitability, or moralize on its legacy.

Balancing the diary with the GAR essay, the reader recognizes the signal importance of the Gettysburg battle to Fulton: it was the crescendo of his military experience and a benchmark to his career as a physician. The diary betrays no careerism or ambition to surpass his colleagues in achieving military rank. Fulton appears to accept the circumstances thrust on him and does his best to manage them. With a few rare exceptions, he focused on the immediate challenges and details, and left the big picture to others. In the belfry of the Catholic church on July 1, rebel officers gleefully pointed out their armies in the distance, forecasting a victory for themselves. Sullenly, Fulton left the belfry and returned to the demands and responsibilities of healing soldiers. Not until Fulton was about to leave the army did he try, writing in the pocket diary, to give form to his Gettysburg experience, but he evidently did not revisit the subject in print until, decades later, he supplied the essay for a GAR newspaper. Gettysburg attracted more newspaper and magazine articles than other battles and Fulton, through his GAR work, stoked his own memories and those of his army compatriots, doubtless working to create monuments to his brigade at the battlefield.[10]

In his diary and memoir, James Fulton never doubts his dedication to the Union cause. In common with other memoirs, he concluded his essay, but not his diary, with his observation about his friendship with Gen. Kemper. This gesture not only fit the zeitgeist of the era, but attests to Fulton's desire to remember, not with horror or recrimination, but with reconciliation, which agreed well with his Presbyterian beliefs.[11] Perhaps a measure of the horror Fulton experienced at Gettysburg and elsewhere in his wartime service might be the very stability and relative calm he sought for the remainder of his life in southwestern Chester County "by returning to familiar places, familiar routines, and resuming family responsibilities."[12] While, in common with other men of the era, Fulton was expected to project a manly ideal shorn of self-doubt and physical and moral weakness, he nevertheless saw and endured much that he did not record. The reader can imagine Fulton reading his diary from time to time as he recalled and shared his experiences—perhaps mainly with other veterans—"remembering them as a time of unity, idealism, and selfless dedication to principle."[13] Fulton's diary may have indeed served a spiritual need, attesting to his "feeling of honorable pride."

NOTES

1. Family data derived from United States Federal Census returns for 1870 (New London, Chester, Pennsylvania, Roll M593_1324, p. 444B); 1900 (New London, Chester, Pennsylvania, Roll 1393, p. 3A); 1910 (New London, Chester, Pennsylvania, Roll 7624_1328, p. 7A); 1920 (New London, Chester, Pennsylvania, Roll 7625_1550, p. 6B); and 1930 (New London, Chester, Pennsylvania, Roll 2020, p. 1A); Hugh R. Fulton, ed., *Genealogy of the Fulton Family* (Lancaster, PA: privately printed, 1900), 97–125, online at https://archive.org/stream /genealogyoffultooofult#page/100/mode/2up, accessed October 22, 2018; J. Smith Futhey and Gilbert Cope, *History of Chester County, Pennsylvania* (Philadelphia: J. B. Lippincott, 1881), 306–10, 555–7, online at https://archive.org/details/cu31924005813518, accessed October 22, 2018.

2. *Daily Local News* (West Chester), November 14, 1882.

3. *Coatesville Record*, June 20, 1907; *Daily Local News*, June 27, 1907.

4. *Daily Local News*, September 27, 1909; Commonwealth of Pennsylvania Certificate of Death File No. 86075.

5. *American Republican* (West Chester) May 6, 1873; *Oxford Press*, May 14, 1873; *Daily Local News*, Oct 10, 1888.

6. *Daily Local News*, October 6, 1875.

7. Brian Matthew Jordan, *Marching Home: Union Veterans and Their Unending Civil War* (New York: Liveright Publishing Corporation, 2014), quotations at 2, 73.

8. *Daily Local News*, March 9, 1900.

9. Daniel Aaron, *The Unwritten War: American Writers and the Civil War* (New York: Alfred A. Knopf, 1973), 328; David Blight comments on the late nineteenth-century boom in war memoirs as "Nostalgia for the heroic and romantic pasts of the battlefield and the plantation [which] found robust markets." Blight, *Race and Reunion: The Civil War in American Memory* (Cambridge, MA: Harvard University Press, 2001), 355.

10. Kathleen Diffley, ed., *To Live and Die: Collected Stories of the Civil War, 1861–1876* (Durham, NC: Duke University Press, 2002), 4. For an analysis of veterans' narratives, see Edward L. Ayers, "Worrying about the Civil War," in *Moral Problems in American Life: New Perspectives on Cultural History*, ed. Karen Halttunen and Perry Lewis (Ithaca, NY: Cornell University Press, 1998), 145–65.

11. Earl J. Hess, *The Union Soldier in Battle: Enduring the Ordeal of Combat* (Lawrence, KS: University of Kansas Press, 1997), ix, 157.

12. Michael Kamen, *Mystic Chords of Memory: The Transformation of Tradition in American Culture* (New York: Alfred A. Knopf, 1991), 89.

13. David Lundberg, "The American Literature of War: The Civil War, World War I, and World War II," *South American Quarterly* 36, no. 3 (1984), 375.

SEVEN

Commentary

CHAPTER 1, DIARY, AUGUST 18, 1862, TO FEBRUARY 19, 1863

Four physicians examined Fulton, two of whom were University of Pennsylvania faculty.[1] Joseph Leidy, MD (1823–1891), one of Philadelphia's most distinguished physicians, served as Professor of Anatomy at the University of Pennsylvania for almost four decades, including during the Civil War era. He had given up the practice of medicine by the end of the 1840s and devoted his research and teaching to human and animal anatomy. By the war, Leidy was famous both for microscopic studies and the field of vertebrate paleontology, which he effectively founded. He was renowned for his exquisitely detailed drawings, and Fulton likely would have studied Leidy's 1861 *An Elementary Treatise on Human Anatomy*. During the war, Leidy not only examined prospective physicians for military service, but consulted at Satterlee (West Philadelphia) Hospital in Philadelphia, one of the war's largest hospitals.

Henry Hollingsworth Smith (1815–1890), Professor of Surgery, second member of the examining panel, had already seen war service from the beginning and had a major hand in organizing the medical infrastructure to meet the demands of the war, particularly managing large numbers of casualties. He led the organization of Pennsylvania's military hospitals, served under one of the Union army's first commanders, George McClellan, and was surgeon general of Pennsylvania during the first two years of war. The two remaining panel members were Dr. Green and Dr. Stewart. The last two names do not appear in the University of Pennsylvania academic catalogues during the war years, but they apparently had been appointed by state authorities to examine candidates for assistant surgeon. James Martin Stewart, MD (1791–1869), in the 1828 graduating class at the University of

Pennsylvania, had been appointed by Pennsylvania Governor Andrew G. Curtin to serve on the Board of Examining Surgeons of Pennsylvania. James Montgomery Greene, MD (?–1871), class of 1823, was a distinguished naval surgeon, although retired by 1861.[2] Fulton's examination at the University of Pennsylvania occurred in July, three months before the academic year's course of lectures began.

Fulton received his orders on August 18 to muster in with the 150th Regiment and did so on August 20, 1862, with the Pennsylvania Volunteers at Camp Curtin near Harrisburg. He may have expected to be sent to Virginia, but evidently stayed home awaiting orders following his examination at the University of Pennsylvania. During the second year of the war, regiments undertook spirited recruitment efforts to replenish numbers lost to expired enlistments, wounds, disease, desertion, or other reasons. Pennsylvania authorities abolished some regiments, amalgamated others, and raised new ones. Fulton evidently expected assignment to Pennsylvania volunteers fighting with McClellan's advance through Virginia. He may have heard that state authorities wished to create a brigade of regiments that absorbed the 1st Pennsylvania Rifles, 13th Regiment Pennsylvania Reserve Volunteer Corps, known as the "Bucktails." Each soldier sported a buck tail attached to his military cap, attesting to marksmanship in hunting. Hunting a buck and securing the tail became the rite of passage to earn membership in the regiment. Major Roy Stone, leader of these riflemen, reported to Lt. Col. Thomas L. Kane, who obtained permission to undertake a recruiting campaign in Pennsylvania to raise more troops exhibiting the same esprit de corps and élan as the original Bucktails. Stone returned to his home state to recruit, accompanied by Capt. Langhorne Wister, both with the ambition of creating a Bucktail Brigade.[3] Stone, who had seen Mexican War service and performed well during McClellan's Peninsular Campaign, and Wister, who also distinguished himself in the same, received appointments as colonels, Stone as commander of the Second Brigade in the Third Division of I Corps, and Wister as commander of the 150th.

At the very time that Fulton underwent the examination at the University of Pennsylvania, his future regiment, not yet designated the 143rd Pennsylvania Volunteers, was recruiting in north-central and northeast Pennsylvania, and soldiers were mustering in Wilkes-Barre (Wilksbarre at the time). Edmund L. Dana, another Mexican War veteran already serving as a militia general, was appointed regimental colonel. The soldiers trained at Wilkes-Barre until early November, and then were sent to Harrisburg. Meanwhile, recruiting for what became the 150th, initially designated the 143rd, began in earnest in Philadelphia in August. The first officers mustered into this new regiment on August 9, Fulton being the third officer to do so. On September 1, the new recruits went to Harrisburg, joining other companies recruited in several counties. While training was in progress and officers attended to myriad administrative tasks, the new regiment dropped its designation as the 143rd and assumed the name of the 150th. The regiment thus encamped, it awaited its chief medical officer, Surgeon Michael O'Hara (mustered September 12, 1862, and promoted from assistant surgeon to surgeon on November 13, 1862). Fulton "was present to relieve such pains and aches as fell to the lot of the men from the miscellaneous food and indifferent shelter of Camp Curtin."[4] From Camp Curtin, the 143rd was assigned to the defenses of Washington, DC. There the regiment remained, drilling and fortifying the city, until it became part of Second Brigade (with the 150th) on February 17, 1863, when the regiment received orders to Belle Plain, Virginia, on the Potomac River. Correspondence between Maj. Stone and state and federal military authorities makes clear an ambition at the creation of the 143rd, 149th, and 150th Pennsylvania Regiments to organize them into a brigade.

The soldiers recruited for the three regiments came from rural counties spanning an arc from Allegheny County in southwest Pennsylvania to Crawford and Clarion counties in the northwest, then eastward to Potter and Tioga counties along the state's northern border, to Luzerne, Wyoming, and Lycoming counties, then south to the east-central Pennsylvania counties of Lebanon, Mifflin, Huntington, Clearfield, and Perry. The central and northeastern regions promoted timber and coal as key industries. North of the Appalachian Mountains, a branch of the Susquehanna River furnished a convenient way for timber procured upcountry to be floated downriver where booms caught it. Timber was stored in man-made structures called cribs—effectively islands—and early in the 1800s, canals linked this region to distant Philadelphia and Baltimore. The canals also served the burgeoning anthracite coal mines, and after 1839, the railroad reached this region. The wide Wyoming Valley, which borders the Susquehanna, attracted a diverse immigrant population not only for farming but also for woolen mills

and factories producing cotton and silk garments and for cigar manufactur-
ing. By the war, towns in the recruiting areas, including Williamsport and
Wilkes-Barre, were in their ascendancy. When war began in 1861, recruiting
was brisk, and pro-Union sentiment ran high. The men took pride in their
hardihood and rifle skills, hence the earning of buck tails in their caps and
the appellation of Bucktail Brigade. Colonel Stone's recruitment broadside
appealed to this regional identity:

> We need not remind our readers of the glory that crowns the original
> Bucktails; the name synonymous with dash and daring. They have conquered
> the adulation not only of their friends but of their enemies . . . [We are orga-
> nizing a] brigade of the same class of men to bear the same name, and wear
> the same badge. It is to be composed entirely of skilled marksmen and young
> men of intelligence who can readily acquire such skill to be armed with the
> most superior weapons, equipped in the best manner, and in every respect
> to constitute a corps d'elite . . . Those young men who enlist . . . can only be
> sustained by steady discipline, stern endurance, rapid marching and hard
> fighting.[5]

Fulton viewed the health of his soldiers from a physiological perspective that embraced their heritage, descent, place of upbringing, occupation,
religion, and moral character. Collectively, these characteristics helped to determine their fighting qualities. The introductory chapter details the army's
requirements for screening recruits.

The men recruited for the 149th and 150th in July were sent to Camp
Curtin near Harrisburg, the largest northern training camp, which opened
in 1861. Eventually, almost three hundred thousand soldiers passed through
Camp Curtin.[6] The recruits experienced brisk training and discipline and
received Enfield rifles. The atmosphere engendered esprit de corps, regimental cohesion, and an identity as special volunteers galvanized by a common
mission and colored by patriotic fervor.

Diary, August 19, 1862

For the first time in the diary, Fulton describes his pleasure in viewing a cultivated landscape. He makes similar observations throughout his diary and
occasionally meditates on land use, topography, his future farming aspira-
tions, and natural beauty. Although the August 19 entry describes Fulton's
view through a train window, most of his other observations were made

while on the march, when entering unfamiliar lands by foot or horseback. In this aspect, his diary parallels a literary genre typified by the lone traveler strolling through a countryside where "nature could be both instructive and virtuous." To a degree, then, the Fulton diary lends itself to analysis within an environmental history of the Civil War.[7]

> we came back to the Hotel where there was an order waiting me from Dr. Smith to meet him at the Beuhler House.

Also known as Beuhler Tavern, Beuhler House was located in Harrisburg at Second and Strawberry streets. In 1860, George Bolton purchased the property, and for decades it remained in use as a hotel under various names.[8] Charles Dickens once spent the night there. The Capitol building Fulton visited (and President Lincoln, too, in 1861) burned down in 1897. The grand edifice seen now in Harrisburg, which emulates the design of St. Peter's Basilica in Rome, was dedicated in 1906.

Diary, August 21, 1862

Fulton for the first time observes the presence of illness among soldiers, in this case, typhoid fever, a bacterial infection spread through contaminated water and food. Although each regiment created a schedule for daily military evolutions, the frequent assignment of soldiers to guard duty at various locations, including hospitals, fractured it. The concentration of soldiers in Washington inevitably furnished opportunities for contagion. A number of soldiers rotated through hospital stays for common illnesses and infections endemic to camp life.

> To Day I have been to the Sol[diers] home seeing the sick.

The Soldiers' Home north of Washington, a house built for a banker in the 1840s, provided a summer retreat for President Lincoln, who used it between 1862 and 1864. Company K of the 150th became Lincoln's bodyguard, and he requested its permanent assignment to him throughout the war.

> the Capitol is the Finest building that I have Ever Seen . . . the paintings in the Capitol are fine one of Genl Washington the father of his country.

The portrait may have been "General George Washington Resigning His Commission" by John Trumbull, painted for the Capitol between 1822 and

1824. Fulton evidently admired the paintings in eight large wall niches, four showing themes of the Revolution and four depicting exploration.

Fulton arrived in Washington, DC, just days following the Union defeat at the Second Battle of Bull Run (August 28–30, 1862). The city was in a state of alarm and fear owing to the proximity of the battle and the Confederate threat to the national capital. Maj. Gen. George Brinton McClellan (1826–1885) failed to take Richmond during the Peninsular Campaign over the previous months and had been relieved of command. President Lincoln appointed Maj. Gen. John Pope (1822–1892) to head the newly organized Army of Virginia which, after a running battle over a few days, retreated. Pope was removed and McClellan assumed command of Pope's forces, now combined with the Army of the Potomac. On September 16–17, McClellan fought Robert E. Lee's forces at Antietam, Maryland, ending in the Confederate withdrawal. McClellan's failure to pursue Lee led to his replacement by Maj. Gen. Ambrose Burnside.

The 150th assumed duty in the nation's capital to strengthen its defenses, under command of the military governor of the District of Columbia. Camp was established at Meridian Hill, a park a short distance from the Potomac River near M and 15th streets. Large open ground furnished an ideal spot for a small tent city and drilling area. The regiment saw much social life while thus encamped. Visitors were constant, especially Pennsylvanians curious to see their own soldiers. Visits were reciprocated, the officers in turn hosting visitors and attending teas, receptions, and dinners. While thus stationed in Washington, the 150th gained Assistant Surgeon Michael O'Hara who, while there, was promoted to surgeon on November 13.

Pennsylvanian Matthew A. Henderson, MD, also appeared in Washington to join the 150th as assistant surgeon shortly after the new year. Almost twice as old as Fulton, forty-nine-year-old Henderson, from Boalsburg, Centre County, achieved a high pass on his examination and, like Fulton, received his degree from Jefferson Medical College, class of 1835. The regimental history of the 150th reports, however, that Henderson suffered from an "indifferent physical condition, and saw little service with the command," and received a medical disability discharge in June 1863. Henderson, however, despite his relatively short military tenure, kept a diary that survives in the collections of the Smithsonian Institution. His account converges with Fulton's, and the two diaries, considered together, may represent the only known instance during the Civil War of two physicians in the same brigade maintaining diaries simultaneously about the same events.[9] Henderson's diary, unlike Fulton's, is a homeopathic "pocket repertory," a combination of homeopathic practitioner's reference guide with ruled pages to record treatments administered. The Smithsonian also holds Henderson's kit of medicines in small bottles, unlabeled, and presumed homeopathic, possibly from the Civil War era. Although Henderson passed the army's examination for assignment as a medical doctor, he evidently maintained interest in homeopathic therapies. Where relevant, quotations from Henderson's diary appear in this commentary.

Fulton transferred from the 150th to the 143rd Pennsylvania on November 18, 1862, having been replaced as assistant surgeon of the 150th by Assistant Surgeon Henry Strauss. He had to travel to Harrisburg to settle affairs. Washington saw much politicking among regimental commanders of state volunteers, state legislators, and federal authorities that influenced the naming, organization, terms of enlistment, and assignment of units. Col. Puleston, evidently Governor Curtin's Washington lobbyist, receives credit for avoiding fracturing the new Bucktail Brigade before it was officially constituted, retaining the 143rd and 150th PA regiments in Washington.[10]

Diary, January 2, 1863

Between December 31, 1862, and January 2, 1863, Union forces under Gen. William S. Rosecrans fought a savage engagement known as the Battle of Murfreesboro or the Battle of Stones River in Tennessee. Both armies retired from sheer exhaustion, but Rosecrans prevailed on the field. In the next diary entry, this fight was clearly the talk of the regiment. The Union campaign to capture Vicksburg, Mississippi, begun in December 1862, and concluded on July 4, 1863, presented a series of skirmishes, battles, maneuvers, frustrations, and delays for Union forces. Fulton and his fellow soldiers would have followed the campaign with eager interest: its success would isolate Texas and Arkansas from the Confederacy and free the entire Mississippi River for Union supply and commerce.

My old horse is doeing fine having a tent for a Stable it protects him from the weather.

Customarily, when in camp, soldiers responded to reveille at daybreak followed by roll call. Soldiers who considered themselves too sick to report for duty presented themselves to the surgeon's tent at six o'clock or six thirty a.m. Fulton visited Harewood Hospital, one of Washington's largest military hospitals, with about two thousand beds, located on 7th Street near the Soldiers' Home. Fulton also enjoyed a visit to Glenwood Cemetery in northeast Washington a short distance away from Harewood, which opened in 1854 as part of the rural cemetery movement, an impetus to create cemeteries featuring bucolic landscapes, peaceful vistas, and tombs of architectural merit accompanied by attractive statuary.

Diary, January 12, 1863

Soldiers of the 150th indeed experienced misery in camp and were later grateful to leave Meridian Hill, having "suffered frightfully from the unwholesome conditions prevailing in that locality." The vicinity had become a town dump: "Various forms of malaria speedily developed among the men, its ravages being especially noticeable in the country companies, nearly one-third of whose numerical strength was presently in the hospitals." Assistant Surgeon Henderson also records expected camp cases of "the ordinary maladies of the season as catarrhs rheumatism + coughs constituting the main."[11]

Diary, January 18, 1863

Ohio Congressman Clement L. Vallandigham (1820–71), an antiwar Midwestern Democrat (popularly termed Copperheads), vociferously and stridently opposed the policies of the relatively new Republican Party, avowed great sympathy for slavery and the Southern cause, and repeatedly attacked the Lincoln administration. See chapter 13 for additional discussion of Vallandigham.

Duty in Washington for almost five months seemed to many soldiers a strange interlude between training and deployment. The regimental history for the 150th records:

> Life was anything but monotonous [in Washington]. As the capital of the republic, the seat of its legislature and of the national treasure-house,—the point to which a majority of the mighty host of volunteers who rose to sustain

the government converged, and to which supplies of immeasurable quantity and almost incalculable value were brought to be distributed among the various armed bodies in the field; the centre where plans of campaign were projected, discussed, rejected, or adopted; from which orders were issued to armies and military departments, and to which reports of all offensive and defensive operations were promptly sent,—Washington, the "City of Magnificent Distances" ... had ... become the scene of more movement, and occupied greater prominence in the eyes of the people, than any other place in the land.[12]

Assistant Surgeon Henderson similarly took advantage of some leisure time in Washington to see the sights in the nation's capital. Neither doctor had evidently visited Washington before, so their diaries include observations on city life, but it was important for both men to witness the functioning of the federal government they had sworn to defend. Henderson's diary includes a mildly eventful amble near the Smithsonian Institution:

The "Smithsonian Institute" occupies a large space near the Potomac + with its towers, domes, + spires constitutes a striking object imposing in its size ɪ interesting for its history + the various uses to which it is appropriated. On returning from my visit ... [I] met the various congregations again, coming from their churches, blacks + whites mingling indiscriminately—at 3 p.m. went to hear "Vespers" in a Catholic church nearby. On entering, found a funeral discourse being delivered over a colored child. The mourning cortege were well + fashionably drest—velvet bonnets with waving ostrich plumes overshadowing a sable brow presented to me an unwonted sight. The first colored Catholics I have ever seen. [13]

Like Fulton, Henderson visited the Capitol to view whatever business was before Congress that day. Viewing republican government in action seemed crucial to affirming patriotic fervor and dedication to the Union cause. Henderson happened on a debate about whether the government should form "negro Reg[iment]ts." After listening to an Ohio Democrat in the House offer "fiery remarks" against the idea, Representative Thaddeus Stevens of Lancaster, Pennsylvania (1792–1868)

then took the floor—The Hall which had been but thinly occupied was soon quite crowded to hear his remarks—The aisles around + the space in front of the Speakers was filled with interested listeners. He read his speech calmly and self possessed taking off the previous speakers, much to the merriment of those standing + sitting around with conclusion after which the vote was to be taken but it drawing near [dusk?] I did not remain. [14]

Henderson then walked to the Senate chamber and heard "a bill to en-
large facilities for the destruction of weevil in grain occupied the time +
attention of the grave + potent seigniors—I walked thru the corridors +
vaulted passages of the magnificent building with feelings of admiration +
its vast size + final[15] will when finished completed be one of the finest edifices
in the world."[16] A few days later, Henderson and Surgeon O'Hara concluded
their tourism by journeying to Georgetown to see the Catholic College (now
Georgetown University) where the college treasurer showed them the forty-
thousand-volume library with books

> memorable for their antiquity dating back to the 12th 13th + 14th Century.
> Some were handsomely "illuminated" throughout their pages an art now un-
> known to us—Saw books written on parchment + vellum—ancient scrolls +
> other manuscripts—Bibles of all ages + nations – works in every department
> in science literature + art—ancient + modern painting + pictures—[The
> library] is a singular-looking room with a rotunda in the centre surrounded
> by pillar + alcoves—Visited also the Museum filled with rare curiosities . . .
> They have a fine set of scientific instruments—pneumatic, chemical,
> philosophical—was invited into the parlor to get a glass of their old Catawba
> wine made within the walls of the establishment[17]

The months of life in Washington came to an end in mid-February. The
new Second Brigade, First Division, First (or I) Corps consisting of the 143rd,
149th, and 150th Pennsylvania Volunteers, was about to assemble in Virginia.
The 149th and 150th regiments marched in snow and slush to the 6th Street
Wharf, where they embarked on the steamer *Louisiana* to Aquia Creek, Virginia, and transferred to smaller boats that took them to Belle Plain, where
they encamped by February 17, the day the 143rd departed Washington for
the same destination.[18]

Diary, February 17, 1863

Henderson recorded the same journey:

> [February 15] Rose, made a hasty breakft, donned blanket + oilskin cover +
> started to walk to boat landing in heavy rain . . . Regt. soon foll[d] [followed] it
> with 149th started in "Louisiana"; passed Alexandria front at C[ourt].H[ouse].
> + Mount Vernon + Fort Washington + near mouth of Acquia @ ch. Stopped
> + cast anchor for the night it being too shallow for our deeply loaded boat to
> go much further—slept on slats in stateroom cold + shivering. [Feb]16 next
> morng started + soon ran aground—A lighter came along + took off troops.

passing Aq[uia] Ch [court house] arrived at Bells Landing—in the midst of
a fleet of vessels unloading troops + govt. stores-soon unloaded + staking
my seat in a U.S. wagon in charge of our medical stores in a train of some 20
started for "Belle Plain" some 2 miles back from the river on a dreadfully sorry
"corduroy" road, the country + heights around being composed to a great
extent of a deep sand into which the teams sink to the hubs in bad weather.
commenced our ascent on a dreadfully jolting road with sharp curves passing numerous camps at each turn + wind of the road + in due time arrived
at the designated spot on the side of a ravine covered with scruffy pine the
surrounding plains showing evidence of cultivation in the furrowed ground
in some of which corn stalks + a scanty growth of rye bore witness to the
attempt to raise some wheat from the sterile soil— As far as the eye can range
around on hilltop + in the vales the country is whitened with the encampments of the U.S. while not a vestige of a landmark is to be seen the fences
having been taken for fuel by the occupying forces—[19]

Diary, February 19, 1863

Winter storms beset the arriving 143rd, inches of snow alternating with rain.
A captain with the 149th wrote, "Snow, snow, snow from morning to night.
Soaked boots, wet stockings, cold feet, smoked faces, swollen eyes make
up the sum of our comforts today." A private in the same regiment added,
"This . . . is a dreadful place. Dead horses and mules and lots of mud would
meet our eyes in every direction."[20] Meanwhile, Col. Roy Stone arrived in
camp on February 19 to assume command of the new brigade.

*"there were several all Sunk into the low form or in other words had Typhoid
Pneumonia.*

Doctors feared the appearance of typhoid and tried to treat cases immediately, but available medicines proved inadequate. Contract Surgeon
John Vance Lauderdale, who served on a hospital ship, expressed resignation
about the problem in a letter to his sister:

I must go through the wards and pour some whiskey down the parched
throats of the Typhoid patient. Nothing else seems to keep them alive . . . I
went to the bunk of a soldier to give him another dose of medicine, and found
him cold and lifeless. There are four or five others, who will hardly live till
daylight. Their mouths are getting dry and their teeth are becoming covered
with black saliva. Their eyes are fixed and they refuse their medicine. It is a
sad sight indeed, but what can we do?[21]

With Col. Stone in place, the chain of command was set: Maj. Gen. Joseph Hooker commanding the Army of the Potomac; Maj. Gen. John F. Reynolds commanding I Corps; and Maj. Gen. Abner Doubleday commanding the 3rd Division. As winter gave way to spring, the brigade trained, developed discipline, and engendered esprit de corps as the Bucktails. Before the regiments arrived in Virginia, the previous December, the Army of the Potomac under Gen. Ambrose Burnside suffered defeat at nearby Fredericksburg. In early April, President Lincoln visited the refreshed, supplied, and trained army, and within weeks Hooker would move his force into battle.

CHAPTER 2, DIARY, FEBRUARY 22, 1863, TO JUNE 28, 1863

Despite the eagerness of the new troops to go on campaign, veteran regiments, especially those who had participated in the disastrous Fredericksburg campaign in December during which the Union army attacked a well-entrenched and fortified Confederate position on high ground, did not exhibit comparable enthusiasm for the spring campaign:

> Of the old troops in the neighborhood, it was painfully evident that many had lost spirit, and that the enthusiasm of the entire army had been seriously tempered by the total failure of the operations under General [Ambrose E.] Burnside. The appointment of General [Joseph] Hooker[22] to succeed him did something to correct this depression, but for several weeks the weather was such that the men were compelled to remain in idleness in their camps, and the influence of the new commander could not be felt. Regimental officers seemed to share in the *moral* [italics in original] fatigue which followed Fredericksburg and the mud march.[23]

Diary, February 22, 1863

the Men Are called upon to go on Picket duty

Picket duty functioned as an early warning system. Soldiers were posted in a loose cordon at some distance from a camp to remain alert to enemy troops. Surgeons took turns on picket duty performing duties described by Surgeon James D. Benton, 111th and 98th New York:

> [E]very day a surgeon is sent out in charge of the picket of each Division and stays until relieved by his successor on the succeeding day. The object of this

is that in case of accident or attack by the enemy he can be at hand or in case of sickness he can send in to camp with a written excuse [for] the person who may be ill. The authority of the surgeon over sick men is supreme and when either officer or man is excused from duty by them no one however high in military authority can with safety interfere with it.[24]

While Fulton performs picket duty during this time, his friend Assistant Surgeon Henderson has a similar routine:

> Rain in the night which continues this day—awakened before day by reveille— rose + breakfasted on pork, potatoes + coffee— attended sick + prescribed—cold feet + general discomfort—Started in rain to visit Head Drs of Med Director in company with several Surg^s of ajoin^d reg^t rode an awful country almost impassable passed the roosting place of [two?] Brig Genl^s + spoke to them was in ones quarters, an outhouse dilapidated, cold + cheerless— Reached Head Qtr of Commands Genl. (Doubleday)[25] was instructed to Dr [possibly Cyrus D.] Hottenstein our chief of Brigade Doctor [assigned to 1st Brigade, 3rd Division, I Corps, and Surgeon, 135th Pennsylvania; mustered out of service on May 24, 1863] [who, apparently with] med director [Dr Bache][26] gave us an exposition of the manner of managing the Med Dep of the army and the arrangements + hygiene of Hospitals—Rode back home in rain; got coffee + meat for dinner and lounged on bed + at fire till evej [evening]—[27]

Diary, March 1863

The weather during this period, colder temperatures alternating with milder ones, periods of intense rain, freezing, and snow, combined to make any movement of troops a "mud march." The 150th PA records:

> [The weather conditions] had converted the camping-ground of the army into a vast mud-hole, which thwarted the plans and intentions of its commanders and doomed the men to almost absolute inaction. The roads over which the supplies for this immense force had to be hauled were like mortar-beds, of such depth and consistency, in places, that both wagons and teams were in danger of being swallowed up; and, indeed, many a poor mule, bearing on his flanks the initials of his country, sank in the red ooze never to rise again.[28]

Diary, April 1863

the object being to make a feint to draw the attention from Fredericksburg

On April 23, Gen. Hooker ordered an expedition to Port Royal, a hamlet on the Rappahannock River, from which the Confederates fled, leaving some supplies and fortifications that the Union army inspected before leaving the area. Union troops reached Port Royal on the south side of the Rappahan-nock, in Caroline County, by ferry from Port Conway on the northern side in King George County. Port Royal is about fifteen miles west/southwest of Fredericksburg. Gen. Doubleday had been placed in command of 3rd Division, I Corps, in January. Lee's Confederate army was dispersed along the southern side of the river, his right flank at Port Royal. Hooker intended this raid as a feint, preparatory to what became the Battle of Chancellors-ville to the east. The raid furnished an opportunity for the brigade to march together for the first time. The raid included setting up artillery positions to cover soldiers who were detailed to construct a pontoon bridge. In any event, the Confederates did not fire artillery at the incoming Union soldiers and the bridge was not built.

Dr. Henderson and myself stoped at King Georges Court House

Assistant Surgeon Henderson also recorded the tale of the sumptuous breakfast at King George Court House:

> On Wednesday on returning back I got ahead of our Brigade + turned off with Dr. Fulton of the 143rd to a small town named "King Geo C House" for breakfast—It is a County seat, now deserted by its inhabitants joining the rebel ranks—We found a house on enquiry where they entertained strangers + soon sat down to a very good meal of fresh fish, biscuits, corn cakes + coffee—I ate ravenously, drinking 3 cups of coffee + doing equal justice to all the other comestibles—During our repast, conversation flowed + our host + his wife entertained us with a history of their griefs how that he built his house for a hotel just as the war fairly commenced + that soon in passing this, the Union Soldiers took away from them their their [*sic*] <u>servants</u> (of which they had six male + female) some of whom they raised. Paying our "greenbacks" 50/100 each) we went on + taking a different road from that the Brigade pursued—reached camp sometime ahead—[29]

for about an hour we were allowed to lie down on our Arms for the night.

The brigade had been on alert for the past few days. Soldiers of the 149th had been ordered on the march with eight days' rations and sixty rounds of ammunition, and they, too, began to throw away blankets.[30] Further, the brigade came under rebel artillery fire as they tried to cross the Rappa-hannock at Pollock's Mill, on Pollock's Mill Creek, which ran north of the

Rappahannock only a few miles from Fredericksburg. Meanwhile, Hooker was deploying troops about twenty miles to the north/northwest to outflank an army half his size led by Lee. Over the first few days in May, however, Lee divided his forces, and Gen. Thomas "Stonewall" Jackson took half the force to attack the Union western flank. Hooker consolidated his troops near Chancellorsville, but his plan deteriorated. On May 2, Hooker summoned the brigade to Chancellorsville, reaching the Union right flank in the early hours of May 3. By this time, however, Hooker had decided to abandon the fight and move his force closer to the Rappahannock. Hooker lost the initiative, and after other battles in the vicinity and at Fredericksburg, by May 7 the campaign was over.

I here took the Ball out of the back of the neck of a wounded Reb

Fulton's brigade was minimally involved in the Chancellorsville fight. Nevertheless, he attended to battlefield wounds in his first look at large-scale combat. Contract Surgeon John Vance Lauderdale, who attended to wounded aboard Union hospital ships, described the horror of battle in a letter to his sister:

> Poor broken down frames of men, some of them were. Some of them must die sooner or later. The exposure of camp life, arduous labor, broken rest, picket duty, excitement of war and the overcoming of that inborn horror of sheding [*sic*] a brotherhood . . . the firing of bombshells into the bodies of men, cutting them down like grass, seeing their heads torn from their bodies, limbs scattered here and there, wounded men groaning with pain, being obliged to wait long, before their wants can be relieved, suffering pain themselves and naturally disturbed by the expression of pain in others, besides other horrid scenes that a battle field strewn with dead men and horses presents, is quite enough to bring a strong man down to the weakness of a child, and render him the victim of disease.[31]

Assistant Surgeon Henderson also comments on his regiment's peripheral role at Chancellorsville:

> Marched all day + just after night passing down a narrow defile in the mountain reached the river at U.S. Ford after dark + crossing over on pontoon bridges proceeded on to the vicinity of Chancellorsville some 8 or ten miles + encamped [May] 3rd dug rifle pits + put up breastworks expecting an attack at once. On Sunday (3rd) occurred the battle of Chanc[ellorsville] at the same also the 2nd battle of Fred[ericksburg] took place—I was ordered to take men

+ stretchers + go to the rear + after the expected action was over send in + bring out the wounded + send them to the Field Hospital.[32]

Diary, May 8, 1863

—the Main and Most Effectual treatment was turpentine Ar. Spt. Am. Brandy. Qn Sul with the External application of turpentine

Diarrhea and typhoid were disabling and often mortal maladies endemic to camp life. Assistant Surgeon Daniel M. Holt, 121st New York, observed in his own regiment, "A great many of them are on the sick list with diarrhoeas and dysanteries [sic], and so reduced that we have to get rid of them as soon as possible by sending them to hospitals. Many of them ought never to have come out, having broken constitutions or bodily defects which entirely disqualify them for the life of a soldier."[33]

About this time the 150th Reg—was blessed with the addition to their Regt. of Dr. [Philip A.] Quinan

Quinan's tenure was short-lived: he was discharged on November 23, 1863. The history of the 150th PA records:

Dr. Philip A. Quinan, who had been assigned as surgeon to the regiment, reached camp and assumed his duties on the 28th of May. He claimed to have had experience as an assistant surgeon in the regular cavalry for several years, and seemed to be well up in his profession; but a natural or studied cynicism, coupled with excessive self-consciousness and a disposition to belittle his superiors in the medical department, failed to commend him to his fellow-officers or secure their friendship. His advent was signalized by an almost immediate reduction of the sick-list from seventy to twenty-nine, whether wisely or unwisely would be difficult to say.[34]

At about the same time, Assistant Surgeon Henderson submitted his resignation (which took effect at the end of June). He links his illness to the sickness of secession, mocking the "sacred soil" of Virginia, the Old Dominion:

I was obliged from fear of entire disability to reluctantly send in my resignation in order to flee to the vital air of old Centre to [recuperate?] (if it so may be) my shattered constitution by the foul + miasmatic atmosphere on the "sacred soil" (cursed secession) of the "ancient Dominion." It has now been 3 days since my resignation was sent up[35]

Diary, May 1863

on they went until they finally got to Falmouth Station there Stoping to wait for the rest of the army

The brigade was disappointed in not having entered the Chancellorsville fray despite its disposition to fight. Marches and countermarches in early to mid-May in the region, coupled with ferocious and persistent rain, caused fatigue and hardship. Nevertheless, the brigade recovered discipline and esprit de corps before marching northwest at the end of the month. Meanwhile, illness—camp fevers, malaria, "nervous debility," and sheer exhaustion—had taken a toll, and several officers and men mustered out due to ill health.

Dr Herd ordered Dr. Humphrey who was at this time Div Surgeon to put me under ~~arres~~ *arrest*

Fulton writes with mild exasperation of the threat to be arrested owing to an administrative matter. His diary is silent on other matters pertaining to military discipline (or the threat of it), but conflicts were most likely to arise when doctors contradicted an operational commander by asserting a preeminent authority over medical affairs. This assertion of authority usually invoked a separate chain of command leading to the surgeon general (see introductory chapter regarding medical and operational chains of command). Assistant Surgeon Henderson experienced an instance of this very conflict:

a misunderstanding between Col. Wister [Colonel Langhorne Wister][36] + myself occurred this forenoon. He ordered me <u>during the action expecting to come off</u> to go between the lines + gather up the wounded for the hospital. Dr. Hottenstein (my Chief) instructed me <u>not to expose myself</u>, but to wait till the action <u>was over</u> + <u>then send in the</u> stretchers, to have them carried out. I told Col. this, + he swore I should <u>obey him</u>. I told him I was a <u>medical</u> officer, only answerable to the Chief Surgeons orders, in the action. He swore again both at Dr. H. + myself, didn't care a damn for Dr. H. + myself, didn't care ad—[?] for D[r] H, This morning rec'd the same instructions as as [sic] yesterday + he swore if I did not obey him he <u>would turn me out</u> of the Reg—[37]

Henderson suffered no consequences other than having offended Col. Wister, but the strain in the relationship between a regimental commander and a physician junior in rank may have persisted.

In a survey of Union courts martial during the Civil War, physicians Thomas P. Lowry and Jack D. Welsh found that, although cases involving physicians occupied a very small percentage of the total, a distinct category emerged involving administrative issues, usually arguments between military commanders and surgeons regarding authority over hospital patients. Relevant to what Fulton and Henderson experienced, one case study examines the court martial of Dr. William Webster over the jurisdiction of doctors over patients. Webster had argued with the commanding officer that surgeons exercised authority over patients in general hospitals, not post commanders.[38]

Diary, June 1[2?], 1863

The cavalry fight, in which the brigade did not participate and the largest cavalry battle of the war, occurred on June 9 at nearby Brandy Station. Union Maj. Gen. Alfred Pleasanton engaged Confederate Brig. Gen. J. E. B. Stuart in an all-day, indecisive fight that many historians regard as the opening fight in the Gettysburg campaign. Fulton's brigade was now on the march to Gettysburg.

Diary, June 13, 1863

The march was arduous. On the march toward Bealton, the 150th PA records that "[t]he march was very trying on account of the intense heat, the dust, and want of water, the column sometimes making four or five miles without encountering even a mud-puddle from which to allay its thirst."[39] The march from Bealton to Manassas Junction on June 14 was no better:

> [It was] one of the most tortuous and torturing marches on record. The heat of the sun was withering. Not a breath of air stirred the leaves; the dust rose like a white cloud, powdering the hair and clothes of the troops and almost stifling them; and, to add to the general discomfort, not a drop of water was to be had at times for a distance of five miles . . . No man was allowed to fall out of ranks, under any pretext, without a pass from his company commander, approved by the regimental surgeon . . . In this march of twenty-seven miles [the soldiers] began to get very footsore, and it was distressing to see them hobbling along, begrimed with dust and perspiration, their tongues almost lolling out from excessive thirst. Stagnant pools, on whose borders lay decomposing horses or mules, and which living animals would not touch, were gladly resorted to by the men in passing.[40]

Diary, June 17, 1863

it tasted good After Eating Nothing but hard tack and meat for so long

Surgeons did not expect the army to supply all of their needs. Sometimes supplies and local foraging secured a welcome diet, and sometimes they did not. Assistant Surgeon John Gardner Perry, 20th Massachusetts, recalled, "I breakfasted this morning on hardtack and coffee; then at noon we dined on boiled beef, without the slightest seasoning of either salt or pepper. Even the water we bathe in, and wash our teeth with, must be left standing for half an hour before using, that the dirt in it may settle; and this same water is all we have for our coffee."[41]

Diary, June 18, 1863

While on the march, the brigade heard cannon fire to the west, along the road to Leesburg. Confederate forces were indeed maneuvering to the west and northwest as Confederate forces under Gens. A. P. Hill and James Longstreet crossed the Potomac River heading north, while Gen. Richard S. Ewell drove Union soldiers from Winchester, Virginia. Maj. Gen. J. E. B. Stuart's cavalry acted as a screen to prevent Union forces from discovering the main Confederate infantry movement north to Gettysburg. Union cavalry clashed with Stuart on June 21 near Upperville, Loudoun County, Virginia. An allied rebel cavalry brigade lurked to the north of Upperville, at Snickersville Gap. Intense fighting between rebel cavalry and Union cavalry and infantry occurred on June 21, which resulted in Confederate withdrawal to the west, but Union forces remained stymied about the location and movements of the larger Confederate force moving north through the Shenandoah Valley.

Diary, June 25, 1863

we marched on untill we came to the Village of Barnesville where we Stoped for the night

A member of the 149th PA wrote of this country, "We have passed through as nice country as I ever saw. It is rich with large wheat fields and the wheat is heavy. The face of the country in the valley is as beautiful as nature could make it."[42]

CHAPTER 3, DIARY, JUNE 29, 1863,
TO JULY 4, 1863

In the absence of a tactical plan left by Maj. Gen. Joseph Hooker, Maj. Gen. George G. Meade concentrated his forces near Frederick, Maryland, and assigned their movements from there.[43] Uncertain about the location and strength of Confederate forces, Meade deployed his troops along a broad arc and had them advance through Maryland into Pennsylvania with the objective of locating Lee's forces. As the brigade marched east over Catoctin Mountain, Capt. John Irwin, Company B, 149th Pennsylvania, observed, "[W]e overlooked a most beautiful valley, flowing with milk and honey, in that highly cultivated section of Maryland, with the town of Frederick in the midst of the valley."[44] Doubtless, many soldiers shared this perception. Local farms along the brigade's march offered the most productive wheat fields in the nation, amid gentle hills punctuated by mills and the creeks that served them. Soldiers heard the rhythmic turn of the waterwheel and the attendant movement of burr grindstones as wheat was shredded into bran, "middling," and flour.

On the whole, the health of the brigade was good, except for the usual complaints of soldiers in camp and on the march: coughing and other breathing difficulties, diarrhea, constipation, and aches and pains of the feet, legs, arms, and back ("rheumatic" disorders). Following the Chancellorsville battle, the 150th saw a few instances of "varioloid" (smallpox), but the removal of afflicted soldiers prevented its spread. Measles also appeared, but again, removal of sick soldiers prevented the spread of the disease. Virtually all soldiers regularly mustered for drill and inspection. The material readiness of the 143rd had suffered due to the wear and tear of the campaign. The soldiers were delighted to receive new shoes on June 27, "for many of the men during their long march had worn out theirs and were nearly barefoot; weary and footsore, they had borne their burdens with little complaint."[45]

Fulton's diary reflects the uncertainty occasioned by a change of command, fortified by rumors and terse communiqués from army authorities that baffled soldiers in the lower ranks. Company officers had a difficult task in maintaining discipline and esprit de corps when orders were issued with unfathomable logic. Soldiers observed their officers closely for inconsistent or irrational behavior and set high expectations for their courage and tactical leadership. Even if officers did not understand their orders, they had to respond as if they were logical and would not result in catastrophe. Regimental medical staff, while they identified with the soldiers in their care, remained aloof to the demanding requirements for drill, picket duty, dress parade (inspections), and many of the other rituals of order-keeping that characterize military life.

Despite this aloofness, medical staff echoed the views of soldiers about their military and political leaders, the general situation of war, and the specific orders guiding the present campaign. Fulton occasionally expresses irritation about those rituals he regards as "military."

Fulton's diary does not follow a strict chronology. Occasionally he departs from events to reflect on political matters, opinions or controversies regarding military leaders, and sometimes returns to an earlier event. He may have written some entries days after the events described, as some entries appear to have been written retrospectively over a few days after the intense experiences of battle. It is difficult to imagine Fulton having the time to write on each day of the Gettysburg battle. He must have carried the octavo pocket diary on his person, as Confederate soldiers stole most of his belongings.

Diary, June 29, 1863

after getting to the Centre of the town we turned to the left passing through the Main Street

Fulton refers to Gens. Rowley and Doubleday, seniors in his chain of command. A native of Pittsburgh and a Mexican War veteran, Gen. Thomas Algeo Rowley commanded the 1st Brigade, 3rd Division, I Corps of the Army of the Potomac from March 28, 1863, to June 30, and from July 2 through July 10, 1863. He assumed command of the division when Gen. Abner Doubleday replaced General John Reynolds as Corps Commander, after Reynolds was killed on July 1 just west of McPherson's farm where the Bucktail Brigade fought. Rowley suffered the ignominy of being accused of drunkenness and was later placed under arrest owing to his conduct during the Gettysburg battle. A West Point graduate and also a Mexican War veteran, Gen. Doubleday had been present at the war's beginning. He is credited for firing the first Union cannon at Confederate soldiers at Fort Sumter. After Gettysburg, Rowley was shunted off to a marginal army position, away from combat, and Doubleday, despite much battlefield experience, was likewise removed from command shortly thereafter (perhaps owing to his reputed slowness and deliberation) and performed administrative duty for the rest of his career.

Soldiers of the 150th, too, enjoyed a warm reception on the march through Mechanicstown (also referred to as Mechanicsville):

> At Mechanicstown several young ladies appeared in dresses made of the national colors, waving diminutive flags, and were enthusiastically cheered. Coffee, tea, and milk were tendered to the men as they passed, and fresh bread, cakes, and pies easily found their way into their capacious haversacks. All that blessed day the hills and woods resounded with patriotic lays which were taken up by regiment after regiment, until the whole army seemed to have been metamorphosed into a vast singing society.[46]

> *when within about 3 Miles of Emettsburg we came in view of that old and well known institution St. Josephs Mary's College for the purpose of Education of Catholic youth for the ministry*

An acute observer of the country about him, Fulton took great interest in the Catholic community of Emmitsburg. During the late eighteenth century, the first Catholics settled in Emmitsburg and founded a parish. The first Catholic church was built in 1793. In 1808, Mount Saint Mary's College and Seminary opened. Elizabeth Bayley Seton, who founded the first sisterhood in the United States (and in 1975 became the first United States–born saint), established the Sisters of Charity of St. Joseph's in 1809. Seton opened St. Joseph's Free School for girls in 1810, the same year that the Saint Joseph's Academy began operation. The community became a leading center of Catholic education in the United States.[47] See chapter 11 for a fuller discussion of the role of Catholic sisters in nursing at Gettysburg.

> *[XI Corps] has a rather a bad odor since the Battle of Chancellorsville—at which place they lost for us the fortunes of that Campaign*

Many others shared Fulton's uncertainty about Maj. Gen. Carl Schurz (briefly the commander of XI Corps), including President Lincoln, who employed him as a way to secure German American support. Born and educated in Germany, Schurz had been compelled to emigrate for political reasons and found employment as a journalist, teacher, lawyer, and pianist, and appointment as ambassador to Spain under Lincoln before he resigned to accept a military appointment. Schurz held strong abolitionist views and became a fervent campaigner for Lincoln among German Americans. Uncertainty about Schurz's abilities was due to his rapid promotion over veteran officers and the widespread belief that political favoritism led to his military appointment. Further, although diligent in his duties, Schurz persistently lost battles at Second Bull Run and Chancellorsville. Although historians agree that these losses were not Schurz's fault, his XI Corps was routed on July 1 as they tried to occupy high ground near Oak Hill just north of Gettysburg. Fulton comments on Schurz's less than inspiring appearance: bespectacled, his look suggested a professor rather than a military leader.

> the country here was quite poor and Stoney and looked poor the people—being
> quite poor and having the appearance of being quite poor and making a bare living

As the Bucktail Brigade reached Emmitsburg, soldiers noticed new behavior in their officers. Pvt. Avery Harris of the 143rd wrote, "The expressions [in the officers' faces] have changed [and they now appear] grave and quiet and very reticent and apparently more thoughtful."[48] The night before the battle, Lt. Col. Henry S. Huidekoper of the 150th had a premonition that he would suffer a wound, so he prepared a tourniquet and secreted it into his saddlebag. Not a few soldiers did the like before battle; many feared bleeding to death under fire.[49] Officers heard that the rebels had taken York, Pennsylvania, and had raided and perhaps occupied Chambersburg to the northwest, west of the South Mountains. Anxiety was high.

For the previous few weeks, marching had been characterized by stops and starts, the frustrating byproduct of moving many soldiers with their knapsacks, supply wagons, ambulances, and livestock in good order. Exhausted soldiers dropped out by the wayside and, once rested, hurried to rejoin their fellows, contributing to more disorder on the march. By June 29, all soldiers had regrouped and were alert that an encounter with the enemy was imminent. They were excited, ready, and now that they had entered their home state, roused to protect it from invasion. Before reaching Emmitsburg, the soldiers of the 149th were delighted to encounter Pennsylvanians who gathered by the roadside to give them food and encouragement.

Diary, June 30, 1863

The brigade bivouacked about four miles southwest of Gettysburg where Willoughby Run separates from Marsh Creek, the latter streaming north while the former meanders north and east along the north side of McPherson's Ridge. The business in the camps of all regiments on June 30 was an odd mixture of anticipation for battle and the administrative ritual of end-of-month preparation and submission of muster reports and financial records.

On July 1, no bugler sounded reveille as the enemy came near; instead, the order was passed from guard to guard. The day dawned clear, "but soon a drizzle came on and it became sultry beyond measure, and, to add to the discomfort, the supply wagons not having come up, it was difficult for the men to make out a good breakfast," according to the regimental history of the 150th. As the 150th's commissary wagons lagged behind the rest of the regiment, officers had to "piece out" a breakfast as best they could, foraging not having been permitted because of the proximity of the enemy. Everyone "had to be satisfied with regulation coffee and hard-tack." Other regiments fared better: the 149th received a three-day meat ration and had the opportunity to cook their breakfast. Orders had been given that directed commanders to provide soldiers with rations for three days and sixty rounds of ammunition each. Circumstances prevented this order from being carried out in all instances.

Stone's Bucktails were not alone in the vicinity. Maj. Gen. Reynolds maneuvered a very large Union force, about one-third of all Union soldiers who would fight at Gettysburg in coming days, and viewed Emmitsburg as a fallback position in case of a massive Confederate onslaught. Nearby, between this advancing force and Gettysburg, Brig. Gen. John Buford's First Cavalry Division was first to fight a major engagement with Confederates, marking the official beginning of the three-day Gettysburg battle.

The 150th records that on July 1 the brigade marched quickly along a road toward Gettysburg, muddied by the infantry force marching ahead of them. The men were

> excited to unusual effort by the frequent boom of field-pieces at a distance of some miles in front. The morning was bright, after an early drizzle, but intensely sultry, the air being charged with moisture, and the men quickly felt the weight of their campaigning outfit, and perspired as they had rarely perspired before. On either hand long stretches of golden grain and luxuriant growths of corn looked beautiful in the sunlight, and it was hard to believe that this armed host was approaching the scene of a battle. Soon, however, citizens were met driving cattle and horses before them in search of a safe retreat, and when, a little later, two children—a boy and a girl—rode past on one horse, crying as if their little hearts would break, it was painfully apparent

that the miseries of war had penetrated to this hitherto quiet pastoral region.[50]

The brigade passed a farmhouse and took a brief break, which allowed soldiers on this warm and humid day to fill their canteens. Soldiers of the 149th noticed perhaps the same nine- or ten-year-old boy and eight-year-old girl on horseback as observed by the 150th, the girl's arms around the boy's waist. The history of the 149th records that "[t]heir anxious and bewildered countenances would have made a fine study for an artist. In reply to the question where they were bounded for, the boy said, 'I don't know; they are fighting on our place over yonder.'"[51]

Diary, July 1, 1863

Col. [Roy] Stone came back and told us that we were needed to the front And to get along as fast as possible.

A mile or two below Gettysburg, along the Emmittsburg Pike, a messenger rode quickly to the officers at the head of the march, ordering them to hasten forward at the double-quick. A short time later, they stopped briefly to hear from their generals:

> When the troops were halted near the seminary, Generals Doubleday and Rowley . . . addressed a few words of encouragement to the several regiments, reminding them that they were upon their own soil, that the eye of the commonwealth was upon them, and that there was every reason to believe they would do their duty to the uttermost in defense of their State. Meanwhile, shells were flying overhead from rebel batteries beyond the ridge to the west, and there was no longer any doubt that there would be trying work that day. The untimely death of General Reynolds had already been whispered to many of the officers, and soon became known in the ranks, occasioning a feeling of profound sorrow.[52]

While he was directing his troops in a wood near the farm where the brigade would engage in furious fighting, a rebel bullet had struck Gen. Reynolds in the upper neck or head, instantly killing him. He had been placed in command of the entire Union left wing, including I, III, and XI Corps and Buford's Cavalry. A Pennsylvania native and graduate of West Point, Reynolds was widely perceived as an exceptional leader. Fulton and his fellow soldiers felt the loss, perhaps fearing the death as a portent of the intensity of the coming fight.

after passing the ravine in front of the Battery the Men passed part way up a
moderate Ascent and there Laid down

As Col. Wister led the 150th forward with the column, he unintention-
ally broke the morning's tension. He ordered the men to unsling and pile up
their knapsacks and

> then gave the command, "Forward!" forgetting that the muskets were not
> loaded. Instantly a score of voices reminded him of the omission, and amid
> some merriment the loading was ordered. Then, with colors unfurled and
> full battalion front, the 150th moved rapidly westward to the brow of the hill
> overlooking the little valley of Willoughby Run, and occupied a part of the
> space between the wood on the left, in which the Iron Brigade lay, and the
> McPherson farm-buildings. The 149th and 143d Pennsylvania took position
> on the right, extending to the Chambersburg road. It was then about eleven
> o'clock.[53]

Fulton later wrote that, before moving into position, the men "threw
away their knapsacks, never to see them again, the enemy getting possession
of them and appropriating everything useful."[54]

Supply wagons had been secured in the rear; ambulances and ammunition stores were kept nearby. The brigade had now reached its fighting position along a fenced, L-shaped configuration presenting a perimeter to the
northwest of a farm owned by Edward McPherson. The soldiers must have
felt relieved to be stationary, covered as they were with sweat and dust. The
McPherson barn had become the First Division hospital. As their officers
contemplated the massed columns of approaching Confederates with awe,
the men of the brigade could not contain their excitement and high spirits.

> [I]n their eagerness for the fray, some of the men indulged in hilarious excla-
> mations which would have sounded strangely enough an hour or two later,
> when the disproportion of the two forces had become sadly apparent . . . After
> taking position in the orchard, and while the shells were flying dangerously
> close to the recumbent line, John S. Weber, of [Company F, 150th PA] stood
> up and yelled: "Come, boys, choose your partners! The ball is about to open!
> Don't you hear the music?"[55]

The spectacle before the brigade was not for the fainthearted: "Then the
whole valley of Willoughby Run and the country beyond was in clear view,
and every man saw for himself what was coming—the Confederates, in a
continuous double line of deployed battalions, with other battalions *en masse*

in reserve. To meet this tremendous onslaught stood one thin line, and not a man in reserve."[56]

The ferocity of warfare mixed moments of sheer terror and panic with comic absurdity. Once the brigade was in position, Lt. Col. Huidekoper and Maj. Chamberlin of the 150th discussed the pending attack when an "antique and most picturesque figure approached." An elderly Gettysburg citizen, John Burns, old musket in right hand and wearing "a blue swallow-tail coat, with brass buttons, dark trousers and a high hat," asked to fight with the troops. After ensuring that Burns had sufficient ammunition, Wister said, "I wish there were more like you," advising the old man to go into the woods and fight where he would be more sheltered. But John Burns was not the kind that looked for shelter, and he fought during the day not only in the open, but in the very front. When evening fell he was still there, but badly wounded.[57]

I met Dr. [White G.] Hunter comeing to the field to order me to the Hospital for Special Duty

Dr. Fulton had entered a dependency of the McPherson farm to see wounded men of Hall's Maine Battery. He later wrote:

> As we went over the ridge to take position we saw a battery stationed on the summit just to the left of the turnpike. Many of the horses had been killed, the guns silenced, and the wounded had been taken into a small stone house to the left of the pike, also on the McPherson farm . . . There was presented a sad spectacle. Spread over the floor the men of the battery lay, wounded and bleeding. There was no one to care for them. I looked around for my Orderly. He was nowhere to be seen. His duty was to carry the instruments, bandages and medicines. I had nothing to work with.[58]

The barn, house, and dependencies attracted wounded men of both sides on July 1, after the battle began, and for days following. Methodist minister Leonard M. Gardner recorded his observations of the wounded at the farm on July 5, after the battle had ended:

> I found the barn above and below, the wagon shed, the tenant house, the pig sty, and the open barnyard were all crowded with badly wounded soldiers . . . In the wagon shed a few boards were laid on some trustles [trestles] and the work of amputations began. I was asked to assist in holding the limbs . . . The heat was intense . . . the odor from the wounds was repulsive. One after another was placed on the scaffold, put under chloroform and while the surgeon performed the operation, I would hold the limb until it was separated from the body![59]

Fulton found his orderly at Seminary Ridge, which was fortuitous because Fulton had just been ordered to go to the brigade hospital in town, where the army "had taken possession of the Catholic church, the Courthouse, and a great many private houses."[60] Fulton also found his hospital steward, so the three of them walked west past the Lutheran Theological Seminary on Seminary Ridge, then downhill and into town.

I found that the Catholic and Presbyterian churches on high Street had been selected as hospitals

St. Francis Xavier Catholic Church was located on High Street between Washington and Baltimore streets; the United Presbyterian and Associated Reform Church was a half block away on the corner of High Street and Baltimore Street. Dr. Fulton assumed command of both and negotiated with—or directed—neighbors of contiguous homes to open their doors to the wounded. Doubtless a red flag had been posted at both churches, the universal marker of a field hospital. Fulton's initial concerns at his field hospital were basic: "At the church we had no means of heating or cooking. It became necessary that we have fire, in order to prepare beef tea. In looking around we went into the house of a Mr. Meyers, where we had full permission to use the stove."[61]

Gettysburg resident Albertus McCreary observed the Presbyterian hospital at work: "The surgeons were at work in the hospital that adjoined our back yard. I spent hours watching them operating on the wounded. On a table out of doors operations of all kinds were performed."[62] Outside St. Francis Xavier, a Confederate officer captured Fulton:

> I went to the front into the street to see what was really going on. The first thing I knew a Confederate Major tapped me on the shoulder and said I was his prisoner. I asked him what was to be done. He told me where I would find Gen. A. P. Hill and report to him. I did so. The General asked me if we did not have a good many sick and wounded. I told him we had, not only our own men but theirs also. He politely told me to go back and do the best I could for them.[63]

Built only a decade before the battle, St. Francis Xavier was an imposing brick church of tactical value because its cupola afforded a view of the fight. An operating table was set up in the foyer just beyond the front door to take advantage of the sunlight. A few doors to the west was the private residence of Peter and Mary Meyers. These citizens, typical of many, took in wounded soldiers to convalesce in their own homes. Confederate soldiers looted some Gettysburg homes and in some cases removed ailing Union soldiers. The Meyerses' daughter, Elizabeth Salome Meyers, known as Sallie, a young teacher home for vacation, entered St. Francis to offer her assistance to wounded Bucktails. She later wrote:

> Then came the order: "Women and children to the cellars: the rebels will shell the town." We lost little time in obeying the order. My home was on West High street, near Washington, and in the direct path of the retreat [of Union soldiers]. From 4 to 6 [p.m.] we were in the cellar, and those two hours I can never forget . . . The noise above our heads, the rattle of musketry, the screeching of shells and the unearthly yells, added to the cries and terror of the children, were enough to shake the stoutest heart.

Sallie Meyers and her family emerged to find "horrible sights."

> The Roman Catholic Church and the United Presbyterian Church, a few doors east of us, on opposite sides of the street, had been taken possession of as hospitals. Dr. James Fulton . . . had been working hard to get things in some sort of shape for the wounded, who were rapidly filling the churches. He asked mother's permission to use our kitchen and cook stove for them. It was gladly given and from that time we knew no rest, day nor night, for many long weeks.
> On Thursday [July 2] morning, Dr. Fulton came to us and said, "Girls, you must come up to the churches. Our boys are suffering for want of attention . . ." I went to the Catholic church. The men were scattered all over it, some lying in the pews and some on the bare floor. The suffering and groans of the wounded and dying were terrible to see and hear . . . I knelt by the first one inside the door and said: "What can I do for you?" He looked up at me with mournful, tearless eyes, and said: "Nothing; I am going to die."
> To be met thus by the first one I addressed was more than my over-wrought nerves could bear and I went hastily out, sat down on the church step and—cried. In a little while, by a great effort, I controlled myself, re-entered the hospital and spoke again to the dying man. He was wounded in the lungs and spine and there was not the slightest hope. He was Sergeant Alexander Stewart of the [149th] Pennsylvania Volunteers . . . He asked me to read the fourteenth chapter of John. His father had read it the last morning they knelt together around their family altar.[64]

Meyers had Stewart removed to her father's home, where she cared for him until he died on July 6. Fulton arranged that all food preparation for the Catholic hospital be undertaken at the Meyers house. Over the next few days, Sallie Meyers performed many nursing tasks, including assisting at amputations.

> *I went down and found that they were all duch [German] and from the 11th Corps."*

Fulton later recounted the episode involving soldiers of the 11th Corps more charitably:

> Being busy we took no note of time until the ladies of the house, who had gone to the cellar for safety, came to me, saying that our men were crowding in upon them, and wanted me to drive them out. I tried to get the poor fellows (Eleventh Corps men) to go on and make their escape to our lines, they being on the retreat. But I could not get them to move, and many were taken prisoners that night who could easily have made their escape. They had, however, done good work; for had the Eleventh Corps not come up and supported the right of the First Corps in that first day's fight ... the rebels certainly would have captured a large portion of our corps.[65]

It is not clear whether Fulton was taken prisoner twice or whether his later account of meeting A. P. Hill was a revision of his diary narrative that he was taken to Ewell. The later account derives from Fulton's "Gettysburg Reminiscences." Fulton's observations of German-born soldiers and glimpses of his nativistic thinking are discussed in chapter 13.

> *I Should have to march again*

On July 1, Fulton left his regiment around 11:30 a.m. and shortly after noon found his two assistants. The three made their way past the seminary and into Gettysburg, the scene of much confusion. Fulton tried to assume control over the makeshift brigade hospital while cannon fire and the frantic movements of troops of both sides scared the townspeople, some of whom tried to leave town. Some hid in their homes or basements, others sought refuge in public buildings. By about four o'clock in the afternoon, following hours of stationary fighting while greatly outnumbered, the Bucktails withdrew, first to Seminary Ridge and then to Cemetery Hill.

Had Fulton remained at McPherson's farm during the afternoon, he would have exhausted himself with the casualties. The brigade lost, overall, about half its men. Virtually no officers were left standing on the field. Another Pennsylvania veteran of Gettysburg, St. Clair Augustine Mulholland (commander of the 116th Pennsylvania Infantry) later recalled the performance of the Bucktails:

> Never in the history of wars did men stand up under like conditions and make such a defence. There they were, one thin line, without a man in reserve, meeting charge after charge, and seeing beyond, as far as the eye could reach, other lines of fresh troops, ready to take the places of those repulsed. Every field officer in the brigade, save one, was shot, and many of them several times. In the One Hundred and Forty-third 36 per cent, were killed and wounded, and 91 missing, many of these being numbered among the dead; the One Hundred and Forty-ninth lost 50 per cent, killed and wounded and 111 missing; the One Hundred and Fiftieth lost 50 per cent, killed and wounded and 77 missing, 25 of whom were afterward found to be dead or wounded . . . Can we ever forget Roy Stone falling away out in front of his line, or Langhorne Wister clinging to his command with mouth so full of blood that speech was an impossibility; or Huidekoper remaining in command of his regiment with shattered arm and a ball through his leg.[66]

As fighting intensified at McPherson's farm and the contending armies maneuvered around each other north and west of Gettysburg, the town came under shelling and small-arms fire, the troops of both sides entering and leaving the town simultaneously. One street might be in Confederate possession while a column of Union infantry marched down the next. The Meyers family, in common with neighbors, hid in cellars until early evening. A local teacher, Sarah Broadhead, whose volunteer nursing at the Seminary in a few days brought her in contact with Fulton, describes the confusion:

> What to do or where to go, I did not know. People were running here and there, screaming that the town would be shelled. No one knew where to go or what to do . . . About 10 o'clock the shells began to "fly around quite thick," and I took my child and went to the house of a friend up town. As we passed up the street we met wounded men coming in from the field. When we saw them, we, for the first time, began to realize our fearful situation . . . All was bustle and confusion. No one can imagine in what extreme fright we were when our men began to retreat. A citizen galloped up to the door in which we were sitting and called out, "For God's sake go in the house! The Rebels are in the other end of town, and all will be killed!"[67]

When Broadhead and her companions—neighbors—emerged later from hiding to find the Confederates in control of the town, they found pandemonium: "How changed the town looked when we came to the light. The street was strewn over with clothes, blankets, knapsacks, cartridge-boxes, dead horses, and the bodies of a few men, but not so many of these as I expected to see."[68]

Lt. Col. Huidekoper's premonition had been prophetic. The brigade commander, Col. Stone, had been shot in the arm and hip. Col. Wister continued to lead his troops despite inability to speak due to a bullet through the mouth that removed a piece of his jaw. Maj. Chamberlin received bullet wounds to the chest and shoulder. A bullet through the leg knocked Huidekoper down, but he resumed the fight. Then a bullet pulverized his right elbow. Both Huidekoper and Chamberlin, following surgery, later recuperated at the Meyerses' home.

Between three and four o'clock, the Union line at McPherson's farm had broken, and the brigade evacuated to Cemetery Hill, periodically regrouping and exchanging fire with the advancing Confederates. By late afternoon, Gettysburg was largely in Confederate hands. On July 1, the Union army I and XI Corps had lost about nine thousand soldiers killed, wounded, missing, or captured. Despite the uncertainty of the battle, many townspeople opened their doors to the wounded, and many went forth to offer help. Fulton was aware of the identity of individual regiments and military leaders among the Confederates, even as the fight continued. He enlisted several citizens to give immediate help, not as a military officer commandeering civilians and civilian assets, but as a negotiator who persuaded citizens to volunteer their assistance in the face of calamity.

> Among those that made themselves the most useful of the citizens was M[r] Meyers and family, Mr [Solomon] Powers and his family, Miss Harriet Schilling—Mrs. R Eyster with Whom I had the pleasure of being for Some time

Mrs. R. Eyster was probably Rebecca Eyster, who ran Rebecca Eyster's Young Ladies Seminary located near the Catholic Church at High Street and Washington Street.[69] Virtually every private home in Gettysburg became a refuge for wounded and escaping soldiers. Another private home on Washington Street near High, owned by James and Catherine Foster, lodged two I Corps doctors on July 1—US Volunteers Drs. Thomas H. Bache of Philadelphia and J. Theodore Heard of Boston, attached to the Medical Director, I Corps—who narrowly escaped obliteration, as Fulton relates. On the spectrum of nursing duties performed by women, see chapter 11.

At the end of July 1, the Union line began to assume a fishhook shape as soldiers occupied high ground south and southeast of the town, the town itself in Confederate hands. The town had become one vast hospital, as public and private buildings now accommodated the wounded from both sides. Union soldiers wore armbands of white cloth to denote their status as medical assistants and found that they could move among the wounded with few restrictions. In many cases, Union soldiers and medical personnel formally surrendered to Confederate soldiers and instantly resumed their medical work: implicit to formal words of surrender was a promise, on the soldier's honor, to behave. Fulton conversed freely with Confederate soldiers and staff officers about the battlefield strategy. These conversations and his mobility attest to the relative immunity of medical personnel from incarceration as prisoners of war. Physicians' assistants such as hospital stewards, orderlies, and ambulance drivers rarely received this courtesy.

After his wounded leg and shattered elbow rendered him unfit for fighting, Lieutenant Colonel Huidekoper walked over a mile to St. Francis Xavier:

> On arrival at the Church (about 5:30 pm) I found an operating table placed in the entry, with the double doors open for light during operations . . . I went into an empty pew on the left hand side of the church . . . [and] asked some men to tear the pew door off its hinges and place it crosswise on the back and front of the pew. On this, I placed my swollen arm . . . About six o'clock . . . I went to the (operating) table and got onto it with my head towards the west. I took some chloroform but not enough, for I distinctly remember having said, "Oh, don't saw the bone until I have had more chloroform.' What I next remember was my saying, "You took my arm off, did you, Doctor?" He was [Surgeon] Dr. [Philip A.] Quinan, Surgeon of my Regiment . . . I then swung off the table feet first and was told to seek a place in the pulpit to lie down . . . stepping carefully among the hundreds of soldiers who were lying in the attic. . . Spying the gallery at the other end of the church, I worked my way back to the operating table and ascended the stairs to the gallery, which, as I had thought was empty . . . The night was a horrible one. All night long I heard from downstairs moans, groans, shrieks, and yells from the wounded and suffering soldiers."[70]

As Huidekoper rested after the surgery, he heard several Confederate officers enter the church, including Gen. Ewell, whose own left leg had been amputated owing to a wound at another battle. Ewell's officers observed the course of the battle from the church belfry. When Huidekoper heard Ewell remark, "We've licked the Yankees," he "spoke up angrily in denial."[71] Fulton's diary is not clear whether Ewell, in Fulton's presence, entered the church and ascended to the belfry: on July 2, other Confederate officers did so, accompanied by Fulton. Fulton's later recollection is that his first and only conversation with Ewell occurred on July 1, yet his meeting while the general ate his breakfast appears in his diary under the July 2 entry.

While Fulton continued his efforts to provide food, water, and medical assistance to soldiers of his brigade and others, the exhausted remnants of the Second Brigade regrouped at Cemetery Hill. William Wright (149th PA) later wrote, "I was nearly dead for water. I happened to see some water a lieing [*sic*] on a rock that had geathered [*sic*] the evening before when it rained. I was so near to give out that I lay down and drank off that rock."[72]

Fulton found lodging with Solomon and Catherine Powers at West High and Washington streets. That he found time to collect his thoughts and write in his diary is remarkable, given his prisoner status (largely unsupervised), yet he clearly felt motivated to record the events of his very full and exciting days. He must have yearned to know what became of his regiment and brigade and must have been aware that the Union lines had changed substantially since the morning. Had he ended the day with the remnant of his brigade at Cemetery Hill, he would have been aghast to learn that Second Brigade had lost 64 percent of its men.[73]

Fulton's anxiety must have intensified early in the morning of July 2 as a fierce cannonade began. Confederates lodged on Seminary Ridge began firing upon Union forces at Cemetery Hill. At the mercy of the Confederates occupying the town, Fulton reported to his captors, asking "what the program for the day was."

Diary, July 2, 1863

there was no way of providing for them unless we could get Some flour And Start our Bakery

Fulton's later reminiscence about Gettysburg elaborates on the encounter with Gen. Ewell, whom Fulton met on July 1.

I found the General eating his breakfast on the bridge-way of a small Pennsylvania barn. I saluted him as politely as I knew how. After looking me over he wanted to know my business. I stated it in as few words as possible. He wanted to know how many sick and wounded we had to feed. I told him I could not tell, owing to the confused condition of things incident to the battle; the wounded were constantly coming in; we had no record, and it was impossible to keep one; but I thought about 2,000. If we could get provisions for that many I believed we could get along.

He replied in a sharp manner that it was a queer way of doing business, wanting bread to feed people and not knowing how many there were to feed. However, he directed me to go back, and the flour would be there. I did go back, feeling fairly good. . . . The flour never came.[74]

Gen Ewell was Sitting upon the Bridge of the Barn Eating his Breakfast in quite a Soldierly like Style.

Fulton later evaluated his assessment of Ewell:

My intercourse with Gen. Ewell did not give me a very exalted opinion of the man. His bearing toward me was that of great superiority, giving the impression that it was to him a great condescension to enter into conversation with an ordinary Yank. I never saw him afterwards, and am unable to say whether the two days following knocked any of the nonsense out of him or not.[75]

Fulton contrasts Ewell with the behavior of other Confederates as "cordial and gentlemanly. Several times the pickets stopped me. They were reprimanded, and told I had the right to go where I pleased inside of their lines. I accordingly did use the privilege when there was a prospect of getting any thing [sic] for our sick and wounded, or those of the enemy in our care."[76]

In the diary for July 2, Fulton has Ewell and his staff visiting the church hospital in order to ascend to the belfry for a look at the battle. Fulton's later reminiscence, however, maintains that his encounter with Ewell while the general ate his breakfast was the only such meeting. The following anecdote about Ewell and his staff appears rather differently in the later recollection. Much of what Fulton has earlier learned about Longstreet's movements, according to the diary, came from conversations with unnamed Confederates in occupied Gettysburg. In the later account, Fulton implies that he observed Longstreet's army from the belfry in company with Confederate officers who explicated the tactics:

In the afternoon, or towards evening of July 2, as the cannonade was progressing, an old Confederate officer with his staff came along by our hospital, the Catholic church. He said "We must go up here," meaning the cupola of the church. The young men looked up, and did not seem to admire the undertaking; they did not make any move toward going. The old gentleman said: "Young men, dismount and give your horses to the Orderly." They did so, and all went up into the gallery of the church, thence to the ladder into the cupola,

I alone of our men going with them. At that time a splendid view was to be obtained of the left of our line as far as Big Round Top. At this time little or nothing can be seen. When we looked out upon the broad expanse laid before us a beautiful but terrible spectacle was presented.[77]

Sending his staff in the church to mount the cupola—that they might get a view of the Battle field

While up in the cupola, Fulton later wrote, when the battle appeared to favor the Confederates, he "was correspondingly depressed. Sick at heart, I left the lookout, went down into the gallery, and lay down upon a bench."[78] Certainly there was little impetus to be cheerful:

The evening and night of July 2 are not readily blotted from the memory of those engaged in the fight of the day. Beaten back with fearful loss in killed, wounded, and prisoners, I had seen the streets raked with grape and canister [shot] after our retreating comrades; the dead, swollen to three times their natural size, lying as they fell upon the thoroughfares of that small town. . . . The hosts of the exultant enemy were around us, declaring that on the morrow they would "clean us out" and go on their way rejoicing to Baltimore and Washington, there to dictate terms of peace of abject submission on our part."[79]

Remarkably, Fulton found time to ruminate about the promise of democracy, unpatriotic citizens, and the conduct of the battle. The diary evinces pride in Fulton's relative independence while moving about an occupied city, and his conversations with the rebels are an odd feature of this war of Americans fighting Americans. Fulton began July 1 on the march toward Gettysburg and certain battle; on this, the next day, he negotiated with the Confederate leadership for food. He must have regarded his own experiences as almost unbelievable.

Although he had a Confederate's-eye view of the Gettysburg battle, by the morning of July 3, with no direct information about his comrades, Fulton must have been apprehensive about the conduct of the fight. Early in the morning of what would be the final day of battle, Fulton might be forgiven for thinking that a calm prevailed, which may have heightened his anxiety about the fate of his brigade. Soon, musket fire awoke both sides to battle. Around 1 p.m. (Fulton records 3 p.m.), the Confederates began a massive artillery barrage preceding the most famous—and costly—attack of the three days, Pickett's Charge. The previous night, the brigade regiments were dispersed for skirmish duty, and this day they were reunited and assigned a position on the Union line south and east of the copse of trees reached by the Confederate soldiers during the attack.

Diary, July 3, 1863

of the citizens during the fight there was but one Killed And She was a young Lady or at Least calling herself such

Mary Virginia—Ginnie or Jennie—Wade, twenty-year-old Gettysburg resident, was making bread at her home when a bullet passed through two doors and struck her dead. Her notoriety began almost immediately. Fulton not only heard of her but somehow developed the opinion that her political sympathies were pro-Southern. Wade's beau was a Union soldier, and possibly she was making bread to give (or sell) to Union soldiers. In recent years, Wade has become a bulletin board for innuendo: she has been depicted as a noble patriot, a hussy, and worse.[80]

The Confederates began their withdrawal from Gettysburg and the long march back to Virginia. Many Confederate field hospitals continued operations, and the departing army abandoned its wounded to the care of Union hospitals and generous townspeople. Fulton frequently mentions Solomon Powers, his wife, Catherine, and their family at the corner of West High and Washington streets. Their daughters went out in search of wounded soldiers to bring back for nursing: "Their wounds had been dressed as skillfully as the attention could have been given by the most expert nurse; nourishing dishes had been prepared such as would appeal to the appetites of fevered and pain-worn men."[81] Daughter Alice Powers later recalled, "On Saturday morning [July 4] Dr. James Fulton came into the room where we were attending the wounded, and told us to come out and sing the 'Star Spangled Banner,' for the rebels had gone. Sure enough when we went to the door, the last gray-coat was seen going out at the end of the street."[82]

Fulton himself later recollected:

I well remember Mrs. Catherine Powers, one of the heroines of Gettysburg, coming and getting an apron full (of hard bread or "crackers") for her "poor fellows" as she styled them. Well were they cared for who had the good fortune to get into her house. The whole family gave their undivided attention to the wounded under their care. . . . They had during the time about 30; one dying, the rest recovering. . . .

After the battle provisions poured in from every quarter. Soon the Catholic church was wanted for service. We sent our patients some to one place, some to another. I went to the Courthouse for duty. It was soon wanted for the purpose of meting out justice. I then went to the Seminary. We there had Gens. [James Lawson] Kemper[83] and [Major General Isaac] Trimble,[84] a number of other Confederate officers . . . Kemper liked to have me talk with him, no doubt feeling lonely. We sometimes had it pretty warm, neither hesitating to utter his sentiments fully and frankly. A warm friendship sprang up between Kemper and me. He was a gentleman of whom I learned to think highly before we were separated by the fortunes of war.[85]

CHAPTER 4: DIARY, JULY 5, 1863, TO DECEMBER 25, 1863

Diary, July 6, 1863

Still I could find plenty to do And Still make my self as useful or more so than before

Fulton's diary entry for July 6 is an extended sketch of his regiment's whereabouts until October, when he again writes regular entries. The demands of hospital work during July and August and the traveling and troop movements during September militated against finding time to write in the diary. Fulton mentions that his work took him from the makeshift hospitals at the Presbyterian Church to the Adams County Court House and then the Lutheran Seminary. The surgeon with whom Fulton would collaborate for a few weeks, Dr. Robert Loughran, had worked at the St. Francis Xavier Church before being placed in charge at the seminary. All of these places presented a common picture immediately after the battle, described by a visitor to the Court House around July 6: "Every available place in the rooms, halls, vestibule and stairway was crowded with suffering heroes. Many had lost an arm or leg. Groans of agony were heard on every side."[86]

At the inception of the battle, the Union leadership recognized the importance of adapting the Lutheran Seminary into a hospital, so it was placed in service on July 1 under the direction of George New, surgeon in chief, First Division.[87] At the conclusion of the battle, on July 4, Surgeon Robert Loughran replaced him. The medical director of First Corps, Surgeon J. Theodore Heard, and Thomas H. Bache, medical inspector, also attended the wounded here and were captured by the Confederates. Fulton related a close call for both of them at their boarding house (see chapter 3, Diary, July 1, 1863). Fulton also encountered Sarah (Sallie) Broadhead here as she attended soldiers "wounded in every conceivable manner, some in the head and limbs, here an arm off and there a leg."[88] By the time that Fulton entered this busy hospital, about six hundred soldiers were receiving treatment, including Confederate captives and instant town celebrities Brig. James L. Kemper, who had participated in Pickett's Charge until wounded, and Maj. Gen. Isaac R. Trimble, a division commander also wounded and captured during the charge. By this time, all of Gettysburg had become "a vast hospital"; "[a]ll the public buildings are given up to their use; the churches, courthouse, college, theological seminary, are filled with the wounded, whilst all around the town for miles in every direction, hospital camps have been improvised."[89] Fulton worked for weeks before finding time to meditate again in the pages of his diary. During these weeks, he evidently formed his friendship with Kemper, later recounted in his only published memoir (see Appendix B).

Dr. Loughran And my self Roomed together And we had quite a pleasant time of it—About the first of August W^m came down to see me in

William T. Fulton, James's brother, previously a major with Purnell Legion Maryland Infantry, was at this time a lieutenant, Co. A, 29th Pennsylvania Infantry, a three-months' regiment that was organized for the defense of Pennsylvania on June 19, 1863, and mustered out on August 1, 1863.

after getting to Washington I went to [Major] Gen[eral Henry W.] Halleck

At this time, Maj. Gen. Halleck was general-in-chief of the Union army. Fulton says that he visited Washington and had an audience with Gen. Halleck, to whom he complained that rebel soldiers took his medical tools at Gettysburg, and whom he asked for an extension of leave. It would have been very unusual for the army's highest general to meet with a junior assistant surgeon to transact business appropriate for a low-ranking person. Could Fulton have named Halleck by mistake? Halleck's name appears nowhere else in the diary.

they visited the House of Dr Stringfellow Brother of the notorious Kansas Stringfellow.

The local Stringfellow family must have provided Fulton and his fellow soldiers much occasion for storytelling. War of 1812 veteran Robert String-fellow operated a farm on the Rapidan River near Culpeper. Son Benjamin Franklin Stringfellow (b. 1816) obtained a law degree and moved west with his physician brother John H. (b. 1819), later becoming attorney general for Missouri. Benjamin became a notorious "border ruffian" who agitated against antislavery or free-soil advocates vying to keep Kansas free of slavery. Another Benjamin Franklin Stringfellow (b. 1840) received a commission in the Confederate army and served under J. E. B. Stuart and John Singleton Mosby, but his most notorious experience was as a spy for Robert E. Lee. Other members of this family served in both Confederate and Union armies. A clergyman, the Reverend Thornton Stringfellow (b. 1788), published *Scriptural and Statistical Views in Favor of Slavery* in 1856. Presumably the house (known to the family as "the Retreat") Fulton visited was that of Dr. John Stringfellow, who had returned to Virginia during the 1850s.[90]

Diary, October 11, 1863

During these past weeks on the march, wounded men from Gettysburg, now recovered, rejoined their regiments, and brigade strength began to improve. Some of the Gettysburg wounded never recovered sufficiently to return to the brigade. Others, who convalesced at home, never returned to the army. Some wounded men recovered and were assigned noncombat roles such as service in the Veteran Reserve Corps. Some men deserted. Soldiers requiring long-term hospital care returned to their states for hospitalization: the states bore huge costs of soldiers' health care. Once at a remote hospital, soldiers were no longer subject to regimental oversight, and some simply disappeared. Most, however, remained with their regiments. Throughout these fall months, the brigade found itself escorting or guarding the supply wagon train or patrolling the railroad. Soldiers of the 149th, for example, manned log-built blockhouses at key places along railroad lines such as bridges.[91] Meanwhile, new draftees arrived to fill the ranks.

Throughout the diary, Fulton occasionally rails against Copperhead Democrats and those sympathetic to the South. Soldiers of the regiments forming his brigade, in common with other volunteer regiments, remained politically aware and frequently conversed about such matters. Just before the Chancellorsville campaign of spring 1863, soldiers of the 150th held a drumhead forum to rebuke Democratic antiwar press and prepared a resolution that was published in the *Washington Chronicle, Philadelphia Press,* and *New York Tribune.* It asserted loyalty and allegiance to the government and concluded:

> Resolved, That our feelings towards traitors, both North and South, is one of implacable hatred, and that, while this army has bullets for those at the South, it has also heels broad enough to crush the vile 'copperheads' of the North if they persist in their insidious attempts to weaken and overthrow the government.[92]

Similarly, during fall 1863, soldiers of the 149th formed political discussion committees and drafted resolutions supporting the re-election of Governor Andrew Curtin. Some soldiers published pro-Democrat letters in their hometown newspapers.[93]

In early October, Lee was on the march again. The previous spring, skirmishes in the same area and the cavalry battle at Brandy Station were intended to shield Lee's main force from its invasion of Maryland and Pennsylvania. Now, Gen. Meade was planning his first major post-Gettysburg offensive against Lee's forces along the Rapidan River. Lee had detached part of his force under General Longstreet to head west. On September 13, Meade's cavalry defeated Confederate cavalry at the Battle of Culpeper Courthouse, thus providing a prelude to what became known as the Bristoe Campaign. Later in September, Meade, too, detached some of his forces to move west, and Lee took the offensive. Battles occurred at Auburn on October 13–14, Bristoe Station on October 14, Buckland on October 19, and Remington (or Rappahannock Station), all in Virginia, on November 7. Confederates were able to take the railroad tracks and force the Union line back northwest along the Orange-Alexandria Railroad, which the brigade had earlier secured. Fulton was near the scene of fighting on October 13–14 at which Confederate Lt. Gen. A. P. Hill precipitously attacked well-positioned federal soldiers firing behind a railway embankment. Hill's soldiers suffered a significant loss. The brigade remained marginal to the battles and skirmishes and assumed the defense of Centreville, Meade's main base.

Diary, October 20, 1863

Reaching that place about Dark we passed through the Gap a short Distance and stoped for the night the night being dark we could not see much

The march through Thoroughfare Gap occurred in the rain, along muddy roads, records the 149th. The weeks on the march had taken a toll, as the soldiers' uniforms were worn, torn, and many soldiers were shoeless, but by October 23, supplies had caught up with the brigade.[94] After advancing as far as Haymarket, in a few days, the brigade returned through the gap to Bristoe, being responsible for guarding the wagons.[95]

Diary, November 6, 1863

Despite Fulton's exultation in the countryside, fall rains and freezing nights had set in. The 149th experienced a bout of typhoid fever that caused five deaths.[96] Although missing action elsewhere, brigade soldiers remained vigilant for Confederates. Soldiers feared guerrillas: partisan ranger John Singleton Mosby and his cavalry threatened troops in relatively unprotected areas, and, indeed, some brigade soldiers were taken prisoner by his men. The Mine Run Campaign consisted of skirmishes and minor battles from November 7 to December 2 between forces under Meade and Lee. Meade tried to secure an advantage over Lee, whose troops occupied a defensive line along the Rappahannock River, but the indecisive warfare in cold, rainy weather accomplished no tactical gains for either side, leaving both commanders frustrated. As winter approached, federal troops created a winter camp near Paoli's Mill, not far from Kelly's Ford.

Diary, "/Warrenton Junction Nov 1863—/,"

What Fulton saw on November 7 is unclear. Union Maj. Gen. John Sedgwick and VI Corps fought the Confederates at Rappahannock Station and forced their retreat from the Rappahannock River to the Rapidan. Fulton appears to admire Sedgwick's brash evening attack that overran fortified rebel positions with hand-to-hand fighting. Shortly after, Meade sent II Corps, III Corps, and V Corps to Mine Run Creek in an effort to flank Lee, but the campaign, which did not involve Fulton's brigade, proved inconclusive. The 3rd Division of I Corps, which included the 143rd, remained on station along the railroad and apparently did not participate in the battle on November 7. Railroad security continued to be the chief occupation of the brigade until it reached winter camp in late November.[97]

Diary, November 8, 1863

Men Sometimes get panic Stricken when no Reason can be assigned or imagined.

Seven men from the Brigade were indeed taken prisoner by Mosby's Raiders at their camp on an extreme end of the railroad line on November 30.[98] See chapter 13 for additional discussion of bravery and panic.

Diary, November 19, 1863

Fulton, refers, of course to the formal dedication of the National Cemetery at Gettysburg and the delivery of the famous address by President Lincoln. The cemetery was organized and funded in only four months, and at its dedication, bodies of Union soldiers were still being removed from temporary graves and reinterred there.

Diary, November 22, 1863

Cap[tain] Rickhard with his Company was left back with at the Bridge nearest Manassas.

On November 30, the 150th Pennsylvania received orders to form a detachment of men to guard nearby Licking Run Bridge, a short distance from Warrenton Junction. Supervising officers worried about Mosby's Raiders, who invaded the camp that very evening and captured several soldiers, including some of the 143rd and 149th Pennsylvania.[99]

Diary, November 29, 1863

The Battle of Mine Run occurred between November 27 and December 2. Fulton probably describes a series of engagements between Union forces of III Corps (joined by II Corps) and Ewell's Corps Confederate troops under Maj. Gen. Jubal A. Early. Fulton's brigade was not involved in the fighting.

DIARY, NOVEMBER 30, 1863

The Mine Run campaign had ended, and the brigade settled in for what soldiers hoped would be winter quarters. One soldier of the 149th wrote in a letter, "We have here a pretty camp, plenty of wood and water and comfortable shanties to live in. These shanties are well built of round logs and covered with clapboards like those of the first settlers, having weight poles to keep the wind from blowing them off."[100]

Diary, December 8–9, 1863

The 150th records more details about Wister's arrest:

> At the mills, not far from the camp, were a number of old wooden buildings, entirely unoccupied, and by permission of Colonel Wister . . . the men of his command helped themselves to the boards, using them as flooring for their tents. The owner of the property entered complaint at General Newton's head-quarters, and by the general's order Colonel Wister was put in arrest. This engendered a storm of indignation throughout the corps, which grew in intensity . . . until its echoes reached the ears of the corps commander. Colonel Wister was very popular among all the officers, by whom his action was thoroughly approved, and, with his Quaker-like views of what was permissible in the enemy's country in time of war, there was no disposition on his part to make any apology for his conduct.[101]

A few days later, Wister was released to resume his duties.

Diary, December 19, 1863

they will be at home just in time to Enjoy Christmas they have ten day's Leave.

Granting furloughs was one of the commanding officer's greatest prerogatives. A furlough held great medicinal significance owing to nostalgia, at the time a diagnosable illness. A homesick soldier might not only decline in personal health and performance, but might infect comrades with the same malady. The only sure remedy for nostalgia was to send the sick soldier home for a short visit. Surgeon Thomas T. Ellis wrote, "Experience had taught me that men suffering from wounds and the long-continued privations of camp life, would recover much sooner under the kind care of home and friends than in a military hospital, and thus return to their duty in far less time than if kept in general hospitals."[102]

CHAPTER 5: DIARY, DECEMBER 26, 1863,
TO JANUARY 29, 1864

Fulton's regiment had seen eight months of continuous frontline duty and finally settled into winter quarters. Until the last few weeks, unrelieved tension and worry must have preoccupied many soldiers as they performed their duties in an unfriendly environment. The regiment had been functioning at approximately half strength for several months despite periodic infusions of new recruits. Fulton may well have thought that he had done laudable service and it was time to go home. He may have been disappointed at an apparent lack of progress compared with campaigns the previous spring. Perhaps Fulton was distressed with the larger political or military scene. His brigade had revisited places in Virginia where his regiment had marched and camped in the months leading to Gettysburg, and now Union and Confederate armies seemed to dance precariously around the same towns, rivers, and creeks. In common with many soldiers and surgeons, his desire to return home may have been his chief motivation to leave the war to others: he gives his reason in the diary as his wife's illness. Fulton's diary ends with a discussion of his own resignation, and he describes other soldiers and their officers who have been examined for disability discharge.

A description of winter quarters for the 150th Pennsylvania probably speaks to Fulton's situation:

[A] model camp was completed, as accurate in its alignments and snug in its construction as a well-ordered New England village. To insure proper drainage, the company streets were cleared of stumps, and surface sewers hollowed out on each side, leading down the slope to the little valley below. Then, by incessant raids on the commissary department, enough empty boxes were finally secured to furnish each hut with a substantial floor . . . When all was finished, the regiment was justly proud of its camp, which in symmetry and picturesqueness was probably not surpassed by any in the army.[103]

Fulton may also have thought that his regiment—his brigade—had changed so much over the previous year that the social order had become less recognizable. An earlier sense of a close-knit regiment and brigade may have been dissolving. A reorganization was in progress. During early 1864, I and III Corps were dissolved and consolidated within II, V, and VI Corps. The Bucktail Brigade remained intact as 1st Brigade, 3rd Division, I Corps until March, 1864, whereupon they became 3rd Brigade, 4th Division, V Corps until June, 1864. Between June and September, they were 1st Brigade, 1st Division, V Corps. After September, Fulton's regiment, the 143rd, was detached from the 149th and 150th Pennsylvania and assigned 1st Brigade, 3rd Division, V Corps until February, 1865, when the 143rd was assigned to Hart's Island, New York Harbor, Department of the East, until the regiment mustered out in June 1865.

While Surgeon C. E. Humphrey, who mustered in with the 143rd just before Gettysburg (May 25, 1863) remained with the regiment until it mustered out in 1865, as did Surgeon Francis C. Reamer (mustered in September 16, 1862), both assistant surgeons left in spring 1864. Fulton and David L. Scott were discharged on April 8. These men were replaced by I. C. Hogendobler (mustered in September 7, 1864) and Edward Brobst (mustered in December 27, 1864).

By February, when the brigade was stirred to action once again, General Meade remained in charge, but Ulysses S. Grant had been placed in overall command as lieutenant general. The brutal Overland Campaign was beginning, and had Fulton remained, he would have found himself at the Wilderness, where many of his old comrades lost their lives.

Diary, December 27, 1863

James Lawson Kemper (1823–1895), a career politician and lawyer from Virginia, was colonel of the 7th Virginia Infantry and later achieved the rank of brigadier general. Wounded at Pickett's Charge in Gettysburg, he was a prisoner of the Union army until September, 1864, when he was released, promoted to major general, and placed in charge of Virginia reserve troops. Kemper's Brigade at Gettysburg consisted of five Virginia regiments, including the 7th. Fulton befriended Kemper while he recuperated from wounds at the Lutheran Seminary in Gettysburg. See chapter 3 and Appendix B.

Diary, December 30, 1863

Night about dark I was Called to See a little daughter of Mrs. Green.

The Green family made an impression. The regimental histories of the 149th and 150th PA record family members. Near Culpeper Court House, the 143rd and 149th PA bivouacked on the property of "a comely widow of most lady-like manners and still in the freshness of her womanhood," Mrs. Green, in whose "delightful old mansion" Col. Langhorne Wister (at this time commanding the 121st, 142nd, 143rd, 149th, and 150th PA) and some brigade staff lodged.[104]

Diary, January 1, 1864

In lieu of reflecting on the past year and wondering what was to come, Fulton's first experience of the new year is admiration of nature and meditating on God's purposes. The day before, Surgeon William Mervale Smith, 85th New York, at this time in North Carolina, recorded in his diary for December 31:

> It is the last day of December—how swiftly has it gone—and the year, too, has gone. One of the most eventful in the history of civilization. To me, it has been one of the hardest, most perilous and diversified with the most extraordinary experiences of my life. It made its record in my intellect, and my physical powers, which will never be effaced. It is scarcely possible that the coming year will bring to me so many & varied and wonderful experiences as the year that is closing."[105]

No More Furloughs will be granted on account of So Many Reinlisting in the Veteran Corps.

In April 1863, the War Department created the Veteran Reserve Corps, originally called the Invalid Corps. Officers and enlisted soldiers too disabled to perform as soldiers in the field but capable of handling light duty were assigned to the corps. Most of these soldiers performed guard or garrison duty or served as clerical personnel or cooks. Many recovering or convalescent soldiers in hospitals, under medical supervision but still carried on the army muster rolls, were detailed to the corps. Soldiers honorably discharged from service could re-enlist in the corps for light duty.

Diary, January 7, 1864

Fulton's associate, Assistant Surgeon Henderson, also records several smallpox vaccinations in his diary for 1863. His diary, written in a "homeopathic repertory," contains a section labeled "Vaccination Engagement," where he lists four soldiers by name and company whom he vaccinated, each with an entry to indicate that the vaccination "took." The vaccination page contains columns for "NAME AND ADDRESS," "DATE OF VACCINATION," "TAKEN OR NOT," and "REMARKS." The successfully vaccinated soldiers are:

- Private Simon Trainer, Company C (mustered August 30, 1862; killed at Gettysburg on July 1, 1863)
- Private "Jery [Jerimiah] Clark," Company H (mustered September 4, 1862, wounded at Spotsylvania on May 12, 1864, and discharged due to wounds)
- "Jos Cundy" [Lundy?] (no record of either name in the 150th)
- "A. [Andrew T.] Harvey," Company H, (mustered August 28, 1862, wounded at Gettysburg and mustered out, June 3, 1865)

Diary, January 8, 1864

we got a detail of 3 Men for Nurses for our Hospital.

The men detailed as nurses did not have medical training. Rather, they were judged incapable of performing combat duty and were therefore assigned as general hospital assistants.

Diary, January 11, 1864

During these days of early January, when Fulton occupied his time in examining soldiers for possible medical discharge and an alarming appearance of smallpox, the weather was brutally cold. The 150th PA records: "Of course, in such weather, with the ground frozen and rough beyond description, drilling was not even thought of, and as both camp and picket details were light, there was ample leisure for reading and reflection, social visits, and card-playing, especially the latter."[106] Despite the cold, as they settled into their winter quarters, the 149th resumed the military rituals of two drills and one dress parade daily, weather permitting.[107]

Diary, January 12, 1864

I think that Wm Porter will have Nothing More than Varioloid.

Now officially eradicated from the planet (except for samples kept at two secure laboratories, one in the United States and the other in Russia), smallpox was characterized by a weeks-long cycle of symptoms that began with fever and malaise, and progressed through vomiting, aches and pains, and the appearance of skin eruptions that became pustules and scabs. People who survived displayed scars or pits that remained after the scabs disappeared. Doctors of Fulton's era characterized the disease as either distinct or confluent. The distinct version involved the aforementioned symptoms. The confluent version observed the same symptoms but with more severity and usually caused death. According to a contemporary medical text, "Both the distinct and confluent small-pox are produced either by breathing air impregnated with the effluvia arising from the bodies of those who labor under the disease, or by the introduction of a small quantity of variolous matter into the habit by inoculation."[108]

Second Gettysburg narrative

And the Brave Color Bearer was Benj Crippen of Co E 143 Pa.

Fulton refers to an article that appeared during 1863 in *Blackwood's Magazine* (published in Edinburgh, Scotland) that featured an account of Gettysburg by a British colonel who accompanied Confederate troops as an observer. The colonel narrates the moment:

> [General A. P. Hill] pointed out a railway cutting, in which they had made a good stand; also, a field in the centre of which he had seen a man plant the regimental colour, round which the regiment had fought for some time with much obstinacy, and when at last it was obliged to retreat, the colour-bearer retired last of all, turning around every now and then to shake his fist at the advancing rebels. General Hill said he felt quite sorry when he saw this gallant Yankee meet his doom.[109]

Today, near the reconstructed McPherson's Farm at the Gettysburg battlefield, a monument stands to the 143rd Pennsylvania that bears a relief sculpture of Sgt. Crippen shaking his fist.

Medical Recipes

"Capt Gimber"

Fulton evidently planned to write a note about or involving Capt. Henry W. Gimber, Co. F, 150th Pennsylvania, as this name appears above the text margin, below which a recipe appears, apparently written at another time.

The recipe(s) that follows may be unrelated to Gimber. Gimber was captured by the Confederates on July 1 at Gettysburg and remained a prisoner of war until March 1865. Gimber's account of his POW experience appears in the regimental history of the 150th.[110] It is unlikely that Fulton would have received any word about Gimber's fate while he was still on active service.

"~~Captain Janey~~"

"Captain Janey" does not appear to relate to the recipe that follows. The only soldier in Fulton's brigade with a similar name was Capt. Benjamin F. Janney, Co. E, 150th PA, who was commissioned captain on September 1, 1862, and resigned the following month on October 16.

"~~Cap. Elsegood~~"

"Cap Elsegood" does not appear to be related to the recipe that follows. According to the regimental history of the 150th PA, William A. Elsegood helped recruit soldiers for the 150th when the regiment was first formed. At the time, he served in the 66th PA, but he transferred to the 99th PA as a lieutenant in Co. H, where he was promoted to captain on March 3, 1862.[111] He resigned his commission on July 4. Fulton may have written the names of Janey, Gimber, and Elsegood during his early service with the 150th, but his intentions in doing so are unknown. He may have wanted to record what he prescribed to fellow officers.

"Orderly Sergeant W. S. Leach"

William S. Leach was mustered in as sergeant, Co. G, 143rd PA on September 18, 1862, and discharged into the Veterans Reserve Corps on November 15, 1863. Perhaps this recipe relates to a medical reason for Leach's discharge. This recipe appears to be the only one in Fulton's diary explicitly linked to a soldier.

"~~——— For Cap~~ Pine"

The above crossed-out entry may have been made when Fulton was first mustered into the 150th during its active recruiting phase. Capt. Pine is Lieutenant William S. Pine, later promoted to captain of Co. E, 150th PA.

NOTES

1. University of Pennsylvania, *Catalog of the Trustees, Officers, and Students of the University of Pennsylvania, Session 1862–63* (Philadelphia: Collins, 1863), online at http://www.archives.upenn.edu/primdocs/upl/upl1/upl1_1862_63.pdf, accessed October 22, 2018.

2. Ewing Jordan, *University of Pennsylvania Men Who Served in the Civil War*, Pt. 1, Department of Medicine Classes 1816–1862 (Philadelphia, 1900), online at https://archive.org/stream/universityofpenn00jord#page/n5/mode/2up, accessed October 22, 2018.

3. Circumstances of the creation of the 143rd, 149th, and 150th Pennsylvania Volunteer Regiments are detailed in: Thomas Chamberlin, *History of the One Hundred and Fiftieth Regiment Pennsylvania Volunteers, Second Regiment, Bucktail Brigade* (Philadelphia: J. B. Lippincott, 1895); Richard E. Matthews, *The 149th Pennsylvania Volunteer Infantry Unit in the Civil War* (Jefferson, NC: McFarland & Company, 1994); and Samuel P. Bates, *History of Pennsylvania Volunteers 1861–65*, vol. 4 (Harrisburg, PA: B. Singerly, 1870). Hereinafter referred to simply as Chamberlin, Matthews, and Bates.

4. Chamberlin, 26.

5. Quoted at Matthews, 4.

6. The size and situation of Camp Curtin can be gauged by a tour of extant landmarks. See Lawrence E. Keener-Farley and James E. Schmick, eds., *Civil War Harrisburg, A Guide to Capital Area Sites, Incidents and Personalities*, rev. ed. (Harrisburg, PA: Camp Curtin Historical Society, 2014).

7. Mart A. Stewart, "Walking, Running, and Marching into an Environmental History of the Civil War," in *The Blue, the Gray, and the Green: Toward an Environmental History of the Civil War*, ed. Brian Allen Drake (Athens: University of Georgia Press, 2015), 210.

8. Cooper H. Wingert, *Harrisburg and the Civil War* (Charleston, SC: 2013), e-book; William Henry Egle, *Notes and Queries Historical and Genealogical Chiefly Relating to Interior Pennsylvania*, vol. 1 (Harrisburg: Harrisburg Publishing Company, 1894), 293–4

9. Chamberlin, 70; Henderson, Diary, 1863, National Museum of American History/Smithsonian Institution, object #MG*M-09670. On Henderson's class at Jefferson Medical College, see "Part I: Jefferson Medical College 1855 to 1865," in *Thomas Jefferson University—A Chronological History and Alumni Directory, 1824–1990*, ed. Frederick B. Wagner Jr. and J. Woodrow Savacool (Philadelphia: Thomas Jefferson University, 1992), 29; online at http://jdc.jefferson.edu/wagner1/17, accessed October 22, 2018. The record of Henderson's examination for assistant surgeon is found in the Record Book of Candidates Examined by Pennsylvania State Medical Board for Surgeons and Assistant Surgeons, 1861–1865, RG 19.169, Pennsylvania State Archives, Harrisburg.

10. Matthews, 31; Chamberlin, 47.

11. Chamberlin, 46; Henderson, February [no day] 1863.

12. Ibid., 49. Henderson also describes Washington similarly as a city of "'magnificent distances' + filled with splendid edifices of marble belonging to Government." Henderson, February 1, 1863.

13. Henderson, February [no day], 1863.

14. Ibid., February 2, 1863.

15. Finial; the dome was still under construction.

16. Ibid.

17. Henderson, February 7, 1863.

18. Matthews, 36.

19. Henderson, February 15–16, 1863.

20. Quoted in Matthews, 40.

21. Peter Josyph, ed., *The Wounded River: The Civil War Letters of John Vance Lauderdale, M.D.* (East Lansing: Michigan State University Press, 1993), 61. Letter to sister, May 2, 1862.

22. On January 26, 1863.

23. Chamberlin, 59.

24. Christopher E. Loperfido, ed., *A Surgeon's Tale: The Civil War Letters of Surgeon James D. Benton, 111th and 98th New York Infantries 1862–1865* (Gettysburg, PA: Ten Roads, 2011), 73. Letter to parents, March 6, 1864.

25. Gen. Abner Doubleday, who would assume command of I Corps on July 1, 1863, at Gettysburg.

26. I Corps, US Volunteers, Surgeon Thomas H. Bache of Philadelphia.

27. Henderson, February 26, 1863.

28. Chamberlin, 60.

29. Henderson, date uncertain.

30. Matthews, 57.

31. Josyph, *Wounded* River, 55. Letter dated April 28, 1862.

32. Henderson, May 2, 1863.

33. James M. Greiner, Janet L. Coryell, and James R. Smither, eds., *A Surgeon's Civil War: The Letters and Diary of Daniel M. Holt, M.D.* (Kent, OH: Kent State University Press, 1994), 24.

34. Chamberlin, 97.

35. Henderson, May 29, 1863.

36. Commander of the 150th Pennsylvania.

37. Henderson, letter to sister, "'Wilderness' near Chancell'ville," May 3, 1863.

38. Thomas P. Lowry and Jack D. Welsh, *Tarnished Scalpels: The Court-Martials of Fifty Union Surgeons* (Mechanicsburg, PA: Stackpole Books, 2000), 183.

39. Greiner et al., *A Surgeon's Civil War*, 101.

40. Ibid., 102.

41. John Gardner Perry, *Letters from a Surgeon of the Civil War*, comp. Martha Derby Perry (Boston: Little, Brown, 1906), 152.

42. Quoted in Matthews, 73.

43. The chief sources regarding the campaign of the Bucktails preceding and during the Gettysburg battle are David G. Martin, *Gettysburg July 1* (Conshohocken, PA: Combined Books, Inc., 1995); Matthews, *149th Pennsylvania Volunteer Infantry*; James J. Dougherty, *Stone's Brigade and the Fight for the McPherson Farm* (Conshohocken, PA: Combined Publishing, 2001); Bates, *History of Pennsylvania Volunteers*; Thomas Chamberlin, online at http://files.usgwarchives.net/pa/1pa/military/cwar/150-bucktails/bucktail-13.txt, accessed October 22, 2018; and Stewart Sifakis, *Who Was Who in the Civil War* (New York: Facts on File Publications, 1988).

44. Quoted in Matthews, *149th Pennsylvania Volunteer Infantry*, 75.

45. James Fulton, "Gettysburg Reminiscences: A Surgeon's Story," *National Tribune* (Washington, DC), October 20, 1898.

46. Chamberlin, 115.

47. The Emmitsburg Historical Society website details the founding and history of its Catholic institutions online at http://www.emmitsburg.net/history/index.htm, accessed October 22, 2018.

48. Matthews, 75.

49. Henry M. Rogers, "Henry Shippen Huidekoper," *Harvard Graduates' Magazine* 27 (March, 1919): 325–6.

50. Chamberlin, 117.

51. Quoted in Matthews, 79.

52. Chamberlin, 118–9.

53. Ibid.

54. Fulton, "Gettysburg Reminiscences."

55. Chamberlin, 120.

56. St. Clair Augustine Mulholland, *The Story of the 116th Regiment Pennsylvania Volunteers in the War of the Rebellion* (Philadelphia: F. McManus, Jr., 1903), online at http://www .archive.org/stream/storyof116thregio2mulho#page/n9/mode/2up, accessed October 22, 2018, 143.

57. Ibid.

58. Fulton, "Gettysburg Reminiscences."

59. Quoted in Gregory A. Coco, *A Vast Sea of Misery: A History and Guide to the Union and Confederate Field Hospitals at Gettysburg July 1–November 20, 1863* (Gettysburg, PA: Thomas Publications, 1988), 6.

60. Fulton, "Gettysburg Reminiscences."

61. Ibid.

62. Quoted in Coco, *Vast Sea of Misery*, 18.

63. Fulton, "Gettysburg Reminiscences."

64. Elizabeth Salome Myers, "How a Gettysburg Schoolteacher Spent Her Vacation in 1863," *San Francisco Call*, August 16, 1903, online at http://chroniclingamerica.loc.gov/lccn /sn85066387/1903-08-16/ed-1/, accessed October 22, 2018.

65. Fulton, "Gettysburg Reminiscences."

66. Mulholland, *Story of the 116th* Regiment, 144. For additional details of the McPherson farm fight, see Dougherty, *Stone's Brigade*.

67. Sarah Broadhead, *The Diary of a Lady of Gettysburg, Pennsylvania from June 15 to July 15, 1863* (privately published, no date), 14.

68. Ibid.

69. "Gettysburg Female Institute Artillery Projectile," *Gettysburg Daily* blog, January 16, 2009, http://www.gettysburgdaily.com/gettysburg-female-institute-artillery-projectile/, accessed October 22, 2018.

70. Quoted in Martin, *Gettysburg July 1*, 456.

71. Henry M. Rogers, "Henry Shippen Huidekoper," 326.

72. Quoted in Dougherty, *Stone's* Brigade, 105.

73. Ibid.

74. Fulton, "Gettysburg Reminiscences."

75. Ibid.

76. Ibid.

77. Ibid.

78. Ibid.

79. Ibid.

80. Wade has been portrayed as a spy, as a woman of loose morals, a hero, an innocent casualty of war, and other characterizations. It would be interesting to learn why Fulton was so dismissive of her. The Wade controversy is recounted and analyzed in Noah Trudeau,

Gettysburg: A Testing of Courage (New York: Harper Collins, 2002); and Ericson, "'The world will little note nor long remember,'" in *Making and Remaking Pennsylvania's Civil War*, ed. William Blair and William Pencak (University Park: Pennsylvania State University Press, 2001), 81–102.

81. Alice Powers, "Dark Days of the Battle Week," *The Compiler* (Gettysburg), July 1, 1903.

82. Ibid.

83. Kemper arrived in Gettysburg on July 2, participated in Pickett's Charge on July 3, and was wounded and captured.

84. On July 3, Trimble assumed command of Pender's Division, 3rd Corps, Army of Northern Virginia, was wounded in Pickett's Charge and lost a leg as a result.

85. Fulton, "Gettysburg Reminiscences."

86. Quoted in Coco, *Vast Sea of Misery*, 22.

87. Michael A. Dreese, *The Hospital on Seminary Ridge at the Battle of Gettysburg* (Jefferson, NC: McFarland, 2002), 72.

88. Broadhead, *Diary of a Lady*, 17.

89. Dreese, *Hospital on Seminary Ridge*, 92, 133, 142, "vast hospital" quotation from the July 16, 1863, edition of *Lutheran and Missionary*, cited at 120.

90. Family details can be found in various genealogical sources including *Portrait and Biographical Record of Buchanan and Clinton Counties, Missouri* (Chicago: Chapman Bros, 1893), 171, online at http://cdm.sos.mo.gov/cdm/ref/collection/mocohist/id/38868, accessed October 22, 2018; and R. Shepard Brown, *Stringfellow of the Fourth* (New York: Crown, 1960).

91. Matthews, 114.

92. Chamberlin, 65.

93. Matthews, 114.

94. Ibid., 116.

95. Chamberlin, 156.

96. Matthews, 116.

97. *Encyclopedia Virginia* features a comprehensive overview to the Mine Run Campaign and related engagements online at http://www.encyclopediavirginia.org/Mine_Run _Campaign#start_entry, accessed October 22, 2018.

98. Matthews, 117.

99. Chamberlin, 165; Matthews, 117.

100. Matthews, 117.

101. Chamberlin, 165.

102. Thomas T. Ellis, *Leaves from the Diary of an Army Surgeon* (New York: John Bradburn, 1863), 80.

103. Chamberlin, 169.

104. Ibid., 168.

105. Thomas P. Lowry, ed., *Swamp Doctor: The Diary of a Union Surgeon in the Virginia & North Carolina Marshes* (Mechanicsville, PA: Stackpole Books, 2001), 107.

106. Chamberlin, 171.

107. Matthews, 119.

108. W. Beach, *The American Practice of Medicine, Revised, Enlarged, and Improved: Being a Practical Exposition of Pathology, Therapeutics, Surgery, Materia Medica, and Pharmacy, on Reformed Principles* (New York: Charles Scribner, 1855), 455–8.

109. "The Battle of Gettysburg and the Pennsylvania Campaign. Extract from the Diary of an English Officer present with the Confederate Army," *Blackwood's Edinburgh Magazine*, 94 (September 1863), 377.

110. Chamberlin, 266–71.

111. Ibid., 16–7; Bates, vol. 3, 540.

PART II

EIGHT

"Examined at the University of Pennsylvania"

Dr. Fulton, His Professional Milieu, and Military Medicine 1862–1864

SHAUNA DEVINE

BECOMING A CIVIL WAR SURGEON

On August 18, 1862, Dr. James Fulton noted in his diary, "To Day at 12 o clock Received orders from Surgeon General H. H. Smith to report to Dr. Nelson at Harrisburg as Soon as possible. packing up in All haste."[1] Thus began James Fulton's service as an assistant surgeon in the 150th Regiment of the Pennsylvania Volunteers. On November 11, 1862, he was transferred to the 143rd Regiment, Bucktail Brigade, where he would doctor until he was honorably discharged from service on April 8, 1864.[2] Fulton had only been in professional practice for two years before entering the service, and his time doctoring during the Civil War profoundly influenced his training and development as a physician.

One month before he received his official orders, Fulton sat for a standardized medical examination, which was required for entrance to the Army Medical Department. His examination was administered by the Pennsylvania State Medical Board for Surgeons and Assistant Surgeons. Four physicians examined Fulton on various subjects, including the distinguished Joseph Leidy and Henry Hollingsworth Smith, both of whom were, in addition to being newly appointed senior officers in the militia, members of the University of Pennsylvania faculty. The two remaining examiners were Drs. Greene and Stewart, appointees of the state authorities to examine candidates for service.[3]

The examining boards had been reformed just weeks earlier as part of newly appointed Surgeon General William Hammond's ongoing efforts to reorganize the Army Medical Department along more scientific and professional standards.[4] Under Hammond's guidance and the new three-year militia act, physicians looking for regular army commissions or seeking promotion were required to sit for a multipart examination, which consisted of a written examination on the basic principles of anatomy, surgery, and the practice of medicine; an oral examination on anatomy, surgery, and the practice of medicine and pathology; another oral examination on chemistry, physiology, hygiene, toxicology, and *materia medica* (the study of the properties of substances used for medicines); a clinical, medical, and surgical examination at a hospital; an examination on a cadaver; the performance of a surgical operation; and an essay (see Appendix A).[5] The exam that Hammond designed was difficult. He reasoned that the Union troops deserved the best care possible and thus the best practicing physicians in the country. When the mixed results of the examinations were revealed in 1862–1863, Hammond began the practice of reaching out to medical reformers and prominent professors with suggestions on how to better structure and reform medical school curricula along more scientific guidelines.[6] Hammond's larger program of reform mirrored the agendas of the leading medical reformers of the day (mostly medical school teachers, journal editors, and physicians with postgraduate experience in the Paris Clinical School or German states who saw firsthand the benefit of more stringent academic requirements), who advocated for more science, clinical knowledge, and hospital instruction in the curriculum, longer periods of study for medical students and physicians, and especially more unity among the profession.[7]

The immediate goals of the medical exams were twofold. On one hand, by placing eminent and well-educated physicians such as Joseph Leidy and H. H. Smith on the boards, military leadership hoped that the highest medical standards would be achieved, since, in their evaluation of the candidates, they were expected to emphasize current medical trends, the most up-to-date scientific knowledge, and professionalism. In the years leading to the war, there was a professional backlash against both the proliferation of proprietary medical schools and some of their graduates, along with complaints about the overall weakness of the apprenticeship system.[8] The tough entrance exam was, in part, seen by some reformers as an opportunity to eliminate those

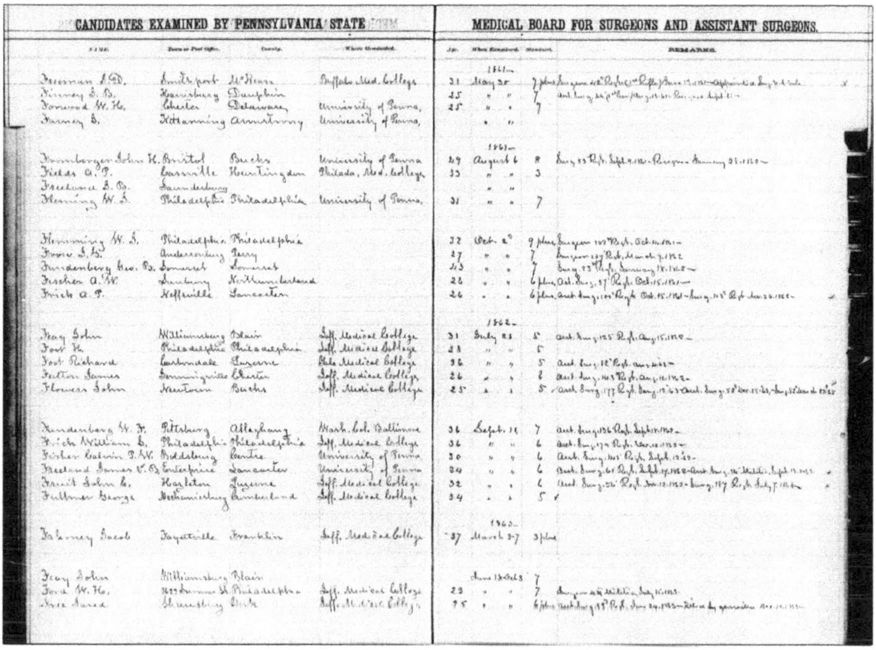

Figure 8.1. The Pennsylvania record of James Fulton's examination pass to become an assistant surgeon in the army. Fulton appears in a group with other candidates whose surnames begin with the letter F who graduated from Jefferson Medical College. Column headings include Name, Town or Post Office, Where Graduated, Age, When Examined, Standard, and Remarks. Under Remarks, it is noted that Fulton has been assigned to the 143rd PA as an assistant surgeon. Credit: 19.174 Reports of Examination Roll 6835, Pennsylvania State Archives, Harrisburg.

deemed less competent due to a lack of formal training or those practicing alternative medicine such as homeopathy. Fulton, a graduate of the prestigious Jefferson Medical College, passed his exam and was appointed in the militia August 18, 1862, at the rank of assistant surgeon.

BECOMING A DOCTOR

Following his earlier education (see chapter 1), from 1855–1859, Fulton studied with a preceptor, his cousin Dr. Thomas H. Thompson of Oxford, Pennsylvania, while also attending Jefferson Medical College, where he earned his MD degree in 1859.[9] He was the type of candidate that Hammond envisioned in the reformed Army Medical Department. Unlike some American physicians during the Civil War, Fulton was well educated. While a number of students entered medical school without having obtained a college education, there were those with means or opportunity, such as Fulton, who obtained a college degree before medical school. However, this was a smaller portion of the students, which represented the class differences in education before the war. Indeed, for an ambitious, wealthy student in the long-settled eastern United States, there were not only considerable educational opportunities in the medical field but also a network of professionals devoted to helping each other succeed, and these social connections became increasingly important during the war years.

There were different paths to becoming a medical doctor prior to the Civil War. Before 1820, the apprenticeship system served as the principal mode of medical training. Numerous medical practitioners, even in leading centers such as Philadelphia, New York, and Boston, practiced medicine without a medical degree. After 1820, however, the number of medical schools in America grew from just six to 47. There were also more than a dozen sectarian schools established in the Jacksonian era. Beginning in 1820, as William Rothstein has demonstrated, the number of medical school graduates grew steadily from 1,375 in 1819 to 17,213 on the eve of the Civil War.[10] The growth of proprietary schools was possible because there was little guidance for each state on a common set of educational and medical standards, since the value of science was debated, and there was almost no professional consensus on what was needed. Thus, in the 1830s and 1840s, the penalties for practicing without a medical license were ignored or removed, coinciding with the withdrawal of state recognition for medical societies.[11] While this led to the formation of a new unregulated medical marketplace, it also intensified the competition between orthodox and unorthodox physicians and elite and rank-and-file orthodox physicians.

Efforts to address the problems compounded by the growth of medical schools along with the desire to institute larger reforms within American medicine took shape in 1847–1848 with the creation of the American Medical Association (AMA). Despite the efforts of the reformers, however, the objectives of the new AMA did not amount to significant change until after the Civil War. In part, this was because the orthodox medical profession had been widely derided by the public for its promotion of heroic medical remedies and grave-robbing scandals.[12] Moreover, medical education still lacked unified standards, and thus there was a general lack of cohesion within the profession. Depending on a practitioner's setting and interests, some thought that scientific medicine was useful, while others did not know how the pathological science coming from Europe would benefit the immediate and daily care of their patients. Further, competing medical sects posed challenges, because some advocated less-intrusive treatments, which resonated with the public. Finally, the competition between medical schools for students, rather than students competing for entrance into medical schools, was fierce, and thus, larger professional reforms were still years away.[13]

Fulton studied in Philadelphia, where the growth in educational facilities was striking before the war. He attended one of the most prestigious proprietary schools, Jefferson Medical College, which was founded in 1825 using the state charter of Jefferson College in Canonsburg, Pennsylvania. Shortly afterward, the Medical Department of Pennsylvania College was formed (1839), followed by Philadelphia College of Medicine (1847) and Franklin Medical College (1847), making Philadelphia the prewar epicenter of medical education. Jefferson Medical College was considered the top among these schools, boasting many notable graduates, including Charles D. Meigs, Robley Dunglison, J. K. Mitchell, Daniel Drake, Austin Flint, Samuel D. Gross, John Brinton, and James Fulton, among many others.[14] The exemplary faculty at Jefferson was a draw for students, as W. W. Keen (and later assistant surgeon) noted in 1860, "I left college in June 1860 and in September began the study of medicine at the Jefferson Medical College. I went there rather than the University of Pennsylvania because the Jefferson Faculty was a far stronger one than that of the University of Pennsylvania because of faculty like Gross, Pancoast and Dunglison."[15]

While medical school curricula varied from school to school, Jefferson's illustrious faculty taught the most relevant subject areas and current scientific methodologies. While Fulton was a student, the curriculum consisted of seven subjects, including anatomy, physiology and pathology; *materia medica*, therapeutics, and pharmacy; theory and practice of medicine; chemistry and medical jurisprudence; principles and practices of surgery; and obstetrics and diseases of women and children. Schooling consisted of two four-month terms, the second term being identical to the first. Though Fulton does not specifically discuss his medical school training in his diary, life at medical school was by all accounts exhausting. Students attended five to six mostly didactic lectures a day, six days a week. Lectures were crowded (the matriculates in Jefferson College numbered 630 in 1859), and students spent long hours studying and were encouraged to read countless books.[16] Despite the good intentions of the faculty, there was constant pressure to add more clinical opportunity and practical training to the curriculum. Jefferson Medical College, like many other top schools of the period, lacked the resources and access to hospitals, patients, and bodies to adequately accommodate the many medical students.

Indeed, just as top centers in Europe were creating opportunities for medical students to work with patients and dissect unclaimed bodies, many American medical students often graduated with very little hospital or anatomical experience.[17] As Thomas Bonner has suggested, "the concern of students was chronic and constant to find a means of learning practical medicine."[18] Thus students with means either traveled to England, Paris, or the German states to augment their medical education, or they turned to private instruction or extracurricular study at home (hospital or dispensary training, anatomical classes, and specialty courses such as obstetrics were particularly popular). While not all medical students took advantage of these opportunities, these avenues were crucially important for supplementing a medical school education prior to the Civil War.

Fulton received his MD degree from Jefferson College in 1859, which meant that he passed a series of brief oral exams administered by his professors, engaged in at least a three-year apprenticeship with a qualified preceptor, and submitted the required graduation thesis, in which he wrote about puerperal peritonitis.[19] Fulton does not discuss extracurricular training in his diary; however, he likely engaged in at least some private courses with a member of the Jefferson faculty.[20] He may have also attended rounds at a local hospital, where possible, so that he could walk the wards with a more senior physician.[21] However, not having had a regular hospital position, he would have had little to no experience performing surgeries, dissecting bodies, or even examining and diagnosing hospital patients. Thus, Fulton, like many of his peers, no matter how well trained and educated before the war, was unprepared for the challenges that lay ahead. Many physicians not only adapted to the wartime medical environment, however, they thrived professionally. The war, then, was a crucially important intervention in James Fulton's medical education and professional development.

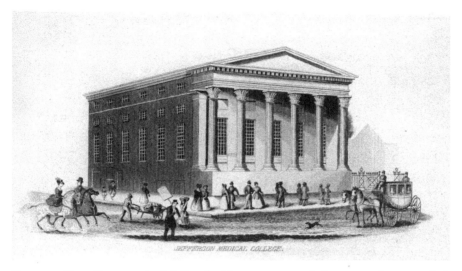

Figure 8.2. The Jefferson Medical College building as it appeared after 1846, with its extended "Grecian façade" (applied to an older 1826 building) by architect Napoleon Le Brun. It was located on the west side of 10th Street, just south of Sansom Street. The Le Brun façade, as Fulton saw it, remained this way until another façade treatment updated it in 1881. Credit: Jefferson Medical College.

ASSISTANT SURGEON FULTON AND THE 143RD REGIMENT

Hammond officially assumed the Office of the Surgeon General in April 1862, and with the support of Congress, began the process of reforming and strengthening the Army Medical Department. He added a medical inspecting corps; increased the number of surgeons, assistant surgeons, medical cadets, medical storekeepers and hospital stewards; collaborated with the United States Sanitary Commission and other civilian bodies to support the hiring of female nurses and civilian hospital workers; issued circulars that provided for the formation of the Army Medical Museum and publication of the *Medical and Surgical History of the War of the Rebellion*; built permanent hospitals along scientific standards; created field aid stations and field hospitals; and paved the way for the development of Medical Director of the Army of the Potomac Jonathan Letterman's ambulance and field relief system. In short, when Fulton was mustered into the service in 1862, the Army Medical Department was transforming from one geared toward the needs of a peacetime army to one that could manage and treat the wounded and sick combatants of war.

Fulton's diary entries are replete with vivid descriptions of what it was like to doctor during the war. Fulton was an assistant regimental surgeon, a position commissioned by state governors. General Order No. 79, issued July 15, 1862, increased the number of assistant surgeons from one to two for each regiment.[22] In the 143rd, Fulton served under Surgeon C. E. Humphrey and Surgeon Francis C. Reamer and alongside Assistant Surgeon David L. Scott, though the physicians from all brigade regiments worked closely together. The Surgeon General's Office monitored the sickness and health of each regiment. As part of Hammond's reforms, all medical data (incidences of wounds, types of diseases, efficacious treatments, deaths, etc.,) were to be recorded and submitted to the Surgeon General's Office for analysis and eventual publication in the *Medical and Surgical History of the War of the Rebellion*.[23]

The main task of the regimental surgeon was to build and foster a regiment. Fulton described many of his activities and duties, which included physically examining potential recruits to determine their health, for entry into the service; examining the men daily and weekly; treating the sick and wounded men; making requisitions for medicines; preparing hospitals to receive the wounded after battles; enforcing proper sanitation in the camps; packing and moving temporary hospitals, and finding locations for new hospitals as the regiments moved with each new campaign; and, beginning in 1863, ensuring that the men were properly nourished and comfortable.[24] A typical day for Fulton began with "examining the sick at morning call," meeting the soldiers, visiting the men in the hospital, prescribing medicines, and determining whether the men were healthy enough to perform their regular duties or reduced duties, or if they needed to be admitted to the regimental or general hospital due to illness.[25] Per the standing orders of the surgeon general, Fulton and the other surgeons in his regiment were then required to write a report that detailed the number of men unable to perform regular duties, along with a list of the diagnosed diseases and injuries. Each regiment was provided with standardized forms for the morning and weekly sick call, and most surgeons kept their own casebooks and diaries.[26]

On January 2, 1863, Fulton remarked that he was exceptionally impressed with the "fine appearance [of] the Reg.," noting after the morning sick call, "The sick list is not very heavy there being no serious cases of disease of any consequence," a welcome state of health for any regiment.[27] Unfortunately, the health of the men did not last long. In February, the regiment moved from established forts in the District of Columbia to tents on Belle Plain, a low stream- boat landing on Potomac Creek in Northern Virginia. On February 19, 1863, Fulton described "considerable Sickness" among the men, including "a number of cases of Measles—this being the most troublesome to treat of all." He went on to detail the preliminary fever and the accompanying "catarrhal symptoms," which he noted "were severe but those cases that had Pneumonia of which there were several all Sunk into the low form or in other words had Typhoid Pneumonia." Fulton was clearly frustrated with the outbreak of measles. He lamented that "in Spite of Every Effort And Remedy us[ed] by us the consequence was that they Sunk and Died." He tried treating the men with "stimulant And Supporting" treatments, but the cases were particularly virulent, erupting "not only upon the External Surfa[ce] of the Body but that the mucus And Serous membranes of [the] lungs and bowels were Equal[ly] Effected" and "exhibiting a high state of inflammation."[28]

DISEASES

Measles was a serious disease among adult men during the war, particularly the first year, in which 21,676 cases were reported, with 551 deaths.[29] The disease remained a problem throughout the war, primarily among "freshly raised regiments and recruits."[30] Exposure to symptoms could range from ten to twelve days; the disease was highly contagious and thus easily spread among the men in the crowded camps. More serious cases of measles (classed as an eruptive fever during the war) were accompanied by respiratory complications ranging from bronchitis or croup to deadly pneumonia, inflammation (most commonly cerebral), diarrhea, and a generalized rash and high fever. Physician Joseph Woodward warned physicians, "epidemic measles generally made its appearance at an early period of each regiment, frequently in its first encampment and swept through the ranks, attacking all those who had not previously had the disease, and occasionally even these did not escape."[31]

As the soldiers crowded together in camps, they became vulnerable to infectious disease, particularly those men from rural areas who had not been exposed to infantile diseases such as chicken pox and measles. This was particularly problematic among the Confederate armies, where more recruits hailed from rural areas. After the battles of spring 1863, and with imperfect understanding of the etiology of measles, Fulton linked the high incidence of measles among the Southern boys with the environmental changes that they endured fighting so far north: "Even of the many, hundreds of Rebs that died with disease no visible sign now remains of the ravage that the Climate Severe made upon them from the far South their Lungs not being able to withstand the rigors of this North Virginia climate the consequence was that hundreds died many, with the measles—And many, more with Pneumonia—And Typhoid Fever so that in this way, the Southern Confederacy lost many of her best men."[32]

Once measles made its appearance in a regiment, it generally lasted from one to two months, with symptoms including fever, rash, diarrhea, and respiratory complications, lasting longer among some men. Most Civil War physicians had either seen cases of measles in civil practice (primarily among children) or read about the disease in medical school; however, it would not be until 1916 that the specific measles antibodies were identified serologically, and not until the 1950s that the measles virus was isolated, followed by a vaccine in the late 1950s and early 1960s. Thus, other than isolation, localized treatments for the rash, and a nourishing diet to help the patient rebuild his strength, there was little that physicians could do for very serious cases of measles. In the best-case scenario, the symptoms would begin to subside on the fourth day of the eruption. In these cases, the eruption and the "febrile symptoms" such as the fever and respiratory affection would "gradually fade" and then disappear altogether.[33] Fulton, however, described the dreaded and particularly fatal form of measles that was usually accompanied by "congestions of the lungs," "Pneumonia," and "catarrhal symptoms," and he lamented that his "patients without an Exception Sinking And Dying—by the reasons that those parts by which the functions of life were to be carried on were unable to act hence inducing inaction—And death."[34] It was always a tremendous challenge and often a sacrifice for the many Civil War physicians who tirelessly doctored the soldiers. While managing his regiment's outbreak of measles, Fulton noted, "we could not keep warm—I suffered More in the Night having to get up three times during the night and visit sick Men in camp—After Each visit it was Still More difficult to get warm . . . I think was the Severest Storm that I have Ever been called to pass through or at Least I think there was more real suffering from the cold than I Ever Experienced in my life before."[35]

Life did not get easier for Fulton as the war progressed. On May 8, 1863, having just concluded the Chancellorsville campaign, Fulton had the task of setting up camp and "imediately set to work to fix up our hospital as there were many Sick Typh. [typhoid cases] Malarial Fever being the prevailing disease with Diarrhea having myself quite a severe time of this uncomfortable disease."[36] Fulton had been treating cases of typhoid fever almost since joining the service, remarking early on, "typhoid Fever Seems to be the prevailing disease."[37] Like measles, typhoid fever, an acute intestinal infection caused by the *salmonella typhi* bacteria and spread by ingesting contaminated food and water or through close contact with someone who was infected, was particularly virulent in the crowded army camps during the first year of the war. [38] Moreover, while Civil War-era physicians increasingly understood that typhoid fever survivors could acquire immunity from subsequent attacks, physicians did not yet understand the "healthy carrier state" (or, more likely, a temporary convalescent carrier)—that is, a seemingly healthy individual who communicated the disease, thus further aiding its spread among susceptible recruits[39]—though they had made some strides in their investigations into typhoid fever before the war, most notably W. W. Gerhard's research, which detailed the clinical differences between typhus and typhoid fever. A preventive vaccine and diagnostic test for typhoid fever would not be developed until the turn of the century. [40] Throughout the war, physicians at the new Army Medical Museum conducted research projects into typhoid fever hoping better to understand the disease; however, the *salmonella typhi* bacillus was not identified until 1880.[41] Thus, in the 1860s, the standard approach to managing typhoid fever was by creating an epidemiological picture of the disease and studying its pathogenesis through the examination of the small intestines at autopsy, which usually displayed the characteristic ulcerations of the Peyer's Patches (accumulations of lymphatic tissue in the small intestine that stem the growth of bacteria).[42]

In the 1860s, physicians still did not agree on a separate and distinct cause for the disease. The English physician William Budd published *Typhoid Fever* in 1871 (a summary of his widely read papers dating to the 1850s), in which he argued that typhoid fever was a specific disease with a specific cause and was spread via contaminated water; however, his views were only beginning to gain currency during the war. For many physicians during the Civil War, typhoid fever was still a "miasmatic" infectious disease transmitted via excremental discharges, contaminated water or food, or by an unknown poison in the air. The disease was not thought to be directly contagious (as in smallpox) but rather infectious. It was believed that excretions, once outside the human body, somehow gained virulence in the soil, air, or from other environmental factors, thus giving rise to the disease.[43] However, the idea of disease erupting *de novo* was still favored by some physicians; thus, the larger debate during the war years, as in Europe, centered on whether the disease was transmitted person to person (whether directly or indirectly) or whether it arose spontaneously.[44] Fulton does not specifically discuss how the disease was transmitted from the sick to the healthy, but rather treatment, which at the time generally consisted of therapeutic measures, including the administration of "turpentine . . . Brandy. Qn Sul" (quinine sulphate), or hygienic measures, "by far the more important."[45] Since the therapeutic remedies offered little relief to the sufferers, physicians were encouraged to perfect their strategies of prevention—particularly cleanliness in the camps and hospitals, properly prepared food, and well-situated latrines.[46]

The contagiousness of smallpox, on the other hand, was well understood by most Civil War-era physicians. On January 6, 1864, Fulton discussed one of his patients, noting "to day, I Saw porter Examined him Carefully, found his tongue heavily furred with a thick white Fur And deeply Marked with the impression of his teeth Nausea So great that he could Retain Nothing in his Stomac great pain in his back—it Seemed Like a Strange Kind of Rheumatism to Me—he also had high fever—I gave him Something to control the febrile action his face was Much Swelled but with No Sign of irruption."[47] Shortly after, Fulton followed up on the case, "again Visited Porter And found him very bad indeed with Evident Symptoms of Small Pox. I ordered him Some Liquor And in the Course of the day the irruptions Made its appearance—we had him Sent as Soon as possible to the Small Pox Hospital of the 2ond Division this Evening Dr Ramsey Sent Me a Small portion of Vaccine Matter with which I will first Vaccinate Company H. then as Many of the others as I can."[48] Although preventative policies during the war were dominated by vaccination (which, if administered correctly, were effective) physicians had the constant challenge of obtaining a pure supply of vaccine material and ensuring that the vaccine matter was potent enough "to take" and that no secondary diseases were transmitted with the vaccine virus. Moreover, although it was strict policy to vaccinate all soldiers before they joined their regiments, it was not always possible to do so.[49]

Fulton noted just one day later on January 8 that "Porter died during the Night—this has been a case of short duration he has been sick only three days the patient dying the day that the rash Made its appearance—this Morning I vaccinated the Most of Company H hopeing if possible to prevent the Spread of the disease"[50] Shortly after the termination of this case, Fulton's superior, Dr. Ramsey, arrived to examine "two cases that have the premonitory Symptoms of Small Pox." While physicians had an imperfect understanding of the pathogenesis of the disease, they understood that there was a premonitory stage, the period of infection, followed by developing symptoms marked by the eruption of pustules. To prevent the spread of this deadly disease, early and correct diagnosis was crucial, and some physicians were ordered to construct research projects with the hopes of developing more effective diagnostic techniques.[51] Fulton's diary reveals the challenges of making a correct early diagnosis: "as yet there is No irruptions And other Symptoms to Mark Clearly that the disease is Small pox." Thus, Dr. Ramsay ordered Fulton to monitor the progress of each suspected case of smallpox, during which time his patients were isolated from the other soldiers and patients. Fulton examined the men and found one suffering from a rash "fully developed upon his body Legs and arms so much as to Satisfy Me that the case was one of Varioloid without any doubt." It was, however, "a Mild Case of Varioloid" classed as variola "confluent," and he was immediately sent "to [the] Varioloid Hospital."[52] For the next few days, "But little of interest transpired Except that we were busily Engaged in beautifying our hospital grounds and takeing precaution against the Sp[r]ead of Small pox." While these labors were often difficult for Fulton, the challenge of managing these cases, some in the advanced stages of disease, was itself a reflection of the tremendous clinical opportunity afforded to physicians during the war.

SURGERY

The field of surgery similarly offered new challenges and practical training for Fulton. In one case, he treated a rebel prisoner who was en route to the hospital after being shot in the eye. Fulton, "took the Ball out of the back of the neck of a wounded Reb who had been shot in the Eye the Ball passing apparently through the Brain—but not killing him." After Fulton removed the ball, the Reb was "taken to the Hospital."[53] In another entry, Fulton described a case in which one of his soldiers, while being treated for typhoid fever, accidently discharged his gun into his leg. Fulton noted that the "ball passing between the tibia and fibula—Severing both the Main arteries as we afterward Learned but no hemorrhage taking place and the bones not being injured." The regimental physicians then had to decide on a course of action. Jonathan Letterman's 1862 directive, which ordered that physicians "in all doubtful cases consult together" so that "a majority of them shall decide upon the expediency and character of the operation" transformed surgical practice during the war.[54] The surgeon in charge of the regiment or hospital put the better-trained surgeon in charge of a group of two or three junior physicians, and the hierarchy of the doctors was entirely "based on their skill and judgement," not on rank.[55] Thus, Fulton in "conjunction with the opinions of others" determined that the leg could be saved. However, shortly afterward, worrying "Symptoms of mortification Manifested themselves."[56] He once again consulted with a Dr. Hottenstein, and they again decided to delay the amputation until "the line of Demarcation would form." Though the boy was not faring well, shortly afterward, the doctors determined that an amputation was the best course. The patient died three days later. Fulton noted that "had his leg only been amputated at first he would without doubt have recovered—but in trying to save the leg we lost they [sic] Boy."[57]

Fulton's last entry regarding this case reveals the important teaching and learning environment stimulated by wartime practice. Since most physicians had little surgical experience before the war, surgical practice during the war became an important training ground. W. W. Keen, similar in educational background to Fulton, summed it up well, noting, "People sometimes imagine that a practicing physician can be transformed into an army surgeon merely by putting a uniform on him. I was not lacking in ordinary intelligence and was willing to work, but I was utterly without training."[58] With amputations, physicians learned through experience that if a primary amputation was performed within 24 to 48 hours of receiving a wound, and done correctly, it could save a soldier's life. A secondary amputation, such as the one performed by Fulton and his team, was generally performed three or more days following the injury, but as the above case illustrates, this could be dangerous, because infection had time to develop and spread. Once infection had occurred, an amputation was essentially performed through infected tissues, thus aiding the further spread of diseases such as pyemia and osteomyelitis. Each amputation and surgical operation was an opportunity to learn how better to judge the severity of a wound, recognize the potential for serious infection, and in consultation, decide on the best course of treatment.[59]

The case of 1st Lt. Charles B. Stout of Company C, 143rd PA (see chapter 2), who was accidently shot with the "Ball Entering the thigh Just Above the Knee cutting the Femoral artery and splitting the Condyles from the Femur," was more clear-cut for Fulton.[60] He noted upon examining the wound that the "action was plain there was Nothing left but to operate we Amputated at the lower third of the thigh he did well but there being so many, cases of Fever he was taken to the Fitzhugh Hospital and there he was left."[61] One can infer a confidence developing within Fulton as he became more experienced. The following month, Fulton described another amputation. His patient, George Muehler, "Shot the End of his Big toe," and it was the first time Fulton "Ever Amputated the great toe." He was proud of the results of the operation, particularly that he succeeded in "getting good flaps—And I think he will have a fine Stump."[62]

GETTYSBURG

Day-to-day life for a regimental surgeon could be filled with long periods of relative inactivity, but during and after major battles, physicians were frantically busy. Fulton participated in some of the war's bloodiest battles, perhaps none more critical than Gettysburg. Upon arriving in town following action at the McPherson farm, Fulton was ordered to create a makeshift hospital. His first task was to find a suitable location for a temporary hospital, and he secured the Catholic and Presbyterian churches on High Street to house the Third Division Hospital.[63] Fulton looked after the injured and dying men and commented often on the men and boys in the wake of the battle: "I could now See that quite a number had been Struck Some wounded others Killed one poor fellow Laying on his back though he had not been killed more than an hour his face was already black and Swelled up as though it would burst."[64] As the first day wore on, he remarked on the "Men falling on Every Side," which "presented a Spectacle sad indeed to look upon—you would see a man fall here a horse there and often the carnage ceased, the Sight presented was a

Sad one the men that had been Killed and that Still Lay upon the Streets were Stripped of their Shoes and Some of them had their pants taken off—and left there to undergo decomposition in the hot Sun."[65]

Fulton's diary provides further insight into the many professional challenges faced by physicians in Gettysburg. On July 5, he noted, "Dr. W T Humphrey and all the Surgeons that could go were taken from the Hospitals to go with the army Expecting an Engagement before they reached the river." Fulton was thus placed in "charge of the third Division Hospital," where he could continue to treat the brigade's wounded. [66] Fulton managed the wounded as they were brought in, and he operated on the soldiers and made them "as comfortable as possible" under the circumstances. On July 6, Fulton appeared to be physically and emotionally drained, remarking, "To day the wounded that had not been brought in from the farm houses round were brought in by the Ambulances we received one hundred and forty—it being difficult to find room in which to place them Many of them had to be placed upon the floor in the doorway And any other place that they could get to lay down."[67]

In what must have been a professional embarrassment for Fulton, he remarked on July 6 that "Dr Taylor . . . made a complaint about the third Div Hospital Stating that I was not fit to have charge of it and that the men were not properly cared for," and he "finally succeeded in getting Dr. Jayne to put him in charge of it and of course left Me Subordinate to [Dr.] P A [Philip A.] Quinan [Surgeon, 150th PA]—the Hospital of course was not in a good condition for the reason that we had not received Any Stores to do it with—And that there was So many that had just been [illegible word] without proper places. for my part I did not care much though I felt capable of performing the duty that had been assigned to Me."[68] There was often confusion and difficulties when evacuating troops from the site of battle, along with preparing temporary hospitals to receive the large number of casualties. Dr. Taylor may have been Surgeon John Howard Taylor, commissioned into the US Volunteers Medical Staff on October 2, 1861 (see chapter 4). He may have been a medical inspector, a position created by Hammond in 1862 for officially inspecting military hospitals or who awaited supplies post-battle if the hospital was not in good order. Taylor may have also been a rival of Fulton's and simply wanted to be placed in charge.[69] The medical world in the nineteenth century was still a small one. The war years offered physicians the opportunity to become known through publications, their efficacious care, research projects, promotion through the ranks, and a good entrance exam, among many other avenues, but as a result, it was a period rife with competitive rivalries. Indeed, professional associations, personal friendships, or a well-placed enemy could make or break a career.[70]

Nevertheless, Fulton continued his work in Gettysburg at the Seminary Hospital under the charge of Surgeon Robert Loughran, where he performed "mostly amputations" on the men belonging to the 148th regiment. He "dressed the men [himself] Every day useing the chlorinated Soda pretty freely in the water with which the wounds were cleansed."[71] His objective was to "stimulate the granulations as well to Keep the odor good—we also used alcohol pretty freely as a Stimulant to the granulations." Fulton was pleased with the recovery of his patients (and perhaps a little defensive), noting that "the stumps all did well under My care and not a single patient died—a fact that was to me quite Gratifying."[72]

CONCLUSION

From James Fulton's early education to his medical education at Jefferson College to his many assignments as a regimental surgeon in the 143rd to his postwar private practice, he took full advantage of the varied educational opportunities available to a medical doctor in the second half of the nineteenth century. It was his time in the war, however, that would have the most profound impact on his practical training as a physician. From managing cases of measles, typhoid fever, and smallpox to performing a number of difficult surgeries and amputations, Fulton had relatively few unstressed intervals during his time in the service. He routinely retrieved medicines for his division; he polished his diagnostic skills as a member of the "Boards of Surgeons," approving sick leaves, discharges, or assignments to invalid corps; he daily inspected the hygiene of the camps and hospitals, and structured them accordingly within the evolving understandings of contagion and prevention; and he was even called to doctor men whose feet "were frostbitten."[73] On occasion, he treated civilians, once remembering, "I was Called to See a little daughter of Mrs. Green. She has an abscess on her Ear And is Suffering Considerably with—I ordered her Morphia—and a flax Seed poultice to the Ear—And promised to see her Again in the Morning."[74] And through it all, he was ever mindful of Hammond's emphasis on policy, procedure, and record keeping, "To day I have been busily in Makeing out My Reports to day we have had to Make a Morning a weekly a Monthly And a yearly Report Making a good amount of work for one day—though by patience And perseverance And diligence we have Succeeded in accomplishing the work—those of them have been sent in and the third the yearly is in Readiness to send to the Surgeon General."[75]

An 1848 report of the AMA noted that medical students viewed American medical teaching as "defective and erroneous, every system of medical instruction which does not rest on the basis of practical demonstration and clinical teaching."[76] For Fulton, the war years went much further in providing the type of practical training and medical education not available before the war. In the process, many orthodox physicians forged a social connection and started to come together based on the more unified standards encouraged by wartime practice. American physicians revealed the potential in the profession's medical and scientific capabilities, thus paving the way for the larger reforms in medical education, science, and medicine that followed the war. Unlike any domestic or foreign educational opportunity before it, the wartime experience of doctoring not only exposed physicians to conditions not often, if ever, seen in civil practice, but provided extensive diagnostic, practical, and clinical training for American physicians.

SHAUNA DEVINE, PhD, is an assistant professor at the Schulich School of Medicine and Dentistry and an associate research professor in the Department of History at Western University. She is the author of *Learning from the Wounded: The Civil War and the Rise of American Medical Science* (2014), which examines the development of scientific medicine during the American Civil War and the impact of the war's events on American medicine.

NOTES

1. James Fulton, Diary, 1862–1864. Entry for August 18, 1862.

2. Fulton had been requesting leaves of absence between January 25, 1864, and April 18, 1864, and two absences had been approved. He may have been suffering from some form of illness that led to his discharge. James Fulton, biographical information, unpublished paper, Society for Civil War Surgeons.

3. For Fulton's examination, see *Record Book of Candidates Examined by the Pennsylvania Medical Board, 1862*, #19.168, RG 19, NARA. See also Fulton's diary, summary for 1863.

4. William Hammond replaced Clement Finley, who was pressured to retire from the service in April 1862. Hammond, with the support of numerous prominent physicians and the politically influential USSC, was officially appointed surgeon general with the rank of brigadier general by General Orders No. 48, April 28, 1862. Mary Gillett, *The Army Medical Department, 1818–1865* (Washington, DC: Government Printing Office, 1987).

5. Shauna Devine, *Learning from the Wounded* (Chapel Hill: University of North Carolina Press, 2014).

6. Hammond to S. D. Gross, May 9, 1862; Hammond to T. M. Markoe, May 19, 1862; Hammond to Valentine Mott, Dec. 12, 1862, Entry 2, RG 112, NARA. Hammond worked tirelessly to improve the quality of physicians in the Army Medical Department while facing considerable backlash from Secretary of War Edwin Stanton, who, as one example, threatened to eliminate the examining boards altogether if more physicians did not pass the difficult entrance exam. Bonnie Ellen Blustein, "To Increase the Efficiency of the Medical Department: A New Approach to Civil War Medicine," *Civil War History* 33, no. 1 (1987), 22–39.

7. John Burnham, *Health Care in America: A History* (Baltimore: Johns Hopkins University Press, 2015).

8. Samuel D. Gross, for example, noted that the instruction he received in the apprenticeship system was merely "a waste of precious time" and was grateful for the opportunity "for attending lectures." Despite the deficiencies in medical school education, most ordinary preceptors did not have adequate resources to provide sufficient clinical training, and many more lacked current medical equipment and textbooks. Samuel D. Gross, *Autobiography of Samuel D. Gross* (Philadelphia: George Burie, 1887), 1:28.

9. Oxford was a typical Pennsylvania farming community. In 1850, it had a population of 186 and by 1860, 482. It was a stage stop on the Baltimore-to-Philadelphia Pike and would by 1860 become a stop on the expanding railroad. Even if Dr. Thomas Thompson was an exemplary preceptor, there would still have been a real limitation to the practical experience that Fulton could obtain in that environment. Thompson received his medical degree at Jefferson in 1838 and practiced at Oxford until 1861. Robert E. Carlson, comp. and ed., "Chester County (Pennsylvania) Medical Practitioners to 1940" (unpublished manuscript: 1986).

10. William Rothstein, *American Medical Schools and the Practice of Medicine: A History* (New York: Oxford University Press, 1987), 98. Burnham notes that the 1860 census accounts for 55,000 medical practitioners. See *Health Care in America*, 116.

11. James Mohr, *Licensed to Practice: The Supreme Court Defines the American Medical Profession* (Johns Hopkins University Press, 2013); David A. Johnson and Humayun J. Chaudry, *Medical Licensing and Discipline in America* (Lexington Books: New York, 2012).

12. Michael Sappol, *A Traffic of Dead Bodies: Anatomy and Embodied Social Identity in Nineteenth-Century America* (Princeton: Princeton University Press, 2002).

13. Rosemary Stevens, *American Medicine and the Public Interest: A History of Specialization* (Berkeley: University of California Press, 1971), 27–30. It was a challenging period for the medical profession—it was really a medical market without either traditional or obvious utility to guide it. In the 1850s, there were clearer reasons to learn physical diagnosis; anatomy and physiology, and anesthesia-based surgery; the pathology of Budd and Snow, Simon and Farr was beginning to suggest the need for change, and with the most recent epidemic experiences (cholera, yellow fever), prescient leaders saw firsthand the need for change, but it was by no means obvious to most of the rank and file. The need was seen by a large number of

physicians during the war. Devine, *Learning from the Wounded*; Dale Smith, "Austin Flint and Auscultation in America," *Journal of the History of Medicine and Allied Sciences* 33, no. 2 (1978): 129–49; Martin Pernick, *A Calculus of Suffering: Pain Professionalism and Anesthesia in Nineteenth Century America* (New York: Columbia University Press, 1985).

14. Frederick B. Wagner Jr. and J. Woodrow Savacool, eds., *Thomas Jefferson University— A Chronological History and Alumni Directory, 1824–1990* (Philadelphia: Thomas Jefferson University, 1992), 89–124.

15. W. W. Keen, "An Autobiographical Sketch by W. W. Keen," Reminiscences for His Children; 1912 with additions 1915, APS, 28.

16. Wagner and Savacool, *Thomas Jefferson University*, 104.

17. John Harley Warner, *Against the Spirit of the System: The French Impulse in Nineteenth-Century American Medicine* (Princeton: Princeton University Press, 1998); Sappol, *A Traffic of Dead Bodies*. Adequate clinical training could come from a knowledgeable and experienced preceptor; however, many preceptors of the era did not fully understand the new anatomic pathology coming out of Europe and physical diagnosis based on it.

18. Thomas N. Bonner, *Becoming a Physician: Medical Education in Britain, France, Germany and the United States, 1750–1945* (New York: Oxford University Press, 1995), 220.

19. These were by all accounts mere reflections of the didactic nature of the lectures. One student wrote that his oral exam at Harvard in the 1850s consisted of one question: "Well White, What would you do for a wart?" Rothstein, *American Medical Schools*, 53. Fulton's graduating thesis on puerperal peritonitis does not survive, but the thesis title appears in the Jefferson Medical College *Register Book & Catalogs*.

20. This was not the case for all medical students, but by the standards of the day, the educational and clinical resources of Philadelphia were exceptional. See Rothstein, *American Medical Schools*; Rothstein, *American Physicians in the 19th Century: From Sects to Science* (Baltimore: Johns Hopkins University Press, 1972); Kenneth Ludmerer, *Learning to Heal: The Development of American Medical Education* (New York: Basic Books, 1985); Ronald Numbers, ed., *The Education of American Physicians* (Berkeley: University of California Press, 1979); Bonner, *Becoming a Physician*; and Stevens, *American Medicine and the Public Interest*.

21. Most private-school teachers were connected with one or more of the hospitals or dispensaries in the city. See, for example, Rothstein, *American Medical Schools*.

22. William Grace, *The Army Surgeon's Manual for the Use of Medical Officers, Cadets, Chaplains, and Hospital Stewards* (New York: Bailliere Brothers, 1864).

23. Circular No. 5, issued June 9, 1862, Washington, DC, Circulars and Circular Letters of the Surgeon General's Office, 1861–1865, p. 38, entry 63, RG 112, NARA.

24. Medical screening of new recruits was abysmal the first year of the war, but pre-enlistment physical examinations continued to improve in the second and third year of the war, in part because the doctors became more experienced at diagnosing illness and because the Union Army improved the physical exams (Hammond and Jacob Da Costa, among others, created and provided a long list of instructions for examiners/physicians). Fulton's diary discusses each of these tasks as he describes his daily activities.

25. Fulton, January 12, 1863.

26. For more on Army and Medical Department Regulations, see Grace, *Army Surgeon's Manual*.

27. Fulton, January 2, 1863.

28. Fulton, February 19, 1863. "Typhoid" was an adjective used in the mid-nineteenth century to describe a particularly debilitating disease, usually with slow fever and gastrointestinal symptoms.

29. Joseph Woodward, *Outlines of the Chief Camp Diseases of the United States Armies as Observed during the Present War* (Philadelphia: J. B. Lippincott, 1863), 267. However, he also notes that "the number of deaths represented by these figures far underestimates the mortality proceeding from this cause." Some physicians, for example, recorded the cause of death as diarrhea or pneumonia, complicating these statistics.

30. Ibid., 269.

31. Ibid., 268.

32. Fulton, June 16, 1863.

33. Woodward, *Outlines of Chief Camp Diseases*, 271.

34. Fulton, February 19, 1863.

35. Fulton, February 22, 1863.

36. Fulton, May 8, 1863. Some physicians used the category typhomalarial fevers, likely a milder form of typhoid fever. The term was introduced by Joseph Woodward in July 1862 and was a controversial category during the war—some physicians (including all Confederate physicians) never adopted the term. See Woodward, *Outlines of Chief Camp Diseases*, 77–149.

37. Fulton, October 14, 1862.

38. As the war progressed and the troops developed immunity to some infectious disease, and cleanliness in camps was more strictly enforced, the health of the men improved. Alfred Bollet, *Civil War Medicine: Challenges and Triumphs* (Arizona: Galen Press, 2002), 259–60.

39. Joseph Jones, "Medical History of the Confederate States Army and Navy," *Southern Historical Society Papers* 20 (1892), 109–66. The "healthy carrier" was crucial in shaping public health policies and scientific research projects as the germ theory became accepted in the later nineteenth century. See, for example, Judith Walzer Leavitt, *Typhoid Mary: Captive to the Public's Health* (Boston: Beacon Press, 1996); Pricilla Wald, *Contagious: Cultures, Carriers and The Outbreak Narrative* (Durham, NC: Duke University Press, 2008); and Mark Harrison, *Contagion: How Commerce Has Spread Disease* (New Haven: Yale University Press, 2012).

40. Dale C. Smith, "The Rise and Fall of Typhomalarial Fever: I. Origins," *Journal of the History of Medicine and Allied Sciences* 37 (April 1982), 182–220; and Smith, "Gerhard's Distinction between Typhoid and Typhus and its Reception in America, 1833–1860," *Bulletin of the History of Medicine* 54 (1980), 368–85. Typhoid fever and typhus were distinguished as two separate diseases, each with its own specific cause.

41. Devine, *Learning from the Wounded*, chapter 2. See also Joseph Woodward's Photomicrographs, 1860s–1880s, RG 83, Otis Historical Archives (OHA), National Museum of Health and Medicine (NMHM); Joseph Woodward Letterbooks, 1864; 1883, RG 28, OHA, NMHM; Joseph Woodward Papers, RG 363, OHA, NMHM.

42. See, for example, Entry 621, Medical Records: Reports of Diseases and Individual Cases, 1841–93, file A and bound manuscripts, Entry 623, Medical Records, 1814–1919, D file, NARA.

43. In the 1840s and 1850s, typhoid fever was thought to be caused by impure air and poisonous "miasmas." However, William Budd's ideas were beginning to gain currency among some of the elite physicians during and after the war. As Elisha Harris noted, "The fact is now well ascertained that this fever is, under certain contingencies, infectious, and communicable through the agency of the bodily excretions of the sick; but the greater truth is, that effete animal and organic matter in a state of putrescence, as in badly policed camps, barracks, and latrines, and especially the mephitic effluvia from sinks, etc., are the most powerful localizing causes of its endemic prevalence." See Elisha Harris, *Hints for the Control and Prevention of Infectious Disease in Camps, Transports and Hospitals* (New York, United States Sanitary Commission, 1863), 20; Margaret Pelling, *Cholera, Fever, and English Medicine 1825–1865* (New York: Oxford University Press, 1978), especially chapter 7; and William Budd, *On the*

Causes and Mode of Propagation of the Common Continued Fevers of Great Britain and Ireland (1839), ed. Dale Smith (Baltimore: Johns Hopkins University Press, 1984).

44. John Simon, like William Budd, was at that time (1850s and 1860s) also researching the origin of contagion, and noted that "while there was little reason to suppose that contagion was frequently 'spontaneously generated,' this was not to say that a contagious disease could not arise without contagion; and there were cases, such as the 'traumatic infections' in which spontaneous generation of the disease was of very frequent occurrence." See Pelling, *Cholera, Fever, and English Medicine 1825–1865*, 264.

45. Fulton, May 8, 1863. See also Woodward, *Outline of Chief Camp Diseases*, 114.

46. Woodward recommended that "scrupulous cleanliness must absolutely be enforced. This must apply to the persons and clothing of patients as well as to the beds and bedclothes, the furniture and utensils, the floors and walls of wards, and the passages, grounds and surroundings of the whole establishment. No point requires more care than the removal of the excreta of the sick; urinals, bed pans, and chamber pots should be removed from the ward or tent as soon as used and should under no circumstances be allowed to remain to contaminate the air with unhealthy emanations," Ibid., 119. Sanitation policies and acquired immunity were responsible for the decrease of typhoid fever cases as the war continued. However, there was an increase in case fatality rates. See Bollet, *Civil War Medicine*, 330–1.

47. Fulton, January 6, 1864.

48. Fulton, January 7, 1864.

49. Joseph Jones, *Circular No. 2, Vaccination: Spurious Vaccination* (Louisiana, 1884); Bollet, *Civil War Medicine*, 290–92.

50. Fulton, January 8, 1864.

51. As one example, Southern physician J. Merrillat began the practice of testing urine with nitric acid, looking for the presence of chlorides, hoping to distinguish between smallpox and rubeola. He found no chlorides present in the first stages of smallpox, but did find them present in all stages of rubeola. J. Merrillat, "On the Absence of Chlorides in the Urine of Persons affected with Variolous Diseases," *Confederate Medical and Surgical Journal* 1 (May 1864), 70.

52. Fulton, January 13, 1864. During the war, physicians classed smallpox as variola distinct, variola confluent, and variola malignant confluent.

53. Fulton, April, 1863.

54. Jonathan Letterman, *Medical Recollections of the Army of the Potomac* (New York: D. Appleton, 1866), 60.

55. Ibid.

56. Fulton, May 8, 1863.

57. Ibid. Post-Chancellorsville was still relatively early in the war for Fulton and his regiment. They likely felt more comfortable taking a conservative approach.

58. Keen, *Reminiscences*, 36.

59. See, for example, Devine, *Learning from the Wounded*, chapter 5.

60. Fulton, May 8, 1863

61. Ibid.

62. Fulton, June 18, 1863.

63. Fulton, July 1, 1863.

64. Ibid.

65. Ibid.

66. Fulton, July 5, 1863.

67. Ibid.

68. Ibid. As George Meade's army pursued Robert E. Lee, taking numerous physicians with them, there were huge challenges for the physicians who stayed behind to doctor the men while they waited for the United States Sanitary Commission and Army Medical Department reserves to show up. See, for example, Letterman, *Medical Recollections*. Dr. Taylor would have understood this, making the motives for his recrimination less clear.

69. Fulton's diary hints at a few competitive rivalries. As another example, he noted that "Dr. Quinan had been Brigade Surgeon since he came to the Reg. but about this time Dr. Reamer having to skedaddle from Windmill point came back to the Reg^t and claimed the position of Brigade Surgeon: Quinan being of course unwilling to give up the position and go Back to the Reg. Stood Somewhat upon his dignity . . . [and] claimed that he merited the position from the fact that he had been an asst Surgeon for Eleven yrs in the Regular Army." Fulton, June 18, 1863.

70. The most famous example was Hammond's contentious relationship with Edwin Stanton, and his professional rivalry with R. C. Wood and Joseph Barnes (among many others). In a series of letters between John Le Conte and Joseph Brown, they not only talk about the Hammond supporters versus his detractors, they also talk about the importance of patronage and social connections in securing good wartime medical appointments. See, as one example, American Philosophical Society, John LeConte Papers, August 1861–July 1864, B L493. A good recommendation could also make a difference: "I write to express my regrets in learning that you have failed to obtain the nomination for the position for which you were an applicant. I spoke with my friend in the senate as to your standing and acquirements as a man of science but my commendation was not available sooner and your name was not presented to them." Joseph Henry to John LeConte, January 12, 1863, Ibid.

71. For more on the use of disinfectants during the war, see Devine, *Learning from the Wounded*, chapters 3 and 6.

72. Fulton, July 5, 1863.

73. Fulton, January 20–29, 1864.

74. Fulton, Dec. 30, 1863.

75. Fulton, January 1, 1864.

76. Bonner, *Becoming a Physician*, 220.

NINE

"We Got Up and Began to Pack our Medicines"

What Dr. Fulton Prescribed

GUY R. HASEGAWA

Every Surgeon has his own treatment; each some favorite remedy he
relies upon, and there are none who have not seen a few inveterate
cases which baffle for months all their pet remedies.

—J. THEODORE CALHOUN, "Rough Notes of an Army
Surgeon's Experience during the Great Rebellion"

PRESCRIBING RESPONSIBILITIES

James Fulton undoubtedly spent a great deal of time caring for soldiers, yet
relatively little of his diary describes the specific treatments that he administered. New military surgeons like Fulton, whose previous experience had
been restricted to civilian practice, might enter the service having never
dressed a gunshot wound, amputated a limb, or treated all of the common
maladies of a fighting army. Because there was so much to learn, it seems
unlikely that Fulton was intellectually bored with the medical aspect of his
army experience. On the contrary, his remarks about measles, for example,
and his detailed descriptions of wounds show him to be a curious and observant man of medicine (see chapter 8). Why, then, did Fulton not record
in his diary more detail about the drug therapy he prescribed? Among the
records that regimental surgeons were required by regulations to keep were
a prescription book, in which the medications for each patient were to be
entered daily, and a case book for detailing the more important cases. Even
if Fulton did not contribute to these records—lack of time and a disdain for
red tape often led new surgeons to neglect the tasks—he had other official

paperwork to attend to. He likely decided that his precious free time was best spent documenting for himself the other aspects of what was probably *the* experience of his life in what he recognized as a period of great historical importance.[1]

Among Civil War troops, disease was about twice as likely as battlefield wounds to be the cause of death, and it was a rare soldier who did not find himself under a surgeon's care at one time or another. Fulton makes clear that illness was common and that he prescribed medicines, but the army's way of providing care differed from what he was accustomed to. As a civilian physician, Fulton saw patients in his office, where he likely kept some medicines, or carried a small selection of remedies with him during house calls. If drug therapy was needed, Fulton could administer or dispense whatever he had on hand or write a prescription to be taken to an apothecary's shop for filling. Commonly used agents might be on the apothecary shelf as premade items, but prescriptions often called for multiple ingredients to be combined by a pharmacist into custom-made pills, powders, liquids, or external preparations.

SUPPLY AND DEMAND

For an army surgeon, the prescribing and dispensing process depended on the number of patients being seen and the relative permanence of the treatment environment. In a general hospital—a structure that was far removed from the fighting and was intended to operate for a prolonged time—a dispensary was established. Surgeons made rounds of the wards and wrote prescriptions to be filled in the dispensary by a hospital steward, a noncommissioned officer serving as an apothecary and all-around physician's assistant. The dispensary carried some remedies in ready-to-use form but also had an array of raw drugs and the equipment to prepare individualized and relatively complex medications; completed prescriptions were then sent to the patient's bedside for administration by a nurse or another hospital steward. Regiments in the field held sick (or surgeon's) call, during which soldiers who were or claimed to be ill presented themselves to a surgeon for evaluation; soldiers too disabled to report could remain in their quarters or be moved to a hospital tent and seen there by a surgeon. Treatment decisions might be made hastily if the number of patients was large or if time was short. Furthermore, surgeons in the field were often limited to prescribing the items

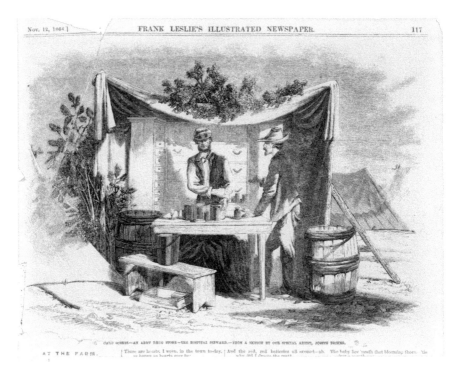

Figure 9.1. Makeshift dispensary established in an army camp by a hospital steward, whose supplies appear to be drawn from the back of a medicine wagon. From a sketch by Joseph Becker, in *Frank Leslie's Illustrated Newspaper*, November 12, 1864. Credit: Library of Congress, Prints and Maps Division, reproduction no. LC-USZ62-119788.

available in a regimental medicine chest small enough to be transported in a wagon or ambulance or carried by a horse or mule. If there was time to set up camp for a few days, a hospital steward would place the chest's items on makeshift shelves for easy access, and when it was time to move on, the chest would be repacked with padding perhaps added to help prevent breakage. A hospital steward could use the apothecary scale and glass measures in the chest to prepare exact doses, but the chest's smaller selection of drugs and pharmaceutical implements limited his ability to prepare complex prescriptions. The amount of effort required to ready the doses determined whether medicines could be administered on the spot or made available to the patient later. During a battle, an assistant surgeon like Fulton might station himself fairly close to the fighting and be accompanied by an orderly or hospital steward carrying a medical knapsack or other container with a small selection of ready-to-use supplies.[2]

Regimental surgeons in the Army of the Potomac replenished their supplies by requesting items from the surgeon in charge of the brigade; Fulton describes his brigade's medicines being transported in an ambulance. In response to one of Fulton's requests, his brigade's chief surgeon, Philip A. Quinan (150th PA), sent "a lot of old trash" in place of what he asked for. It is unclear exactly what Fulton found unsatisfactory about the items received other than their being useless. Since surgeons were accountable for wasted drugs, Fulton had good reason to resent Quinan's suggestion that he (Fulton) discard the unwanted items and report them lost; disposal of Quinan's unwanted items was clearly that surgeon's own responsibility. Surgeons in charge of brigades requisitioned supplies from a medical officer called a medical purveyor; Fulton describes traveling to Brandy Station to pick up supplies for his division from Assistant Surgeon Jeremiah B. Brinton, a medical purveyor.[3]

Fulton likely encountered unfamiliar ailments, but even if he was perfectly confident making diagnoses and formulating general treatment plans, he then had to make do with the medicines on hand. The specific medicinal agents and the amounts available to surgeons were dictated by the surgeon general in the form of a standard supply table. During his army service, Fulton was first subject to a table approved in August 1861 and subsequently to revisions effective in October 1862 and May 1863. The tables included a wide array of drugs, but there was a realization that surgeons who had recently been in civilian practice might prefer other agents. Surgeon Charles S. Tripler, medical director of the Army of the Potomac from August 1861 to June 1862, acknowledged that many new surgeons had been "country doctors, accustomed to a village nostrum practice" and were unable to "readily change their habits and accommodate themselves to the rigid system of the army in regard to their supplies." Tripler's response was "within reasonable limits to disregard supply tables, and to give the surgeons articles of medicine . . . to suit even their caprices" if he thought they might be of some benefit. Tripler found it difficult to be as accommodating as he wanted, since his requests for nonstandard items were often countermanded by then Surgeon General Clement Finley, who retired in April 1862. Finley's successor, Surgeon General William A. Hammond, shared Tripler's liberal attitude and stated that "it is not the design of the Department to confine medical officers absolutely to that [standard supply] table ... but only to establish a standard for their guidance in making requisitions for supplies, leaving individual preferences to be indulged at the discretion of the Medical Director or the Surgeon General." Hammond restated this stance when he appointed Tripler's successor, Surgeon Jonathan Letterman, in June 1862: "You are authorized to call directly upon the Medical Purveyors in Washington, Baltimore, Philadelphia, and New York, who will be directed to furnish you with every thing you may ask for, regardless of tables or forms."[4]

Most medicines prescribed by surgeons were ingested orally in the form of pills, powders emptied from paper wrappers into water, or liquids taken directly or diluted in a beverage. External remedies could be in the form of liniments, ointments, or plasters. Hypodermic injections were rare, but some medicines were administered rectally as an enema or placed into the urethra with a syringe. The "vaccine matter" that Fulton used to immunize soldiers against smallpox was usually made from the scabs or fluid from lesions of persons who had recently been vaccinated with cowpox. Vaccination was accomplished by introducing a small amount of vaccine matter by lancet into the skin of the upper arm. "Vaccine virus," as it was called, was listed in the instruments section of the standard supply tables and was available as needed from medical purveyors and sometimes from sources such as the United States Sanitary Commission. Fulton got his supply from an army hospital dedicated to the isolation and treatment of smallpox patients.[5]

Given his educational background, Fulton could hardly be called a country doctor who favored village nostrums, but his ability to use the remedies he preferred would nonetheless seem ensured by Hammond's liberality. For Fulton to obtain a nonstandard medicine, however, he would have to go through the proper channels, starting with Surgeon Quinan, whom he viewed with contempt. Even with supportive superiors, approval by Letterman or Hammond and then receipt of the requested items might take many days or even weeks, by which time Fulton's immediate need may have passed. J. Theodore Calhoun, another surgeon in the Army of the Potomac, described the de facto situation: "The army surgeon must in his prescriptions keep within the field table. We cannot drag over Virginia roads the assortment to be found in a city drug store, and I doubt not that it is much

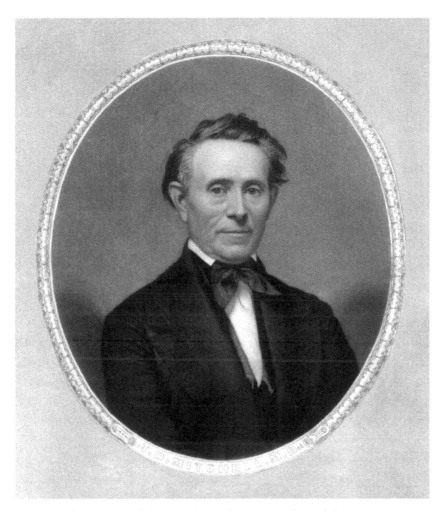

Figure 9.2. Thomas D. Mitchell, MD, who taught *materia medica* and therapeutics to James Fulton's class at Jefferson Medical College. From James F. Gayley, *History of the Jefferson Medical College of Philadelphia*, Joseph M. Wilson, Philadelphia, 1858. Credit: Image courtesy of the Historical Medical Library, The College of Physicians of Philadelphia.

better for our patients that we cannot." There were ways, other than going through bureaucratic channels, for Union surgeons to procure nonstandard medicines. Some states, for example, provided their regiments with medical stores, including drugs not on the standard supply tables, and surgeons could bypass the usual supply chain by purchasing items locally from drug merchants or using medicines donated by civilian relief agencies.[6]

MATERIA MEDICA

Fulton's usual aim in prescribing medicines was not so much to cure ailments—the true cause of most disorders was unknown and thus could not be corrected—as to reduce symptoms and correct imbalances in the body until the patient improved through nature taking its course. Diarrhea, for example, an extremely common disorder that was frequently of infectious origin, was thought to be a manifestation of bowel inflammation. Thus, Fulton might first prescribe a cathartic to rid the sensitive gut of irritating matter and follow that with opium to reduce the frequency of watery stools—all this while hoping that the body would return to its healthy state. When symptoms waned or disappeared unexpectedly, the improvement could be attributed to the influence of the treatment even if it amounted to no more than a placebo effect. Drugs used to correct supposed imbalances often caused obvious effects, such as flushing, vomiting, urination, defecation, or perspiration. Fulton anticipated these but was unaware of the mechanism through which they occurred. "How is it," asked Thomas D. Mitchell, Fulton's professor of *materia medica* and therapeutics at Jefferson Medical College, "that opium contracts the pupil, while belladonna dilates it? How does digitalis induce its special action on the heart? What is the *modus operandi*,—not by conjecture, but in reality? It is utterly impossible to answer." By today's standards, most drugs prescribed during the Civil War would be considered ineffective or too toxic, but a few were unquestionably useful. The anesthetics ether and chloroform were employed for almost all major surgical operations, and opium and morphine lessened pain and helped relieve coughing and diarrhea. Quinine was effective for the prevention and treatment of malaria.[7]

Professor Mitchell also taught that the treatment of patients should not be formulaic:

> The governing maxim . . . should be to treat the case not in reference to the name of the disease, but according to the existing state of the system as developed by the pulse, skin, tongue, countenance, the excretions, &c. &c. . . . . While physicians all over the country have their panaceas and stereotyped prescriptions, we know of none. . . . As the nature of diseases is a subject of constant change in many respects, we are precluded from the adoption of any uniform plan of treatment.

If Fulton took his instructor's teachings to heart, he would have wanted to treat each of his soldier patients individually and with careful deliberation.

In light of the number of patients Fulton might have to see and his limited selection of drugs, he may not have been able to live up to that ideal. Mitchell's
teachings were at odds with some surgeons' practice of prescribing the same
remedy for most or all patients with a certain diagnosis. Oral turpentine, for
example, was often used as standard treatment for typhoid fever, and quinine
was standard therapy for malaria.[8]

FULTON'S PRESCRIPTIONS

Soldiers' expectations of medical encounters probably depended on their
previous interactions with practitioners and what had been heard from
acquaintances. Some soldiers feigned illness in hopes of duping a surgeon
into excusing them from duty—in which case medicines would probably
be prescribed—while others dreaded the prospect of being under a surgeon's care. "An ordinary army surgeon can, by a course of treatment," said
Pennsylvania soldier A. F. Hill, "bring the stoutest man to the grave; and
they seldom fail to do it." This cynicism was reinforced by some surgeons'
perceived habit of using the same medicine—often quinine or mercury
pills—for all ailments, no matter how dissimilar. According to Surgeon
Calhoun, some patients were "loudly clamorous for medicines" and thought
it was "one of their duties to be prescribed for and take medicines at stated
intervals." The opposite could also be true, for Calhoun warned that soldiers
should be witnessed taking their medicine because some would discard it if
given the chance. It seems safe to say that sick soldiers would not be surprised
to be prescribed a remedy that would probably cause noticeable and often
unpleasant effects.[9]

 What Fulton prescribed to sick soldiers was surely influenced by his
medical training, professional experience, reading of medical literature, and
consultation with other physicians. Although he did not consistently record
in his diary the treatments or their rationale, they can be inferred to some
extent. In treating typhoid pneumonia associated with measles, Fulton tried
to counter the debility and loss of vitality with stimulants, which probably
included alcohol in the form of whiskey or brandy. (Alcohol was classified
as a stimulant because of its initial effects of causing warmth and flushing
and speeding the heart rate.) Other agents that Fulton prescribed—copaiba,
carbonate of ammonia, and camphor water—also had stimulant effects, and
copaiba was also deemed useful in disorders of the mucous membranes,

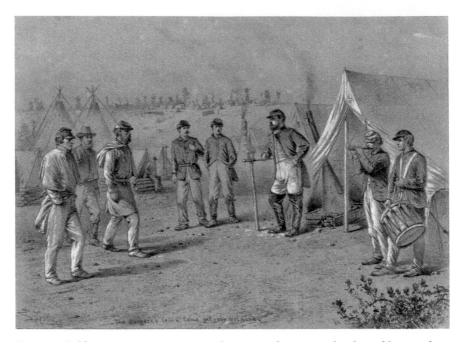

Figure 9.3. Soldiers reporting to a regimental surgeon to be examined and possibly treated, as depicted in "The Surgeon's Call" by Edwin Forbes. The inscription "Come get your quinine" refers to the real or imagined propensity of surgeons to prescribe quinine regardless of the patient's complaint. Credit: Library of Congress, Prints and Maps Division, reproduction no. LC-USZ62-15485.

which Fulton believed were present in typhoid pneumonia. He also used chlorate of potassa, probably given to combat inflammation of the lungs and bowels. Fulton ordered external application of mustard, croton oil, and turpentine to cause local blistering or redness, an effect thought to help remove toxins or draw inflammation away from diseased areas.[10]

Fulton treated the debility and prostration of malaria with turpentine, which could be a stimulant when taken orally. External application of turpentine for malaria, as he described, was not commonly prescribed by Union surgeons, but Confederate surgeons used it when quinine was unavailable. Used in this way, turpentine was thought to affect the nervous system and interrupt the periodicity of fever. Other agents Fulton prescribed for malaria included aromatic spirits of ammonia, probably given as a stimulant, and quinine, whose usefulness in the disease was well known.[11]

Fulton describes cleansing stumps from recent limb amputations with chlorinated soda to stimulate healing and keep the wounds from developing a foul odor. This was a well-recognized use for this chemical, although its antimicrobial actions were not then appreciated. Fulton evidently knew that the same effects were attributed by some physicians to alcohol, which he also used. Army surgeons sometimes treated civilians, and Fulton describes prescribing morphine and a flaxseed poultice for a little girl with a painful abscess on her ear; the morphine was for analgesia, and the poultice was a soothing application to the lesion. All of the medicines that Fulton mentions in the main portion of his diary were or could be prepared from items in the 1861, 1862, and 1863 standard supply tables and, shortages notwithstanding, would be available to regimental surgeons like Fulton.[12]

Fulton compiled a collection of medication formulas at the end of his diary, much as a cook might collect recipes for favorite, recommended, or tasty-sounding dishes. At least one entry, for Cholera Cordial, appears to have been written in a hand other than Fulton's. There is no definitive evidence that Fulton ever used the recipes, and it seems improbable that he would have recorded formulas that he prescribed frequently enough to know by heart. The formulas bear no dates, but attributions on two of them point clearly to their sources. The antimonial and saline mixture, labeled "Proff. Gross," was meant for inflammatory disorders and appeared in Samuel D. Gross's *Manual of Military Surgery*, described by the author as "a kind of pocket companion for the young surgeons who were flocking into the army, and who for the most part were ill prepared for the prompt and efficient discharge of their duties." Gross, Fulton's professor of surgery at Jefferson Medical College, also wrote the two-volume *System of Surgery*, which was issued to some general hospitals and regimental surgeons and contained a variation of the recipe. The other clearly attributed recipe, labeled "Practice Bennett," was for oxaluria (calcium oxalate crystals in the urine) associated with dyspepsia and is from John Hughes Bennett's *Clinical Lectures on the Principles and Practice of Medicine*, which was also available to army hospitals and surgeons. When Fulton writes, "We got up and began to pack our medicines and Books for the march," he may be referring to one or more of these texts.[13]

The recipe for one formulation, which is likely to have been used for gonorrhea, is followed by the name of W. S. Leach, a sergeant in Company G of the 143rd Pennsylvania Regiment during Fulton's service. The clear implication is that the medicine was prescribed for Leach, although Leach, if he had medical experience, could also have provided the formula. (Many physicians, dentists, and apothecaries served in the ranks as combat soldiers.) The name of D. L. Scott, Fulton's fellow assistant surgeon, appears after two agents for checking hemorrhage. Fulton describes his colleague treating wounded soldiers and being ill himself—although not suffering from bleeding—so Scott is more likely to have recommended the hemorrhage-control agents than to have been treated with them by Fulton.[14]

Among the remaining formulas, one is labeled for use in gonorrhea and six, all containing some form of mercury, appear under the written heading of secondary syphilis. Other ailments linked to recipes include cholera, upset stomach, and sore throat. It seems that having recipes for specific maladies contradicted the claim of Thomas Mitchell, Fulton's former professor, that "panaceas and stereotyped prescriptions" did not exist; perhaps Fulton had come to accept that the realities of wartime medicine necessitated some standardization of treatment. There are two strychnia-containing formulations, one apparently intended for the treatment of severe constipation and the other evidently a tonic—an agent producing gentle and persistent excitement of the system—for use in patients with debility and prostration. Fulton includes an ointment and liniment that may have been helpful for scalds, skin ulcers, or excoriated skin surfaces. One unusual recipe calls for zinc oxide, morphine, alcohol, and water to be administered via syringe, probably into the urethra. The most likely indication was gonorrhea, and the formula is unconventional in specifying zinc oxide, for which the reported experience was scant, rather than the more commonly used zinc acetate or zinc sulfate.[15]

There is no certainty about the intended uses of the back-of-diary formulations when Fulton does not state them explicitly. Ideally, a physician wrote the constituents of a prescription in a specific sequence, with the most important therapeutic agent (the basis) first. The basis was followed, in order, by ingredients that enhanced the effect of the basis, those that helped correct undesirable effects of other ingredients, and those (e.g., excipients, diluents, vehicles) that gave proper form to the whole preparation in its final form as, for example, a pill, powder, or ointment. Thus, the first ingredients in Fulton's recipes might suggest their probable use, but most drugs had many possible indications, and writing the most important ingredient first was a nicety only and made no difference in how an apothecary might compound the prescription. Thus, attempts to determine the disorders for which the unclassified recipes were meant are educated guesses at best.[16]

It should not be assumed that the back-of-diary recipes, if Fulton pre-scribed them at all, found use during his army service. Many of the auxiliary recipes call for ingredients that were not ordinarily available to Fulton as an army surgeon. For example, the sore throat liniment contains oil of sassafras, and two of the recipes for secondary syphilis call for compound tincture of gentian. The army's standard supply tables did not list either ingredient, al-though they did include another form (fluid extract) of gentian. Even the pre-scription that appears meant for a specific soldier, Sergeant Leach, contains ingredients absent from the standard tables: powder of cubebs (rather than the available oleoresin of cubebs) and anise seed. The recipes' inclusion of nonstandard ingredients does not suggest that the disorders they supposedly treated were rare and necessitated uncommon medicines. On the contrary, army surgeons predictably encountered such ailments, and their reasonable treatment was allowed by the ingredients in the tables, which were probably just as effective as the nonstandard drugs in the back-of-diary recipes. The presence of nonstandard components in the back-of diary recipes likely re-flects the individual preferences of the recipes' originators with no particular concern about what was available in the army. If it were necessary to surmise whether the back-of-diary recipes, as a group, were used by Fulton during his army service, the most likely scenario would be that they were not.[17]

Fulton's diary provides only glimpses of the ailments he faced and their corresponding treatments, but it is reasonable to assume that the variety, frequency, and severity of illness and injury he encountered in the army dif-fered from what he saw in civilian practice. As an army surgeon, he also had to deal with a limited selection of drugs, superiors looking over his shoulder, a military bureaucracy, and the confusion and stress of combat. Soldiers could be particularly challenging to treat because certain common factors—crowding, fatigue, poor nutrition, exposure to the elements—predisposed them to illness. Possibly Fulton had little time or inclination to record the details of routine cases in his diary, but it is more difficult to guess how cer-tain activities happened to qualify for entry into his personal chronicle. The availability of official prescription books and case books containing Fulton's entries would help in forming a more complete view of the challenges that Fulton confronted as an army surgeon.

The diary also provides little fodder for determining Fulton's thoughts or evolution as a prescriber. He must have learned that his civilian methods were not entirely workable for a surgeon in a fighting regiment and adjusted accordingly. It is also likely that Fulton's military experience influenced how he practiced medicine when he returned to civilian life. His expanded knowledge probably made him a more confident practitioner, but one must wonder whether he retained, for example, the army's way of making do with a limited variety of remedies or quickly took advantage of his regained freedom to prescribe whatever medicines he wished.

Fulton's experience as a civilian physician made him well familiar with prescribing medicines, so doing the same as an army surgeon was probably less worthy of recording in his diary than other, more novel aspects of his service. It is not surprising, then, that the diary offers only a tantalizing glance at what was certainly a vital and time-consuming activity.

GUY R. HASEGAWA, PharmD, is Senior Editor of the *American Journal of Health-System Pharmacy* and an independent scholar of Civil War medicine. He is the author of *Mending Broken Soldiers: The Union and Confederate Programs to Supply Artificial Limbs* (2012) and *Villainous Compounds: Chemical Weapons and the American Civil War* (2015).

NOTES

1. James Fulton, Diary, 1862–1864, entries for February 19 and May 8, 1863; United States Army, *Revised Regulations for the Army of the United States, 1861* (Philadelphia: J. G. L. Brown, 1861), 284; United States Surgeon General's Office, *Medical and Surgical History of the War of the Rebellion* (Washington, DC: Government Printing Office, 1875–1885), pt. 2, 1:102.

2. *Medical and Surgical History*, pt. 3, 2:899–966; J. Theodore Calhoun, "Rough Notes of an Army Surgeon's Experience during the Great Rebellion: Camp Diarrhoea—Continued," *Medical and Surgical Reporter*, n.s. 9 (November 1, 1862): 123–4; Charles Beneulyn Johnson, *Muskets and Medicine, or Army Life in the Sixties* (Philadelphia: F. A. Davis, 1917), 130.

3. Jonathan Letterman, *Medical Recollections of the Army of the Potomac* (New York: D. Appleton, 1866), 52–6; Fulton, May 8, July 1, and December 10, 1863.

4. US Army, *Revised Regulations*, 281–340; *Directions Concerning the Manner of Obtaining and Accounting for Medical and Hospital Supplies for the Army, with a Standard Supply Table* (Washington, DC: Government Printing Office, 1862); *Directions Concerning the Duties of Medical Purveyors and Medical Storekeepers, and the Manner of Obtaining and Accounting for Medical and Hospital Supplies for the Army, with a Standard Supply Table* (Washington, DC: Government Printing Office, 1863); *War of the Rebellion*, ser. 1, 5:76–93; Bennett A. Clements, "Memoir of Jonathan Letterman, M.D.," *Journal of the Military Service Institution of the United States* 4 (September 1883): 252–3.

5. US Army, *Revised Regulations*, 281; *Directions Concerning Manner*, 10; *Directions Concerning Duties*, 11; Elisha Harris, "Vaccination in the Army—Observations on the Normal

and Morbid Results of Vaccination and Revaccination during the War, and on Spurious Vaccination," in *Contributions Relating to the Causation and Prevention of Disease, and to Camp Diseases*, ed. Austin Flint (New York: Hurd and Houghton, 1867), 142; Fulton, January 7, 1864.

6. J. Theodore Calhoun, "Rough Notes of an Army Surgeon's Experience during the Great Rebellion: Camp Diarrhoea—Continued," *Medical and Surgical Reporter*, n.s. 10 (May 30, 1863): 68

7. Thomas D. Mitchell, *Materia Medica and Therapeutics* (Philadelphia: J. B. Lippincott, 1857), 31.

8. Ibid., 47; Johnson, *Muskets and Medicine*, 159.

9. J. Theodore Calhoun, "Rough Notes of an Army Surgeon's Experience during the Great Rebellion: A Sick Call," *Medical and Surgical Reporter*, n.s. 9 (October 25, 1862): 99–100; A. F. Hill, *Our Boys: The Personal Experiences of a Soldier in the Army of the Potomac* (Philadelphia: John E. Potter, 1864), 229–30; Calhoun, "Rough Notes: Camp Diarrhoea," 68; Calhoun, "Rough Notes: Dispensary," 123.

10. Fulton, February 19, 1863; George B. Wood and Franklin Bache, *The Dispensatory of the United States of America*, 11th ed. (Philadelphia: J. B. Lippincott, 1858).

11. Fulton, May 8, 1863; Wood and Bache, *Dispensatory of the United States*; "On the External Application of Oil of Turpentine as a Substitute for Quinine in Intermittent Fever, with Report of Cases," *Confederate States Medical and Surgical Journal* 1 (January 1864): 7–8.

12. Fulton, July 6 and December 30, 1863; Wood and Bache, *Dispensatory of the United States*; W. H. Triplett, "Improper Treatment of Wounds in Some of the United States Hospitals," *Boston Medical and Surgical Journal* 71 (September 15, 1864): 136–9; *Revised Regulations*, 292–309; *Directions Concerning Manner*; *Directions Concerning Duties*.

13. Fulton, medical recipes (see chapter 5); Samuel D. Gross, *A Manual of Military Surgery* (Philadelphia: J. B. Lippincott, 1861), 166; Samuel W. Gross and A. Haller Gross, eds., *Autobiography of Samuel D. Gross, M.D.* (Philadelphia: George Barrie, 1887), 1:142; Samuel D. Gross, *System of Surgery; Pathological, Diagnostic, Therapeutic and Operative*, 2nd ed. (Philadelphia: Blanchard and Lee, 1862), 1:103; *Directions Concerning Manner*, 12; John Hughes Bennett, *Clinical Lectures on the Principles and Practice of Medicine*, 2nd ed. (New York: Samuel S. and William Wood, 1858), 430; Fulton, December 24, 1863.

14. Fulton, medical recipes; Fulton, December 22, 1863. It is also possible that Dr. Scott himself wrote the recipes that display his name.

15. Fulton, medical recipes; Mitchell, *Materia Medica and Therapeutics*, 47; Wood and Bache, *Dispensatory of the United States*; C. L. Sommé, "Notes sur l'Emploi Nouveau ou Peu Usité de Queíques Médicamens dans Plusieurs Maladies," *Archives Générales de Médecine* 1 (April 1823): 481–87.

16. Jonathan Pereira, *Physicians' Prescription Book*, 14th ed. (Philadelphia: Lindsay and Blakiston, 1865), 2–3.

17. Fulton, medical recipes; *Revised Regulations*, 292–309; *Directions Concerning Manner*; *Directions Concerning Duties*.

TEN

"We Soon Concluded to Operate"

Dr. Fulton's Tools and Methods

JAMES M. EDMONSON

INSTRUMENTS AND IDENTITY

When James Fulton became a military doctor, he had access to army-provided tools. Army regulations decreed what tools were standard issue for hospitals. Instead of carrying army-issued instruments in the field, Fulton could have emulated the practice of other physicians and used his own. The diary gives no evidence that Fulton carried his own tools. Indeed, doing so would have been risky, because if he was captured, the Confederates would likely have confiscated his tools. Then, as now, a surgical instrument set from the Civil War era was a much sought-after thing. If a surgical artifact has provenance (the life history of an object) connecting it to that conflict, its interest is significantly enhanced (as well as its value to a collector of medical antiques). If linked to a doctor known to have served, so much the better. These associations transform the artifact into a piece of historical evidence, something that gives us a sense of what surgeons could accomplish with such tools at hand.

Surviving surgical instruments also convey a sense of what they might have signified to their owners. They clearly were calculated to impress, presented as they are in mahogany and rosewood cases, lined with plush velvet in a variety of hues ranging from bold red to rich olive. The instruments within are beautiful to behold, with each nested in a unique recess. The high-carbon steel of cutting tools rarely rusts unless abused, and some blades still glisten with a mirrorlike finish and can hold an edge sharp enough to shave with. Instrument blades and shafts were invariably nicely fitted with handles of dark ebony or ivory, with brass ferrules and checked surfaces. These instrument sets clearly had significant performative value, calculated to flatter their owners and impress their patients. Some sets, given in thanks by grateful patients or as prizes by approving mentors, were silver-plated and gilt. Such embellishment transformed the instruments from utilitarian objects into honorific trophies, perhaps never actually intended for use.

INSTRUMENTS AND MEANING

What did these instruments mean to the surgeon on active duty ministering to the wounds and infirmities of soldiers? Where did these instruments come from, where did the medicos get them, and how did they carry them? Diaries and letters like those of Fulton and others best answer these questions, because they carry passing comments and observations upon the surgeon's tools. These sources complement the descriptions and depictions of instruments in period surgical manuals. These descriptions hint that among American surgeons, there was something of a cult of celebrity. Leading surgeons never patented their procedures or innovative instruments; to do so was deemed crass, ungentlemanly behavior and was thoroughly disdained until after 1900. They did aspire, however, to having their names associated with a particular selection of instruments.

Consequently, in the pages of surgical manuals and trade catalogues issued by surgical instrument makers at the close of the Civil War, one finds "Dr. Frank H. Hamilton's Field Case," or "Dr. James R. Wood's General Operating Set."[1] Each selection carried the authority and imprimatur of a leading surgeon, several of whom figured as prominent professors of surgery on the eve of the war, and some of whom served in uniform during it. This practice began earlier in Britain and France, where leading instrument makers marketed selected sets of instruments recommended for a particular procedure by a renowned surgeon. In the United States, the surgical instrument trade had come of age in the decades before the Civil War, and now it promoted the celebrity of American as distinct from European surgeons.

INSTRUMENT MAKERS ON THE EVE OF THE CIVIL WAR

The remainder of this essay explores how American surgical instrument makers met the unprecedented demand for their wares in the Civil War and

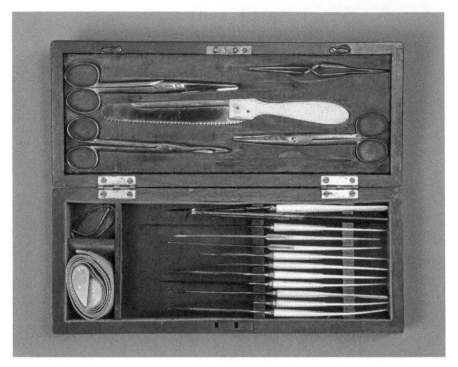

Figure 10.1. This minor surgery set, made by Hermann Hernstein of New York around 1861, belonged to Gustav Weber, a prominent Cleveland surgeon who served as surgeon general of Ohio in 1862. Instrument maker Hermann Hernstein immigrated from Germany to New York in 1841 and made and imported surgical instruments. The instruments in this set appear to be French made, resembling the Charrière instruments depicted in J. M. Bourgery and N. H. Jacob, *Traité complet de l'anatomie de l'homme, comprenant la médecine opératoire ...* *(1832–51)*. Tools included a variety of knives to cut muscle and tissue preparatory to amputation, bone saws, and chisels. Specialized tools included a drill (a trepan or trephine), catheters, and various probes or sounds. Surgical kits of this size and complexity may have been personally owned by army doctors or provided by the army. Credit: Dittrick Medical History Center and Museum, Case Western Reserve University. Photographer: Laura Travis.

how instrument makers collaborated with their clientele, the medical pur-veyor of the United States Army. Collections of letters, including, notably, those of Fulton, Jonah Franklin Dyer (surgeon, 19th Massachusetts), Daniel M. Holt (assistant surgeon, 121st New York), John Gardner Perry (assistant surgeon, 20th Massachusetts), and Maj. William Watson (surgeon, 105th Pennsylvania), are mined to unearth mention of instruments and convey in surgeons' own words how they perceived the tools of their trade.[2] The essay concludes with a look at some surviving examples of Civil War-era instruments, both army issue and civilian, to make a connection to Fulton's experience. Through these tools, we can grasp what comprised the ordinary and banal among instruments, the day-to-day armamentarium of the surgeon. In some surviving artifacts, we glimpse more sophisticated and complex surgical instruments that emerged after but might have originated during the war.

The Civil War placed an enormous strain upon the medical and surgical resources of the combatants. Soon after the war began, it became apparent that the Medical Department of the United States Army was woefully ill equipped to meet the burden placed upon its services. As the Civil War proceeded, the Medical Department increased its manpower, reorganized ambulance and hospital services, and purchased medical supplies and equipment through a system of medical purveyors (also discussed in chapter 9).[3] Particularly for Philadelphia and New York instrument makers, the vast scale and prolonged duration of hostilities generated an enormous demand for their products. Surgeon Richard S. Satterlee oversaw the contracts for supplies, including instruments, during his tenure as medical purveyor of the United States Army (purveyors were usually medical doctors). Satterlee placed contracts with approximately twenty or so instrument makers for the fabrication of cased instrument sets and related surgical equipment for the military.[4] During the course of the war, he requisitioned purchases of over 4,900 amputating and general operating cases, 1,150 cases of trephining, exsecting (removal), post mortem, and "personal" instruments, 12,700 minor surgery and pocket cases, and 65,000 tourniquets.

In April 1862, the War Department secured $5,705,984 to meet the needs of the army's Medical Department. That budget was intended to cover all aspects of the department's staffing and equipping, and for the latter, it made specific reference to "the purchase and repair of surgical instruments." It also included a similar provision for paying private or contract physicians and surgeons in the department's employ, as well as equipping them with surgical instruments as needed. As the war proceeded, the Surgeon General's Office drew up a standard supply table enumerating the officially approved supplies and equipment for the Medical Department. A curious and revealing document, it lists a surprising variety of instruments and appliances. Circular No. 7 describes just the kind of surgical instruments that one would expect a military surgeon to need: "Amputating, trephining, exsecting, general

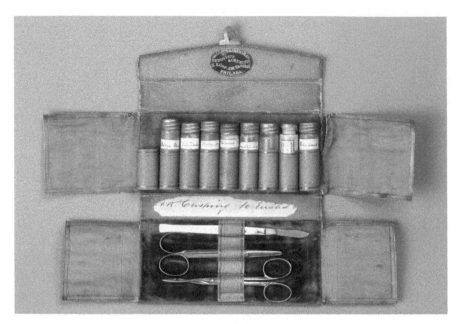

Figure 10.2. In 1854, Charles Bullock and Edmund Crenshaw issued a catalogue advertising surgical instruments as well as pharmacy supplies and drugs. This pocket case made by Bullock and Crenshaw around 1855 belonged to Henry Kirke Cushing (1827–1910), who graduated from Union College in Schenectady, studied at the Cleveland Medical College, and completed his MD at the University of Pennsylvania in 1851. A decade later, on June 19, 1861, Cushing entered military service as the original surgeon of the 7th Ohio Volunteer Infantry. (James A. Garfield also served in the 7th OVI, which fought at Antietam, Chancellorsville, and Gettysburg.) Cushing's youngest son was Harvey Cushing, America's most distinguished brain surgeon. Fulton likely carried a kit such as this one for essential and frequently used tools and medicines. Credit: Dittrick Medical History Center and Museum, Case Western Reserve University. Photographer: Laura Travis.

operating, and pocket instruments." The following year, the Surgeon General's Office issued a revised and expanded version of the supply table featuring a detailed listing of the contents of sets "for capital operations, for the field case, for minor operations, and for the pocket case." In addition, however, one finds new items, including "dissecting case, obstetrical case, pocket case for hospital, teeth-extracting case, medicine case, and medicine panniers."[5]

The supply table also lists the old—lancet, cupping glasses, and scarificator for bloodletting (a therapy increasing regarded as obsolete)—and the new—in the form of the stethoscope, today a commonplace tool, but then still a novelty to some. Circular No. 7 expressly held the medical purveyor accountable for assuring the quality and condition of surgical instruments furnished to doctors in the ranks. At the same time, surgical instrument makers were held accountable for the goods they furnished to the medical purveyor. Circular No. 7 also made provision for scientific investigation: "Applications for microscopes by medical officers in charge of general hospitals will be favorably considered, provided the evidence is satisfactory that the officer will use the instrument for the benefit of science, and will report the results of his observations to the Surgeon-General." Although antiseptic surgery lay a few years away and had no impact upon the conduct of operations at this time, the circular presciently made available carbolic acid (phenol), the mainstay of Listerian surgical protocol. In a curious oversight, the supply table did not include prosthetics, particularly artificial limbs for amputees. This omission was amended by General Order No. 40 (Feb. 11, 1863), which included an appropriation "For artificial limbs for soldiers, for the regular army, and seamen, forty-five thousand dollars."[6] In retrospect, this sum proved completely inadequate for the great numbers of soldiers who had limbs amputated in the Civil War.

INSTRUMENTS IN THE FIELD

Nothing could be more incongruous than the contrast between the regimented and ideally ordered world prescribed in official United States Army regulations pertaining to surgical instrument procurement (and loss) and the absolutely chaotic realities of life in the midst of war. Military service consisted of mustering, bivouac, decampment, deployment, and marches and countermarches. Regiments of soldiers in the Civil War were seemingly always on the move, gaining ground, losing it, and regaining it, and the occasions for supplies to go astray abounded. Despite the rigors of the march and combat and duties of the camp, some surgeons managed to keep diaries or compose letters to loved ones. In these writings, we find mention of instruments, the essential tools that made their craft possible. Such comments sometimes appear offhandedly, as when Daniel Holt wrote to his wife that "I am at this time sitting upon a canister of black tea, with a surgical case upon my lap for a desk."[7] In other circumstances, incidents involving surgical instruments stood out as memorable events. For example, John Gardner Perry recounted such a tale:

> I hear that the surgeon who served before me, while dressing a [captured] soldier's wound, laid the knife for a moment on the bed. The man seized it and made a lunge at the doctor, but, instead of killing him, as he had intended, only ran it into his arm; where upon the doctor instantly shot him. I suspect that the surgeon may have been rough in this instance, possibly intentionally so; I am careful, however, not to leave my instruments within reach of these prisoners, although they seem friendly and I do not fear them.[8]

Most often, surgeons discussed instruments in diaries or correspondence when their personal effects disappeared in the confusion of events. Surgeons accompanying regiments routinely lost baggage and personal effects, including their instruments. Some, in the interest of traveling light, laid aside their more cumbersome equipment, just as enlisted men routinely jettisoned heavy knapsacks (as ordered) when they went into combat. On other occasions, they lost gear consigned to baggage trains that went missing, either from misdirection or seizure by enemy forces. Of course, in the midst of battle, instruments could go astray without warning. At Gettysburg, for example, Fulton's tools disappeared when he became separated from his orderly. Fulton described the scene at the McPherson farm, where he attended to the wounded of a Maine artillery battery: "Spread over the floor the men of the battery lay, wounded and bleeding. There was no one to care for them. I looked around for my Orderly. He was nowhere to be seen. His duty was to carry the instruments, bandages and medicines. I had nothing to work with."[9]

Surgeons' mode of travel further complicated the transport of their armamentarium. Although Union forces implemented ambulance service in August 1862, surgeons were expressly forbidden from catching a ride on them; they were reserved exclusively for the wounded and sick. Daniel Holt, for example, suffered severe rebuke from Major General William B. Franklin when he was accused (unjustly) of riding in an ambulance.[10] As officers, surgeons had to secure their own horses at their own expense, or be compelled to walk on foot with their troops. Carrying a heavy, wood-cased set of amputating instruments, weighing several pounds, posed a problem. Surgical instrument makers sometimes sold sets with a leather carrying case for suspension from a saddle, perhaps in the manner of carrying a brace of

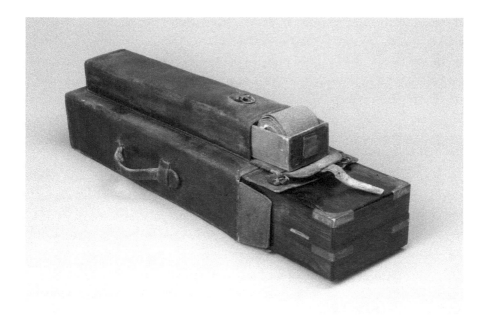

Figure 10.3. Capital surgical set in leather carrying case, c.1861. Gustav Weber (1828–1912) immigrated to America from Germany in 1848 and completed his medical degree at the University of St. Louis (now known as the School of Medicine of Washington University). In 1856, he became Professor of Surgery at the Medical Department of Western Reserve College and taught there and at other schools in Cleveland for forty years. In January 1862, Governor Todd appointed Weber as Surgeon General of Ohio. In this post, Weber organized a system to care for troops in the field and improved the condition of camps and hospitals in the state. Weber also saw action with Ohio regiments on October 8, 1862, in the battle at Perrysville, Kentucky, which ended Confederate efforts to establish a presence in that state. This rare carrying case attests to conditions Fulton found in the field: variable and occasionally harsh weather and the stress and fatigue of the campaign. Credit: Dittrick Medical History Center and Museum, Case Western Reserve University. Photographer: Laura Travis.

pistols across the horse's withers. More commonly, surgeons left such sets in hospital facilities, and when in the field, just kept the essentials of a pocket case on their person. Even if a surgeon managed to find a way to transport his instruments on his mount, in the chaos of battle, the horse might go astray, leaving him empty handed.[11]

Surgeons in the field may have relied on pocket instrument cases for most of their ex-hospital work. Pocket cases were just that, leather roll-ups containing slots for an assemblage of much-used small instruments. The army did not prescribe the contents of pocket cases. These expendable cases deteriorated through use. Doctors may have assembled their own choice of tools, discarded some over time, and replaced them with other varieties, but in any event, they represented a doctor's idiosyncratic determination of what was essential to carry on one's person. Tools thus carried may have included types of forceps, a scalpel, lancet, scissors, a small bistoury (curved-bladed knife), probes, suturing needles, catheters, and a tenaculum (a hook to separate tissues and blood vessels). Dr. Fulton does not refer to a pocket kit in his diary.[12]

Theft or seizure of a surgeon's tools remained a constant threat in time of conflict. In one instance, the appropriation of presumably abandoned apparel had dire consequences for surgeon Daniel Holt. As he recalled in a letter penned at Brandy Station (Virginia) in November 1863, "Quite a serious calamity befell me here; and it was no less than the loss of my overcoat and pocket case of instruments. I had been dressing the wounds of those who were hurt and brought to the rear, when wishing greater freedom of my arms than could be had in such cumbersome folds, I took it off and laid it on the ground beside me . . . some good soldier appropriated it to his own use." Surgeons also might be captured by the enemy, at which time their possessions could be confiscated. Holt recalled being taken prisoner and having all his accoutrements and horse seized; his Confederate captors wanted to swap and barter goods, and curiously, "more than one was after my green sash [denoting his surgeon's status] which happened to be upon my person at the time of capture." Occasionally, a surgeon's fortune could run the other way, and he might recover surgical instruments lost by others in the field. This happened to William Watson, who recalled, "I captured on the march one of the finest Amputating case of instruments I have ever seen. It was made by Kolbe and certainly did not cost less than 60 or 75 dollars." Perhaps this set resembled that of James Fulton, which went missing at Gettysburg. A month after that battle, Fulton proceeded to Washington and reported to Major General Henry W. Halleck that "the Rebs had captured all My Equipment."[13]

JAMES M. EDMONSON, PhD, is Chief Curator of the Dittrick Medical History Center and Museum of Case Western Reserve University, and Associate Professor of History. A historian of medical technology and a Fulbright Hays Fellow, he has curated over thirty exhibitions on medical history, notably on the history of contraception, surgical instrumentation, and diagnostic technologies and the physician-patient relationship. His publications include *American Surgical Instruments* (Norman Publishing, 1997) and *Dissection: Photographs of a Rite of Passage in American Medicine, 1880–1930* (co-author with John Harley Warner, Blast Books, 2009).

NOTES

1. See Stephen Smith, *Handbook of Surgical Operations*, 4th ed. (New York: Baillière Brothers, 1863), 9–12.

2. These surgeons' experiences also illuminate other aspects of Fulton's diary. Chapter 7 features commentary on the diary chapters in which these surgeons' observations appear.

3. See Mary C. Gillett, *The Army Medical Department, 1818–1865* (Washington, DC: Center for Military History, United States Army, 1987). See also General Orders No. 43, War Department, Adjutant-General's Office, Washington, April 19, 1862: "The following Act of Congress is published for the information of all concerned: AN ACT to reorganize and increase the Efficiency of the Medical Department of the Army." Full presentation of the content of the Orders is to be found in William Grace, *The army surgeon's manual: for the use of medical officers, cadets, chaplains, and hospital stewards: containing the regulations of the Medical Department, all general orders from the War Department, and circulars from the Surgeon-General's Office from January 1st, 1861, to July 1st, 1864* (New York: Baillière Bros., 1864), 40–41.

4. The surgical instrument makers that met this demand included virtually all the leading firms in the North, namely, Philadelphia surgical instrument makers Jacob H. Gemrig, Louis V. Helmold, Horatio G. Kern, D. W. Kolbe, Martin Kuemerle, Frederick C. Leypoldt, Snowden & Bro., and A. H. Wirz; New York makers V. W. Brinkerhoff, Hermann Hernstein & Son, Otto & Reynders, George Tiemann & Co., Julian Tiencken, and Wade & Ford; Boston maker Codman & Shurtleff; and Cincinnati makers Max Wocher and William Z. Rees. Surviving examples of their work are to be found today in museums and private collections throughout the United States. For more information on these firms, see James M. Edmonson, *American Surgical Instruments: An Illustrated History* (San Francisco: Norman, 1997).

5. Details of the army's medical budget are found in General Orders No. 77, War Department, Adjutant-General's Office, Washington, July 11, 1862: "The following Act of Congress is published for the information of all concerned: AN ACT to reorganize and increase the Efficiency of the Medical Department of the Army." See Grace, *The army surgeon's manual*, 51–2. Full "purchase and repair" quotation found in Grace, 51: "For the medical and hospital department, including pay of private physicians, purchase and repair of surgical instruments, purchase of extra hospital bedding, clothing, ice, pay of male citizens as hospital attendants; the maintenance of sick and wounded soldiers placed in private houses or hospitals, and other necessary comforts for the sick and convalescing in the various military hospitals—five millions seven hundred and five thousand nine hundred and eighty-four dollars."

On the Standard Supply Table: *Directions Concerning the Manner of Obtaining and Accounting for Medical and Hospital Supplies for the Army, with a Standard Supply Table, Circular No. 7*, May 7, 1863 (Washington, DC: Government Printing Office, 1863); Grace, *The army surgeon's manual*, 121–27. Detailed lists of tools appear in *Directions concerning the Duties of Medical Purveyors and Medical Storekeepers, and the Manner of Obtaining and Accounting for*

Medical and Surgical Supplies for the Army. Standard Supply Table. Revised edition of Circular No. 12, October 20, 1862 (Washington, DC: Government Printing Office, 1863).

6. From Circular 7: "Medical Purveyors will be responsible for the quality of the medical and hospital supplies purchased by them, and they are directed to have surgical instruments made in the best manner, of the best materials, and according to patterns approved by the Surgeon-General. Each instrument is to be inspected, and each chain-saw tested on fresh bone by them, or under their supervision, before being paid for or issued.

"31. Medical officers will report to the Surgeon-General and to the issuing officer all defects observed in the quality, quantity, or packing of medical and hospital supplies, or in the material or construction of their surgical instruments, giving the name of the vendor or maker, and of the officer by whom they were issued.

"Carbolic acid (Bower's), sulphate of iron, nitrate of lead, chlorinated lime, permanganate of potash, or charcoal, will be furnished as antiseptics or disinfectants, when required." On the purchase of artificial limbs, see Grace, 63.

7. James M. Greiner et al., eds., *A Surgeon's Civil War: The Letters and Diary of Daniel M. Holt, M.D.* (Kent, OH: Kent State University Press, 1994), 37.

8. John Gardner Perry, *Letters from a Surgeon of the Civil War,* comp. Martha Derby Perry (Boston: Little, Brown, 1906), 4.

9. James Fulton, "Gettysburg Reminiscences: A Surgeon's Story," *National Tribune* (Washington, DC), October 20, 1898. (See Appendix B.)

10. Greiner, *A Surgeon's Civil War,* 12–3.

11. J. Franklin Dyer remembered that "All we had was what was carried in hospital knapsacks, and I carried my instruments strapped to my saddle." Michael B. Chesson, ed., *The Journal of a Civil War Surgeon* (Lincoln: University of Nebraska Press, 2003), 24. William Watson recalled that "Many of the Surgeons [at Chancellorsville] lost their Horses, instruments and everything they had. I lost nothing but my sword." in Paul Fatout, ed., *Letters of a Civil War Surgeon* (Purdue, IN: Purdue Research Foundation, 1961), 61. Similarly, Dyer wrote, "I have very little baggage to trouble me now . . . Thinking it highly probably that our baggage train would be captured or destroyed on the retreat, I packed all my best articles of clothing in a bundle, which I strapped to my saddle, and which I lost at Savage Station." Chesson, 29.

12. Dr. Samuel D. Gross wrote a handy manual for military surgeons at the outbreak of the war, *A Manual of Military Surgery* (Philadelphia: J. B. Lippincott, 1861), which describes and recommends several small tools for versatility of use.

13. Holt quotations in Greiner, *Surgeon's Civil War,* 156–7, 94, respectively. Watson quoted in Fatout, *Letters of a Civil War Surgeon,* 94. That amount could equal the price of a horse. James Fulton, Diary, 1862–1864. Entry for July 6, 1863.

ELEVEN

"The Christian Commission Also Brought in a Wagon Today"

Dr. Fulton, Voluntary Relief Associations, and Women in Hospitals

BARBRA MANN WALL

—to day, we got a detail of 3 Men for Nurses for our Hospital—we will get about 3 More And that I think will be Enough—

JAMES FULTON, Diary, January 8, 1864

INTRODUCTION

In 1864, Fulton wrote these words about men serving as nurses. At the beginning of the Civil War, the armies had no trained nurses or sick-diet kitchens. Men typically were the nurses in military hospitals, and they often were recuperating soldiers. Indeed, military men disdained accepting women as nurses. Nursing had not yet shed its stigma as a job for untrained workers, many of whom were workhouse inmates or almshouse workers, and nursing as a profession for women did not become well established until after the war. Although he names women who volunteered to aid the wounded at Gettysburg, Fulton does not mention women as army nurses, and he describes a voluntary relief association only once. All around him at Gettysburg, however, and at other battle sites, women provided care to wounded or ill soldiers in makeshift hospitals, or they roamed the battlefield to deliver food, water, or blankets, or appeared on behalf of voluntary relief organizations such as the US Sanitary Commission. They either volunteered or were paid by the army to provide vital nursing care and relief work, often under trying circumstances. Only recently established in his profession, Fulton likely would not have recognized women as nurses in military facilities at all. Throughout his diary, he mentions men such as Josiah Lewis, who served as his hospital steward.

WOMEN NURSES

There is no simple description of nursing in the Civil War, and both trained and untrained nurses worked in the midst of wartime situations. Historian Jane E. Schultz found that as many as twenty thousand women worked in general hospitals, army hospitals, hospital ships, field hospitals, and local battlegrounds for both the Union and Confederacy. Women included enslaved or former enslaved laborers, free blacks, elite white women, farm women, and Catholic sisters. Yet many physicians perceived unskilled female volunteers as useless and their delicate natures as unsuitable for wartime nursing. One Union physician wrote, "Our women appear to have become almost wild on the subject of hospital nursing . . . With the best intentions in the world, [they] are frequently a useless annoyance . . . As a rule, [they] have not the physical strength necessary." Another physician viewed women as "quarrelsome, meddlesome busybodies." On their part, many women viewed army officers as incompetent and resisted their authority.[1]

In 1861, Dorothea Dix acquired authority from the War Department to hire nurses when she offered her services to the Union government in Washington, DC. Although she had no formal nurse's training, she was well known as a reformer for mental hospitals. She became Superintendent of the United States Army Nurses on June 10, 1861. Dix was very strict: she required her nurses to be older than thirty-five, plain looking, and wear dull uniforms, preferably brown, gray, or black, with no hoop skirts. Her nurses' duties typically included housekeeping, cooking, feeding the ill or wounded patients, changing bandages, supervising wards, and assisting with surgery. They were paid $12 a month as army nurses, compared to the $13 a month that privates in the Union army received.[2] Dix's nurses initially worked in the Washington, DC, hospitals and, later in the war, divisional hospitals.

That Fulton did not mention women's work in such public spaces is not surprising. Historian Jeanne Boydston labels the "growing social invisibility of labor" that women performed in their homes as "the pastoralization of housework." She asserts that by the 1830s, women's work had separated from that of men, who were viewed as the productive laborers. The erasure of women's work was part of an economic transition at a time of uncertainty with the rise of industrialization.[3] At this time, nursing was seen as an extension of women's roles in the home. In this context, it would not be surprising that Fulton took this work for granted.

Yet at the start of the war, many women were eager to extend their moral virtues and domestic skills to serve their country. How nursing was defined was a contested issue during the Civil War, and duties complicate the very meaning of the word "nurse." Historian and physician Margaret Humphreys has taken a gendered approach in her argument that perceptions of what were masculine and feminine activities affected much of the medical and nursing care during the war. Sometimes nursing included cleaning or taking care of children, while at other times it involved tending the sick and injured. White middle-class women believed they had a monopoly on knowledge about caring for the sick, and they quickly sensed the need to nurse the sick and wounded. Nursing care also involved the idealized womanly virtues of compassion, tenderness, and selflessness, yet women also actively engaged in medical care. For example, they treated patients already seen by physicians and surgeons and gave medicines, changed dressings, and assisted surgeons in their operations.[4]

While some women provided direct patient care, others were hospital administrators, laundresses, or cooks, and their duties frequently overlapped. A woman might cook or clean hospital wards, while "cooks" might give medicines and bathe people. "Matrons," or women in charge of hospital wards, might do all of these things at one time or another. On January 12, 1863, Fulton mentions a "contraband camp doeing the Hos [Harewood Hospital's] Washing." "Contraband" typically included blacks who had fled the Confederacy and who unofficially worked for the Union army. It was quite common for them to do the washing, yet many who did the laundry also performed nursing duties such as feeding the sick special diets.[5]

Schultz notes that more black women and white working-class women performed the domestic tasks of cooking, washing, and scrubbing, while the higher prestige jobs of nurse and matron went to elite white women. Although certain women were hired to do laundry, when they were not available, the nurses chipped in and did it themselves or found men to help them. Certainly cooking and doing laundry were not highly valued tasks, and the more valued roles were making rounds with the doctors. These assignments also reflected common class distinctions.[6]

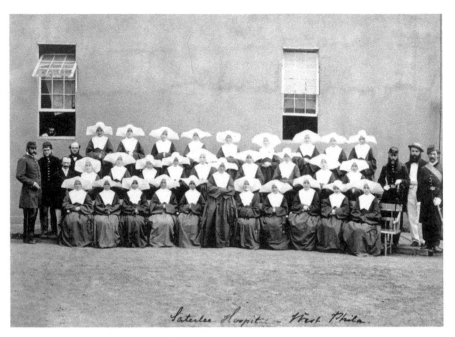

Figure 11.1. The Sisters (Daughters) of Charity pose at one of the largest hospitals during the war, Satterlee (West Philadelphia) Hospital. Union physicians praised these women, who also administered to wounded soldiers at Gettysburg. Credit: Daughters of Charity Province of St. Louise Archives, Emmitsburg, Maryland.

Of equal note is that prominent among women nurses were those connected to the Catholic Church. Close to six hundred Catholic sisters worked as nurses in both the North and South. Whereas most women were not formally trained as nurses, some Catholic sisters were educated in nursing—not according to the understanding of nursing today, but nevertheless, trained in some aspects of the role.[7] Fulton did not mention any nursing sisters in his diary, but they were all around him when he traveled. For example, the Sisters of St. Joseph from Philadelphia worked as nurses at the military hospital at Camp Curtin in Harrisburg, Pennsylvania. When he first went to Harrisburg in August 1862, Fulton reported to Camp Curtin under the orders of Henry Hollingsworth Smith, Surgeon General of the Pennsylvania Volunteers:

> in the Evening at 3.30 we arrived in Harrisburg went to Herrs. Hotel deposited our Baggage—left immediately for camp Curtain in a [illegible word] the dust rising in cloud[s] And being almost insupportable—but not being any worse on the way than it was at camp.[8]

At this time, various regimental companies were mustering in and getting outfitted for the war. In the evening, Fulton walked round town in the company of a senior physician:

> the first time in My life that I Ever Saw market at night—the Capitol of
> the State is quite a fine looking [buil]ding though not what [I ex]pected to
> See—the Court House and insane asylum are fine buildings—after looking
> round untill nine o clock we came back to the Hotel where there was an order
> waiting me from Dr. Smith to meet him at the Beuhler House doeing So he
> appointed me to the 143ᵈ regiment Bucktail Brigade to Report to Col Rough
> Phila to be mustered into service—⁹

Whether or not Fulton toured the hospital at Camp Curtin is unclear, but had he done so, he would have seen the Sisters of St. Joseph. This might have been the first time he ever saw women as nurses. His superior, Dr. Smith, however, not only had recruited physicians such as Fulton but also had obtained the services of the Sisters of St. Joseph. Eight months earlier, on January 9, 1862, Smith had asked Mother St. John Fournier, the superior of the congregation, for sisters to serve as nurses at the Camp Curtin hospital. Sisters did not volunteer individually for nursing service; instead, medical and army authorities such as Dr. Smith or priest superiors specifically requested them. The Sisters of St. Joseph had worked with Dr. Smith at St. Joseph's Hospital in Philadelphia, and he was aware of their good reputation as nurses. On January 22, Smith wrote Mother St. John, "Whilst beset by applicants, every female nurse has been refused, Dr. Smith being unwilling to trust any but his old friends the Sisters of St. Joseph."¹⁰ Smith's preference for Catholic sister nurses acknowledged the image that many physicians held of lay women nurses who were untrained. With their history of firm discipline and obedience to authorities, sisters dispelled physicians' suspicions of women as "meddlesome" nurses, and army physicians often preferred them. At the time of Fulton's arrival at Camp Curtin in August, the sisters were already well established in their nursing roles.¹¹

Fulton's diary comments on the chaos at Camp Curtin, with many men clogging the roads and city. "I have often Seen the roads dusty but never in My life have I Seen Anything to this. Bodies of Men continually on the March and counter March Kept the [dust] flying in clouds all the time."¹² The sisters at Camp Curtin experienced this confusion as well. Conditions were constantly changing, and an epidemic of measles and typhoid fever had erupted. Smith was pleased with the sisters' disciplined work. He wrote their superior that "everything is now neat, orderly and comfortable." Hinting at relationships among the sisters, their male helpers, and the surgeons, Smith described the arrangements of the sister nurses in military language: "Sister Philomene is *Captain of the Ward* in the Camp Hospital and has a drummer boy to attend on her . . . Sister Camelia (Mother) is the *Major* & commands the Surgeons, keeping them in good humor & order by sewing on their buttons & other kind acts . . . [E]verything is in excellent order."[13] On April 14, 1862, Governor Andrew Curtin of Pennsylvania wrote Mother St. John, extolling the sisters who were "sacrificing all personal comfort, ministered faithfully & truly to the comfort & welfare of the sick."[14] Reflected in both of these letters are the romantic notions of the roles of nursing sisters, including self-sacrifice, compassion, obedience, and a sense of duty to care for the sick. Additionally, many of the nuns' nursing tasks included the sort of domestic housekeeping, cleaning, and sewing that some Northern doctors viewed as low status.

GETTYSBURG

The battle of Gettysburg was a pivotal event in the nation, and Fulton's diary reveals that he was fully conscious of participating in the great event of the day. This is the only section of the diary where he mentions women by name. Fulton also had indirect experience with the Daughters of Charity of St. Vincent de Paul as he marched passed their "female school St. Josephs' College" on the road to Emmitsburg, Maryland, just before the battle:

> within about 3 Miles of Emettsburg we came in view of that old and well
> known institution St. Josephs Mary's College for the purpose of Education of
> Catholic youth for the ministry . . . after passing this place and goeing about
> 3 Miles we Came to the celebrated town of Emettsburg here the main item
> of consideration being the Female School St. Joseph's College in which they
> have from one to three hundred pupils under instruction all the time . . . after
> passing this we passed on untill we Came into the town—the Seminary being
> out and to the south of the town—about half a mile near a fine Stream the
> Sisters have quite a fine farm upon which to support those under their care
> they being mostly orphan children and of course having nothing upon which
> to live have to depend upon charity—.[15]

The sisters to whom Fulton referred were Elizabeth Seton's Daughters of Charity of St. Vincent de Paul, and their farm supplied food for the army. As early as 1823, this congregation had worked as nurses at the Baltimore

Infirmary. Thus, by 1861, many of the sisters had more than thirty years of experience in American health care. During the Civil War, 232 Daughters of Charity worked at one time or another in Northern and Southern hospitals, in field hospitals, and on hospital ships.[16]

Although the Daughters of Charity had been running hospitals in the United States for decades, their first work in battlefields came with the Civil War. As Fulton passed through the town of Emmitsburg, he commented on the Daughters' female school, St. Joseph's College. He did not stay in the town, but the Daughters' archives leave a written record of the Union soldiers who did camp on the sisters' property beginning June 29, 1863. When the Union army reached Emmitsburg, Maj. Gen. George Gordon Meade and the other officers occupied the priest's house in town while the rest of the army camped at the Daughters' school grounds, which also included a "White House." The army had placed the entire town under military law, and generals and soldiers desperately needed food. The sisters took on the responsibility of providing meat, bread, coffee, and milk for the hungry men. These were tense times: their land, which Fulton notes had been secluded from the bustle of town, was now filled with men encamped everywhere space would allow, their bayonets shining and their guns moving along the sisters' windows. All day long, every day, the sisters fed the men. On July 1, the army left in the middle of the night for Gettysburg. "In fifteen minutes the Army was gone," wrote an annalist for the sisters, "and St. Joseph's Valley relapsed into quiet." Another sister wrote, "Not a vestige of the great Army was to be seen . . . Glad we were to get rid of them."[17]

The battle of Gettysburg commenced July 1, 1863, and according to his diary, that day, Fulton's unit began the march to the town of Gettysburg. Upon arrival, they came to the house of Mr. Meyers while looking for a place to eat. The diary adds further insight into Fulton's role in medical care during the battle. He reveals that he and other men in his unit were:

> Soon closely Engaged in Meeting the wants of the poor fellows who had been Brought in wounded and were greatly in need of Something to support and nourish them we made up Soup as fast as possible begging Bread And apple Butter for those that could Eat it until we had them pretty well Supplied.[18]

The July 1 entry also mentions some women who eventually tended the wounded on the battlefield. "Among those that made themselves the most useful of the citizens was M[r] Meyers and family, Mr Powers and his family,

Miss Harriet Schilling—Mrs. R Eyster with Whom I had the pleasure of being for Some time—"[19]

Fulton also offers observations during and after the battle. The chronology is not clear, and he appears to group events of several days under a single entry. For example, the July 3 diary entry noted:

> on the morning of the third day M[r]s Powers thought She would go out on the field of Battle and See if there was not some poor men there who were Suffering for the want of attention She found two and gave them Some water And Soon had one of them brought in And cared for As she best could her and her girls doeing all in their power for the comfort of the poor fellows—[20]

Women opened their private homes to receive the injured. Just as Fulton provided "comfort" for the wounded, similarly, women gave water, shelter, and wound care. To them, they were doing what women had done in their homes long before any military hospital system was well established. White middle-class women such as Ms. Powers volunteered their time, and they used their identification as caretakers in the home as justification for working as nurses, despite the fact that men also were nurses.

On July 4, as Confederates were pulling out of the town, Fulton walked over to the Seminary hospital. He noted:

> [T]he Cemetery Seemed to be one Mass of guns it Seemed to Me as though they could not have placed another gun had they wanted to do so . . . but no dead were to be seen Laying upon the field all having been buried—or taken away, the Men Seemed to be takeing it quite cool[l]y resting themselves as best they could after Such hard work as they had had—[21]

Fulton does not mention any encounter with the Daughters of Charity at the battlefield site or in any of the hospitals. Yet the Daughters' motherhouse at Emmitsburg was only thirty miles south of Gettysburg, and on July 4, they left to care for the wounded. Accompanied by their priest superior, Father J. Francis Burlando, fourteen Daughters of Charity took bandages, linen, sponges, and refreshments, intending to do what they could to help. The sisters were distinctive with their large white cornettes (winged head-dresses), which were very conspicuous to the Union soldiers along the road to the town. As one sister recalled, Union scouts met them and, mistaking their carriages for the enemy's ambulances, came close to firing on them. The sisters' entourage halted so that the soldiers could see their large white cornettes while Father Burlando "got a stick and putting a white handkerchief on it, holding it high, walked towards the Soldiers. They watched him closely for they had resolved to refuse flags of truce if offered. But seeing the cornettes removed their doubts." Protected by their religious habits and under Union escort, the sisters finally came to the battle site and saw "thousands of guns, swords that lay scattered around. Going on we came to that part of the B[urial].Ground from whence all the dead had not yet been removed . . . The roads were still filled with water from the rain." Added to the mud was blood, through which the carriage wheels had to roll. The writer mentioned seeing surgeons on horseback who held council in whispering voices "as to what was to be done."[22]

Sister Camilla O'Keefe left a moving account of the devastation the sisters encountered. She wrote, "On reaching the Battle grounds, awful! To see the men lying dead on the road—some by the side of their horses. O, it was beyond description! Hundreds of both armies lying dead almost on the track [so] that the driver had to be careful not to pass over the bodies. O! this picture of human beings slaughtered down by their fellow men in a cruel civil war was perfectly awful!"[23]

When the Union army followed Lee after the battle, most of the surgeons marched with their regiments. Fulton's regiment, the 143rd Pennsylvania, had two assistant surgeons, however, so that Fulton was spared to stay in Gettysburg to treat the brigade's wounded. At the beginning of the battle, he had been placed in charge of the Third Division Hospital, the Catholic and Presbyterian churches. Fulton again does not mention the Daughters of Charity, but they worked as nurses at the St. Xavier Church, the Catholic Church that had become a makeshift hospital under his charge. Fulton concentrates on the surgeons' work, not nurses: "the Surgeons being busily Engaged with the Sick—And wounded most of the operations being performed upon those that were in the Hospitals in town—." Sister Matilda Coskery, a Daughter of Charity who nursed at the St. Xavier Church, recalled an account from the standpoint of nursing. The sanctuary held the most distressing cases "of very worst amputated limbs." The sisters bandaged the wounded and provided drinks and nourishment. Tents and farmhouses extended for three miles outside the town, and ambulances took the sisters out to the area where they provided clothing, jellies, and combs that were needed to clear men's heads of lice. The Confederate wounded who had been abandoned by their army also received care.[24]

At this time, every Daughter of Charity who could be released worked in improvised hospitals in and around Gettysburg, which included not only St. Xavier's Catholic Church but also the Methodist Church hospital and the Seminary (Lutheran) hospital. Interestingly, the sisters' documents fail to mention any cooperation with lay women, nor do they mention any physician by name.[25]

These sisters came to the hospital with a clear knowledge of needed nursing skills. They had been taught by other sisters at the bedside as well as with texts written by sister nurses. Sister Matilda, who at sixty-two years of age nursed soldiers at six different military sites in addition to Gettysburg, was one of the teachers. In the archives is a document entitled *A Manual for the Care of the Sick*, thought to be written by Sister Matilda, probably sometime in the 1840s. She gave instructions on many areas that were considered "nursing," including how to maintain ventilation and a quiet environment, how to make a bed, procedures for treating blisters, what to do if relapse occurred, and how to treat fevers with fluids.[26] Sanitation was almost nonexistent in Civil War hospitals, and the lack of ventilation and basic cleanliness contributed to a high rate of illness. Thus Sister Matilda's instructions were in line with basic care that was needed, which Fulton also advocated. On January 10, 1864, for example, he ordered his men to "Either put their Blankets out to Air or fold them up Nicely And Lay them away, then Sweep or Clean the houses wash their hands and faces—And after Breakfast their utensils used in Cooking And Eating Must be Cleanly washed and put Carefully away—."[27] Sister Matilda would have approved.

RELIEF AGENCIES

Fulton frequently commented on the need for stores for his regiment, and he would have benefitted from relief organizations that were highly instrumental in collecting money and medical supplies for hospitals and battlefields. Thousands of women's aid societies in the North had members who sewed quilts, rolled bandages, and sent food. White Protestant women formed most of the soldiers' aid societies, but so did black, Jewish, and Catholic women.[28]

Clara Barton ran her own relief service independent of other women's groups and organizations. She had not applied to Dix's nursing corps; indeed, she disliked authoritarian women like Dix, and Barton's is an example of the blurred boundaries between official and unofficial nurses and relief workers. Barton often felt distressed when her services were not needed because Dix's nurses were working in divisional field hospitals. Dix appointees supervised diet kitchens and nursing personnel, which Barton viewed as her domain. Yet Barton eventually broke through the male military bureaucracy as she served as a relief worker at makeshift hospitals and hospital ships. She was present in Culpeper in 1862 (before Fulton's arrival in 1863) and brought stimulants, salves, bandages, and hospital clothing. The army was frequently short of these items as it established dressing stations near battlefields. While overworked surgeons and their attendants operated on patients, they did not clean the floors, and Barton spent much of her time tending to that task herself. It was at this time that she began her "course of labor" in an "unoccupied place" between the battlefield hospitals and general hospitals in the rear. To protect her work and avoid trespassing on the US Sanitary Commission's domain, Barton went to the commission's headquarters in Washington, DC, and obtained a letter of introduction, which she frequently showed Sanitary Commission agents in the field. Barton's efforts, however, frequently raised suspicion, since she worked outside official channels of Dix, the Sanitary Commission, or the Medical Department. On their part, Dix and the Sanitary Commission, whose work was often hampered by strict rules, developed a distrust of Barton and her authoritarian ways.[29]

The US Sanitary Commission had formed in 1861 as a voluntary organization whose mission was to provide Northern troops with supplies and medical care. Women were major financial supporters, and they formed a significant part of its workforce. The commission employed male and female nurses, physicians, stewards, and medical students. It did not discriminate against women on the basis of religious denomination, and Catholic sisters also nursed. Much of its work was considered women's work because of the cleanliness and order that women could bring. Women's nursing also included tending to wounds, cooking soups and cereal, and serving tea and coffee. Among the Sanitary Commission's lay female nurses were Protestant women of the middle and upper classes, such as Georgeanna Muir Woolsey, Eliza Woolsey Howland, and Katharine Prescott Wormeley. It was not unusual for class tensions to flare up on both sides when women of privilege had to do custodial labor. Some women hired to nurse did not like mending soldiers' clothing or doing the laundry. Elite women on Union hospital ships were upset when they had to do heavy labor when contraband or immigrant women could not be found to do it.[30]

Fulton's diary mentions a voluntary relief association on July 3, 1863:

> By this time the wounded that had been brought in from the first days had all been operated upon that required an operation most of them being pretty comfortable or as much so as they could be made under the circumstances— we not being able to get up the Hospital Wagons And neither the Gov nor any of the Sanitary Commissions being able to get through the Enemys lines— the men of course had no beds but then there was Straw Brought in and they were made as comfortable with that as it was possible to make them under the circumstances.[31]

Here Fulton mentions the importance of the hospital steward, Josiah Lewis, and the work of a relief organization that provided supplies when the army could not:

> On the Night of the first of July, Dr. Reamer dispatched Joe out on the ~~turnpike~~ road from Gettysburg to Millerston to help to take care of some of our wounded that were among the Rebs . . . To day the people out in the country began to Bring in things for the Sick and wounded Some would Bring in Bread Butter and apple Butter—others again preserves Milk And various things good And useful to those unable to go for them. the Christian Commission also brought in a wagon to day And Supplied Some things for the comfort of those they could accomadate until such times as they would be—Supplied through the Regular channels—which will likely be Sometime as the Rebs burned the Bridge at or near the town as well as doeing much damage ~~also~~ at Hanover Junction—[32]

As noted, the Sanitary Commission could not get through enemy lines, but delegates of the Christian Commission could. The Christian Commission came into operation after the first battle at Bull Run in 1861 with the purpose of providing supplies, medical services, and religious readings to Union troops. It worked alongside the US Sanitary Commission, and both organizations became the most significant agencies for charitable relief during the war. Supplementing Fulton's diary are Christian Commission documents, which note that on July 2, a delegate arrived in Gettysburg and found the wounded lying under every tree. The woods and roadsides were full of them, and only a few could be accommodated in ambulances. The Christian Commission representative began constructing stakes with bedding placed over them for shade, but rain came later in the evening: "We did the best we could, but few escaped the water that night." One soldier recalled the care he received from a member of the Christian Commission: "Without waiting to waste words, [he] supplied me with a feather pillow—the first I had had in a year—a quilt, a draught of wine, some nice soft crackers and a cup of warm tea." The soldier lay on the field until July 15, mainly tended by agents of the Christian Commission.[33]

In the meantime, Fulton's responsibilities to the wounded continued as those who had "not been brought in from the farm houses round were brought in by the Ambulances." On July 6, 1863, he wrote: "we received one hundred and forty—it being difficult to find room in which to place them Many of them had to be placed upon the floor in the doorway And any other place that they could get to lay down—."[34]

CARE OF THE DYING

Fulton and the many caretakers—nurses, other physicians, hospital stewards, and representatives of relief commissions—all played significant roles in caring for the dying. Drew Gilpin Faust argues that as men fought in the Civil War battles, they contemplated death—it was all around them.[35] Similarly, Fulton wrote,

> [T]he Army cannot be Said to be religious though all Seem to have a profound Respect for religion—And talk of death as a something not [Do] unlikely to cross their path and stop their Earthly cares but with little fear— there is a calusness [callousness] and resignation manifested that is truely to be admired—"[36]

As Faust notes, at a time when people still died at home, the four years of the war challenged all the soldiers' expectations as they died amid strangers. A "good death" was very important to soldiers, who wanted comfort and peace of mind and help with what lay ahead. A major role for any caretaker in the war, then, was to comfort soldiers when they were dying, to provide them a Bible if they wanted or relics and crucifixes if they were Catholic, and to notify their families back home that they had, indeed, died well. Witnesses reported soldiers' deathbed conversions, and family members of the soldiers eagerly awaited evidence of salvation.[37]

CONCLUSION

Fulton's experiences with nurses and relief workers highlight the complex nursing world of women and men that developed during the Civil War. Fulton appears grateful for the help that women provided during the Gettysburg crisis, and to be sure, his seeming indifference to them during the bulk of his experiences might simply have been an indication of more pressing matters on his mind to which he had to attend. It is clear, however, that women assumed important roles as relief workers, caretakers, and medical assistants during the period of national emergency. Some surgeons actively employed women, including Catholic sisters, while others did not allow women at all, viewing them as useless. Both women and men shared the goal of helping soldiers to recover or to die well. Fulton's diary does not mention any of these details. While this likely speaks to his view of women as having marginal status within the military and medical realms of the Civil War, their work, nevertheless, was significant.

BARBRA MANN WALL, PhD, RN, FAAN, holds the Thomas A. Saunders III Professorship in Nursing at the University of Virginia School of Nursing, where she is Director of the Eleanor Crowder Bjoring Center for Nursing Historical Inquiry. She has been funded by the National Institutes of Health and by university and private grants. She has published three books: *Unlikely Entrepreneurs: Catholic Sisters and the Hospital Marketplace, 1865–1925* (2005), *American Catholic Hospitals: A Century of Changing Markets and Missions* (2011), and *Into Africa: A Transnational History of Catholic Missions and Social Change* (2015).

NOTES

1. Jane E. Schultz, *Women at the Front: Hospital Workers in Civil War America* (Chapel Hill: University of North Carolina Press, 2004). First quotation was published in *American Medical Times*, July 18, 1861, 25–6, as quoted in *America's Working Women*, ed. Rosalyn Baxandall, Linda Gordon, and Susan Reverby (New York: Random House, 1976), 75–6. Second quotation is in George W. Adams, *Doctors in Blue: The Medical History of the Union Army in the Civil War* (New York: Henry Schuman, 1952), 182. Other sources on relationships between female nurses and male physicians include Katherine Prescott Wormeley, *The United States Sanitary Commission: A Sketch of Its Purposes and Its Work* (Boston: Little, Brown and Company, 1863), 246; Ann Douglas Wood, "The War Within a War: Women Nurses in the Union Army," *Civil War History* 18 (1972): 197–212; Estelle Brodman and Elizabeth B. Carrick,

"American Military Medicine in the Mid-Nineteenth Century: The Experience of Alexander H. Hoff, M.D.," *Bulletin of the History of Medicine* 64 (1990): 63–78; and Scott McGaugh, *Surgeon in Blue: Jonathan Letterman, the Civil War Doctor Who Pioneered Battlefield Care* (New York: Arcade Publishing, 2013).

2. D. L. Dix, Circular No. 8, 24 July 1862, reprinted in Philip Kalisch and Beatrice Kalisch, *The Advance of American Nursing*, 3rd ed. (Philadelphia: J. B. Lippincott Company, 1995), 40; Kalisch and Kalisch, *The Advance of American Nursing*. Regarding pay, see Mother M. Angela Gillespie, notebook, handwritten MS, Archives of the Congregation of the Sisters of the Holy Cross, Saint Mary's, Notre Dame, Indiana. Mark Boatner, *Civil War Dictionary* (New York: David McKay Company, Inc., 1959). The army private received $16 per month by the middle of 1864 after the last raise was given by the government.

3. Jeanne Boydston, *Home and Work: Housework, Wages, and the Ideology of Labor in the Early Republic* (Oxford, UK: Oxford University Press, 1990). Quotation is on p. xx.

4. Margaret Humphreys, *Marrow of Tragedy: The Health Crisis of the American Civil War* (Baltimore, MD: Johns Hopkins University Press, 2013). See also Schultz, *Women at the Front*.

5. Schultz, *Women at the Front*; James Fulton, Diary, 1862–1864, entry for January 12, 1863.

6. Schultz, p. 34; Judith Ann Giesberg, "In Service to the Fifth Wheel: Katharine Prescott Wormeley and Her Experiences in the United States Sanitary Commission," *Nursing History Review* 3 (1995): 43–53; and Kristie Ross, "Arranging a Doll's House: Refined Women as Union Nurses," in *Divided Houses: Gender and the Civil War,* ed. Catherine Clinton and Nina Silber (New York: Oxford University Press, 1992), 102.

7. Ellen Ryan Jolly, *Nuns of the Battlefield* (Providence, RI: The Providence Visitor Press, 1927), 133, 13; and Sister Mary Denis Maher, *To Bind Up the Wounds: Catholic Sister Nurses and the U.S. Civil War* (Baton Rouge: Louisiana State University Press, 1989).

8. James Fulton, Diary, 1862–1864, entry for August 19, 1862.

9. Ibid.

10. Henry H. Smith to Mother St. John Fournier, 9 January 1861 [2]; and for quote, 22 January 1862, Archives of the Sisters of St. Joseph at Philadelphia Mount St. Joseph Convent, Chestnut Hill, Philadelphia (hereafter cited as ASSJP).

11. On January 23, three sisters arrived at Camp Curtin Hospital. They could not go to a wartime hospital without the consent of Bishop James F. Wood of Philadelphia, however, who granted them permission.

12. Fulton, August 19, 1862.

13. Henry H. Smith to Mother St. John Fournier, 2 February 1862, ASSJP. See also Barbra Mann Wall, "Called to a Mission of Charity: The Sisters of St. Joseph in the Civil War," *Nursing History Review* 6 (1998): 85–113.

14. A. G. Curtin to Madam St. John, 14 April 1862, ASSJP.

15. Fulton, June 29, 1863.

16. Elizabeth Seton had established the Sisters of Charity in Emmitsburg, Maryland, in 1809, although St. Vincent de Paul and Saint Louise De Marillac had begun the mission in seventeenth-century France. In 1850, after Seton's death and subsequent to events brought about by the French Revolution, the sisters at Emmitsburg united with the Daughters of Charity of St. Vincent de Paul, who were based in France, and the American sisters assumed the name Daughters of Charity. Jolly, *Nuns of the Battlefield*; and Sister Betty A. McNeil, DC, "The Daughters of Charity as Civil War Nurses, Caring without Boundaries," *Vincentian Heritage Journal* 27, no. 1 (2007): 133–68, online at http://via.library.depaul.edu/vhj, accessed October 22, 2018.

17. The Daughters of Charity nursed at battlefield sites at Antietam and Boonsboro, Maryland; Gettysburg, Pennsylvania; and Vicksburg, Mississippi. They worked on hospital ships up and down the Mississippi River, the Potomac, and Chesapeake Bay. They also worked with the ambulance corps at Manassas, Virginia, and Harpers' Ferry, and they nursed in isolation camps and in improvised hospitals in New Orleans, Pensacola, St. Louis, and Richmond. On the Gettysburg campaign, see *Annals of St. Joseph's*, p. 523. The *Annals* are typewritten and handwritten manuscripts that are located in the Archives of the Daughters of Charity Province of St. Louise, Emmitsburg, MD (hereafter cited as ADOC). First quotation is on p. 524. Second is on p. 534.

18. Fulton, July 1, 1863.

19. Ibid.

20. Ibid., July 3, 1863.

21. Ibid., July 4, 1863.

22. "Gettysburg." This handwritten account, written by a Daughter of Charity, is located at ADOC. This likely was written in retrospective when Father Burlando requested this information so he could submit a report to their general superiors in Paris, France.

23. Sister Camilla O'Keefe's Notes, 1863, Box 7-5-1 (1), folder 6, "Battle of Gettysburg," ADOC.

24. Fulton, July 1 and 4, 1863; *Annals of St. Joseph*, pp. 537, 539–40.

25. The Civil War, 1861–1865, typed copy in ADOC.

26. Sister Matilda was born in 1799. From Frederick County, Maryland, she entered the Sisters of Charity of Saint Joseph's, in August 1828. She worked in numerous nursing roles, primarily in Baltimore. Maryland. She is particularly known for her psychiatric nursing. She died in 1870. See McNeil, "The Daughters of Charity as Civil War Nurses"; Sister Matilda Coskery, *A Manual for the Care of the Sick*, ADOC.

27. Fulton, January 10, 1864.

28. Jeanie Attie, *Patriotic Toil: Northern Women and the American Civil War* (Ithaca, NY: Cornell University Press, 1998).

29. Stephen B. Oates, *A Woman of Valor: Clara Barton and the Civil War* (New York: The Free Press, 1994). Quotation is on p. 63. Elizabeth Brown Pryor, *Clara Barton, Professional Angel* (Philadelphia: University of Pennsylvania Press, 1987).

30. Judith Giesberg, *Civil War Sisterhood: The U.S. Sanitary Commission and Women's Politics in Transition* (Boston: Northeastern University Press, 2000). For a description of the different personnel the Sanitary Commission employed and their job descriptions, see Jane Stuart Woolsey, *Hospital Days* (New York: D. Van Nostrand, 1870); Wormeley, *The United States Sanitary Commission;* Schultz, *Women at the Front,* 34–6.

31. Fulton, July 3, 1863.

32. Ibid.

33. The idea of Christian relief had begun earlier, however, within business men's prayer meetings, and both women and men helped raise funds. The five thousand commission delegates were unpaid volunteers. See the Rev. Lemuel Moss, *Annals of the United States Christian Commission* (Philadelphia, PA: J.B. Lippincott, 1868), Digitized at https://books.google .com/books?id=HrKbf1YQvewC&printsec=frontcover&dq=the+christian+commission& hl=en&sa=X&ved=0CBoQ6AEwAGoVChMI67mR79vixwIVTJUeCh2iCgi5#v=onepage& q=the%20christian%20commission&f=false, accessed October 22, 2018; Edward Parmelee Smith, *Incidents of the United States Christian Commission* (Philadelphia, PA: J. B. Lippincott, 1871), digitized and online at https://books.google.com/books?id=cKk8AAAAYAAJ&pg=P

A159&source=gbs_toc_r&cad=3#v=onepage&q&f=false, accessed October 22, 2018; John C. Chamberlain and the Christian Commission, Middletown, MD, July 11, 1863, online at http://www.edinborough.com/Lean/Commission/Camberlain.htm, accessed October 22, 2018; Smith, *Incidents of the United States Christian Commission*, 161.

    34. Fulton, July 6, 1863.

    35. Drew Gilpin Faust, *This Republic of Suffering: Death and the American Civil War* (New York: Random House, 2008), 4.

    36. Fulton, November 18, 1863.

    37. Faust, *This Republic of Suffering*.

TWELVE

"We Made Up Soup as Fast as Possible"

Nutrition and the Nineteenth-Century Male Body

MARGARET HUMPHREYS

FOOD AND THE LANDSCAPE

As James Fulton left home for the war, he gloried in the sight of the "great Chester Valley," which offered "the broad Expanse of highly cultivated and fertile land Stretching for Miles before the Entranced Vision of the beholder." Little did Fulton know it, but what lay before him, "the highly cultivated farms with Excellent buildings finely fenced," would play an enormous role in the war that was just beginning.[1] Food would win the war; Lee only surrendered in 1865 when he could no longer feed his men. Fulton saw that fact in microcosm during his time in Virginia, Maryland, and Pennsylvania while in uniform. He may have been trained as a doctor, but he looked at his environment through the eyes of a farmer. Food was always on his mind.[2]

He repeatedly commented on how unimproved many Southern farms appeared to him. In June of 1863, near Broad Run in northernmost Virginia, he noted that "the land that was clear looking as though it was too poor to keep a Whiporwile from starving." In contrast, an area in Maryland "seemed as though we had got into the garden of Eden itself," with fields full of good-quality grain. Aside from a general scorn at the laziness of Southerners and the impact of slavery on poor husbandry, Fulton also recognized the destruction war itself had wrought on the food supply. As the army moved toward winter camp near Manassas, he noted "the Army has not been through this part of Virginia and of course the fences had not been disturbed and there had been pretty good Crops." More land could be "made Beautiful if it only had the Enterprise." Still, there was enough local produce that "we could trade Sugar and Coffee for butter And Eggs, Poultry And in fact almost any-thing that a soldier might want in the way of Eating."[3]

Fulton witnessed the deficiencies of the Southern landscape as a pro-ducer of food firsthand when he met with Confederate troops taken prisoner of war. In November 1863, he saw a group of rebels awaiting transport to a prisoner of war camp: "[T]hey presented their usual ragged and dirty appear-ance doubtless Many of them glad to be taken as they will now get plenty to Eat and have nothing to do." He observed local people, too, previously prosperous, who were begging for bread from the Union army. Fulton told an anecdote about the Confederate prisoners that was meant to illustrate just how desperately hungry they were. The Union army issued a sort of hard cracker called hardtack (about which, more below) as a form of ration to take on marches when there would be no time for baking or cooking. He came upon a group of ragged and barefoot prisoners. "[T]here was a pile of Broken hard Bread that had been thrown out and they soon began to put it in their haversacks . . . [They] Seemed quite hungry"—so hungry that they would scrounge dirty crackers from the mud in order to fill their stomachs.[4] Little could he know that the rebel soldiers were well fed compared to the Union prisoners in Southern hands.

RATIONS AND SUPPLY

Fulton rarely commented on his own men going without adequate nutri-ment. The Union army ration dictated that each man should have a fixed daily amount of fresh beef (20 oz.) or salt pork (12 oz.). With that, he was to be served 22 oz. of soft bread or 16 oz. of hardtack or alternatives. Dried peas, beans, rice, or hominy supplemented this base. In an attempt to el-evate the nutritional value of these rations, the army supplied dehydrated vegetables, with the idea that they be rehydrated to give variety to soups. The ration promised fresh potatoes as well, and sometimes soldiers received them. Union troops had a regular coffee ration that was the envy of the Con-federates, who generally had only ersatz brews for their morning cup. The assumption was that this diet would supply more than the needed amount, so that the officers could spend some of the budget for food purchases on other comestibles available locally. When a man went into the hospital, his ration was to follow him, but in the chaos of wound care and patient transport after a battle, he might often end up with no one responsible for drawing his ration and hence feeding him.[5]

An army in the field poses particular problems in terms of food supply. Imagine an army of, say, twenty thousand men (ninety-four thousand Union troops fought at the Battle of Gettysburg). First, none of those men is at home, plowing fields and raising crops. Even if their families could cover the lost labor with the work of women, children, and the elderly, still, the creation of an army means a likely decline in food production. Second, the government is feeding all of those men. The government has to acquire, transport, and distribute the food to the men. Decisions must be made about whether each man or unit cooks its own food, or whether a central kitchen of some sort cooks and distributes it. Fulton was pleased when his mess—a group of officers who decided to cook and eat together—acquired a stove for six dollars; this meant that they would be able to bake bread for the group, and perhaps for the sick, if there was adequate flour. Since the food has to be shipped in, it must be preserved in some way. Barrels of flour, salt, and yeast were not a major challenge in this regard, although flour could get wet and rot, or be full of worms. Harder was the ration of meat. It could be salted, which staved off rotting at the expense of high salt content. Or the meat could be brought to the army "on the hoof"—if the army was able to efficiently muster animals and their transportation.[6]

ON THE MARCH

To a greater or lesser extent, the army expected to live off the countryside. The army had funds to buy local foods, where available. Officers like Fulton had money (when they were paid) to buy individual meals to supplement their army supplies. For example, Fulton bought breakfast near King Georges Court House. "[W]e had quite a good meal for 50 cts," he crowed. "[W]arm Biscuit hoe cake Shad and coffee—So that we could go on our way rejoicing." On another occasion, he could not find food to buy in the vicinity of camp, but he went into town and rented a bed for the night, a bed that turned out to be too soft for comfort. But the next morning, "I had quite a good Breakfast," again for only fifty cents total. These forays into the food of normal life made for memorable meals after stretches of nothing but "hard tack and meat for so long."[7]

Holidays, with their associations of feasting, were particularly difficult. Fulton complained that Christmas 1863 was grim, with nothing in camp but hardtack and raw pork. He went into a hotel, and was grumpy that instead of the turkey, mince, and geese pies he expected, he had to make do with boiled cabbage and potatoes and roast beef. He did get his mince pie, though. Still, it was hardly a Christmas feast in his eyes. Some of the officers bought treats for New Year's Day—barrels of apples from some, and extra canteens of whiskey from others.[8] The fact that Fulton records these various meals or celebratory foods in detail speaks to how important such dining opportunities were to him, both in satisfying his hunger and exemplifying some approximation of regular life.

Living off the land was often problematic, both for Fulton and the common soldiers. Officially, the men were not allowed to take food from locals without compensation. We see just such an infraction, and its adjudication, when the men of Fulton's regiment stole hay and fence rails from a farmer. The man put in a bill to the officers that finally had to be paid out of the regimental payroll. This camp was probably near Washington, DC, and the owner a loyal Union man. As the Union army moved deeper into rebel territory, however, scruples about stealing faded. Fulton saw foraging en masse for the first time in June 1863. He heard "the crack of the rifle" coming from all directions. As there were "fine flocks of Sheep in the neighborhood—the Boys improved their time by getting Some mutton . . . it was but long [a long time] until might be seen a quarter of Mutton—or veal hanging up by almost Every tent indicating that fresh meat was at least abundant one Evening."[9] Elsewhere. the troops justified their theft by proclaiming that the chicken or pig or sheep was an unrepentant "secesh" who would not take the oath of allegiance. Once the animal refused, then it was traitor and subject to forfeiture of all its property—namely its chops and drumsticks and hams. Mostly Fulton applauded the acquisition of local food, although in one instance he pitied a poor woman who had lost her last onions to Union scavengers.[10] The men were also able to supplement their food with fish and clams from neighborhood waterways, or persimmons picked at ripeness.

When the army went on the march, the men had to carry their rations on their persons, and cook when possible on the road. They were advised to cook their rations ahead of time, so that they could be easily accessible. With meat, this might mean cold bacon or something akin to beef jerky. Instead of soft bread, the men carried a pound or more of hard crackers called hardtack. Baked in faraway Milton, Massachusetts, and other Northern towns, this product was shipped to the camp, giving it plenty of time to dry out and become riddled with vermin in its passage. It was too hard to bite off and chew, and required soaking to be digestible. Men made a sort of stew with their cooked meat, hardtack, and available water, when there was the luxury of a campfire and a cup or pan was available. Fulton's associate in the 150th Pennsylvania, Assistant Surgeon Matthew A. Henderson, describes such a meal: "I have breakfasted, mercy what a breakfast half raw, dirty, bloody gritty tough bull beef, half boiled coffee + hardtack—but I tear it apart + suck the juice + drink my muddy coffee with an appetite, coming sometimes only once in 24 hrs."[11]

The men called hardtack "tooth dullers" or "sheet-iron crackers" and joked about using them for paving stones. The men sang derisive songs of their unpleasant fare, and in mockery extolled the protein value of the worms found therein. One story told of men in the trenches during the sieges of Richmond and Petersburg who tossed their wormy crackers to the trench floor in disgust. When rebuked by an officer for the mess they had made and told to clear out the cracker debris, the men claimed that "we've thrown it out two or three times, sir, but it crawls back."[12] These are the very same crackers that the rebel prisoners were gouging out of the mud.

FOOD AS MEDICINE

Fulton revealed his attitude toward food and health in both general terms and in specifics with regard to the wounded and ill. Food and drinking alcohol were important for energy, energy that was evident in high spirits and enthusiasm for the task at hand. As his troops marched toward Gettysburg, they passed through villages of Union sympathizers, "[T]he people generally manifesting much Patriotism the Ladies more Particularly by the waving of Flags And singing of Patriotic Songs." Fulton was pleased by the effect on the men: "[T]hese demonstrations Seemed to do the Boys much good the cheering of the Ladies in particular here." And not only cheering—"they began to get apple butter and good Bread And thing[s] of this character that Strengthened up the Boys And Kept their Spirits good." Mind and body were one in this consideration of mental and physical health. When patriotic songs lagged, alcohol could similarly elevate energy. On one climb over the mountains of Maryland, "the Boy's [sic] learned that a little log house by the wayside had Something for Sale that would Stimulate and the result was that a great running was kept up for a time."[13] General health depended on adequate stimulation—emotional, spiritual, and physical.

All Civil War surgeons knew that wounded men especially needed stimulants to rouse their failing constitutions. Thus alcohol—whiskey or brandy were the best—was genuinely seen as an essential therapy for wounds, especially in the setting of prolonged exposure and dehydration such as might follow a battlefield wound. And wounded men also needed dense, palatable liquids, such as cream-based drinks, or puddings. Fulton was desperate to find such items in the chaos after Gettysburg; nearby, another early responder on the field at Gettysburg, Cornelia Hancock, answered just this need. She found many wounded men piled up near the train station, with no one tending to their needs. Nearby were wagons of supplies, probably from the United States Sanitary Commission (USSC) (see chapter 11). With no one in charge, she took it upon herself to make jelly sandwiches, accompanied by a punch made from whiskey and canned condensed milk. This is the sort of food that Fulton wanted for his wounded, but the "Sanitary" wagons had not penetrated to his location. In the weeks that followed, the USSC used refrigerated cars to move in crates of lemons and oranges, and thousands of bottles of whiskey, brandy, and wine to support the men in recovery. Lemonade was a common treat in Northern hospitals, which no doubt contributed greatly to wound healing.[14]

Would Fulton, trained as a physician, know more about the dietary needs of the sick and wounded than Cornelia Hancock with her homemaker's knowledge? What did science and medicine know about the healthy diet in 1861? One illustrative essay published at the end of the war divided foods into proteins (albuminoids), carbohydrates (starches), and fats. Its author, Dr. Sanford Hunt, drew on the latest of European biochemistry research to describe the best diet for the average man, said to weigh 140 pounds; by the time I was in medical school, such measures related to the "average 70 kg male (155 lbs)." People were, on average, shorter then; the average Civil War soldier was 5'7". Hunt argued that proteins contributed to muscle growth and repair, while the carbohydrates and fats were most important for generating heat and energy. Vegetables and fruits were key as well, although their precise contribution was unclear. He also acknowledged the importance of minerals such as potash, iron, and magnesia, which he deemed essential for proper digestion, and likewise recognized the role of artificial stimulants such as alcohol, coffee, and tea. Hunt's essay features percentages, tables, and chemical analysis; if Fulton studied this sort of account in medical school, it is unlikely that it was at the top of his mind as a Civil War doctor. Rather, he likely thought mainly in terms of basics, such as, "a man needs bread and meat." There is nothing in his diary to display a more technical understanding of the latest in physiology research.[15]

Like Hunt, Fulton probably was aware of the concept of "anti-scorbutics," although he makes no overt reference to scurvy or anti-scorbutic foods here. The specific understanding of vitamins and their contribution to health would not become clear until the twentieth century, but familiarity with foods that fended off scurvy was widespread. Still, getting fresh fruit and vegetables to an army on the move was difficult. "Fresh" implies a high water content, and thus a heavy weight. Lucky men could forage fresh fruit in the vicinity of camp, but it didn't take long for that source to be exhausted. Conveying fruits and vegetables to the men was a major task of the USSC. It supplied delicacies in the forms of jams and fruits to the general hospitals safely behind the lines; it sent pounds of potatoes and barrels of sauerkraut to the front lines. Aside from the situation of the black troops, whose diet was poorly administered by uncaring officers, scurvy was relatively rare among Union men as a result. It was much more of a problem among the Confederates, who had to contend both with an inadequate transportation system and the Union blockade.[16]

GETTYSBURG

Fulton's ideas about the proper feeding of the sick were most evident in the wake of the Gettysburg battle, when he struggled to not only set up a proper hospital for the care of the wounded, but find the supplies to feed them. He was separated from his assistants, his equipment, and even his horse. He found that the wounded who immediately came under his care "had given most of their Bread to our soldiers as they passed in the morning of the 1st of July— that which was left the Rebs took." So the immediate need was food: "Engaged in meeting the wants of the poor fellows who had been Brought in wounded and were greatly in need of something to support and nourish them we made up soup as fast as possible begging Bread and apple Butter for those who could Eat it." To support and nourish is the core of Fulton's healing philosophy.[17]

An immediate problem was the lack of bread, even hardtack, although Fulton was desperate to get the wounded soft bread to eat. He acquired the equipment and knowledge of baking from a local baker, but lacked flour. At this point, the town was occupied by the rebel army, so he visited Confederate Gen. Richard Ewell and explained that the wounded needed bread and asked if they could spare some flour. Ewell promised that it would be done, but no flour ever came. Fulton found the town "so stri[p]ped that no one had anything to give away." And to compound the problem, they could not "get up the Hospital Wagons And neither the Gov nor any of the Sanitary Commissions being able to get through the Enemys lines."[18]

Things began to improve on July 4, as the Confederates retreated and "people out in the country began to Bring in things for the Sick and wounded Some would Bring in Bread Butter and apple Butter—others again preserves Milk And various things good And useful to those unable to go for them." The Christian Commission brought in a wagon, and other supplies, such as "chickens for the wounded" began to arrive. Fulton acquired the drinking alcohol he needed to treat the sick, as he reported "we also used alcohol pretty freely as a Stimulant to the granulations" (a tissue formation in the healing wound). He was pouring the liquor down men's throats, not dousing the wounds with it.[19]

James Fulton recognized food as central to the soldier's lot, whether he was on the march or knocked down by illness or wound. Fulton's viewpoint drew from common knowledge about the supportive power of food, and especially alcohol, more than from any specialized medical knowledge. It is unlikely that he would have differed much in his approach to food from Cornelia Hancock or the women of the Sanitary Commission. He knew hunger and dietary monotony during his time in the army, and thus appreciated his occasional good meals. The abundance of the Pennsylvania farm country, visible on his departure if a bit slow to arrive after the battle of Gettysburg, indeed made all the difference in the fighting strength of the Union men under his care and observation.

MARGARET HUMPHREYS, MD, PhD, is the Josiah Charles Trent Professor in the History of Medicine, Professor of History, and Professor of Medicine at Duke University. She is author of *Marrow of Tragedy: The Health Crisis of the American Civil War* (2013) and *Intensely Human: The Health of the Black Soldier in the American Civil War* (2008).

NOTES

1. James Fulton, Diary, 1862–1864. Entry for August 19, 1862.

2. Fulton's descriptions of the environment can be illuminated through his politics (chapter 13), environmental history (chapter 7), and medical ideology (Introduction and chapter 8),as well as diet.

3. Fulton, quotations from diary entries for June 18, 1863; June 26, 1863; October 21, 1863; and October 24 and 25, 1863, respectively.

4. Ibid., quotations from November 14, 1863, and November 8, 1863, respectively.

5. Sanford Hunt, "Army Alimentation in Relation to the Causation and Prevention of Disease," in *Contributions Relating to the Causation and Prevention of Disease, and to Camp Diseases,* ed. Austin Flint (New York: US Sanitary Commission by Hurd and Houghton, 1867), 73.

6. Fulton, January 12, 1863; William C. Davis, *A Taste for War: The Culinary History of the Blue and the Gray* (Lincoln: University of Nebraska Press, 2003).

7. Fulton, quotations at April 1863, June 27, 1863, and March 22, 1862, respectively.

8. Ibid., December 25, 1863, and January 1, 1864, respectively.

9. Ibid., quotations at March 1863, and June 18, 1863, respectively.

10. Davis, *A Taste for War*, 47; Fulton, June 29, 1863.

11. Davis, *A Taste for War*, 41–2; Matthew A. Henderson, letter to sister, "'Wilderness' near Chancell'ville," May 3, 1863. Collection of the National Museum of American History/Smithsonian Institution.

12. Davis, *A Taste for War*, 43.

13. Fulton, June 26 and 28, 1863.

14. Margaret Humphreys, *Marrow of Tragedy: The Health Crisis of the American Civil War* (Baltimore, MD: Johns Hopkins University Press, 2013), 125.

15. Hunt, "Army Alimentation," 69–94.

16. Humphreys, *Intensely Human: The Health of the Black Soldier in the American Civil War* (Baltimore, MD: Johns Hopkins University Press, 2008), 119–24.

17. Fulton, July 1, 1863.

18. Ibid., July 2, 3, 1863.

19. Ibid., July 4, 1863.

THIRTEEN

"Such Is the Character of Many Men"

Dr. Robert Fulton's Politics and the Moral and Political Consciousness of Soldiers

RANDALL M. MILLER

JAMES FULTON, MD, OF CHESTER COUNTY, PENNSYLVANIA, JOINED the Union war effort in 1862 to serve his country and practice his calling as a doctor. As his diary reveals, the war made him a soldier as much as a surgeon, more committed to his country and sure of his calling. It also matured him politically and morally as he essayed the character and purpose of the Union and the meaning and necessity of men fighting, and dying, for a noble cause. Like the American people, Fulton had to learn about war. In doing so, he learned about himself and discovered an America in fact that had only been an abstraction before he went off to war. In all that, he was like so many other young men who rallied to save the Union and in the end came to appreciate the nation by seeing it in action, defending its foundation and purpose as what Abraham Lincoln famously called "the last best hope" of mankind for democracy and freedom. In his diary, Fulton did not articulate particular political ideologies or align explicitly with a political party or interest, but his values were those of the Republican Party and his morality that of the Protestant ethos that ruled America during his day. His experience during the war reaffirmed those values and that ethos. His diary tells us so.

—✺—

Fulton's discovery of America and himself began with the land. Heading south into the war in summer 1862, Fulton sometimes rhapsodized about the beauty of the mountains and vales he saw in passing through Maryland and Virginia. Like so many other young men of his day, he did not travel much and knew the "America" beyond his home orbit more through story, history, and travel accounts by foreign visitors rather than his own observation and experience. And like many Union soldiers, his movements southward impressed him with the majesty of God's handiwork and the potential bounty Providence had laid before them from the first English settlements in the "New World" to their own time. Throughout his diary, he commented on the land he was coming to know as both a place of wonder and of prospect.

REPUBLICAN IDEALS

The beauty of the land struck him as proof of God's favor for the American people. In 1863, for example, while returning north from Virginia, he wrote upon sighting South Mountain, near Antietam in Maryland, that "it Seemed as though the Author of nature had been more than lavish in his dispensation of beauty—and with which this part of creation had been adorned." He continued, "the love[r]—of nature could here feast his Eyes upon the rough and rugged Mountain, crowned with forest, brought in direct contrast with the richest and loveliest of vallies Spread out beneath like a carpet of richest hues with the Serpentine rivulet meander[ing]." And in a burst of national pride, he concluded that "we Americans go to the Alps to see beauty . . . yet Know nothing of the rich beauty of our own country."[1] And again, on New Year's Day, 1864, amid frustration that the war continued, Fulton felt the spiritual power of nature when viewing the snow-capped Blue Ridge Mountains "Reflecting the Suns Rays in all their beauty." The scene made an impression "rarely felt And only at such times as the mind is Strongly And Solemnly impressed with the beautiful in Nature" that it was "well Calculated to bring Man in communion with his God" and to stand in awe "of the great Superiority of the being that has brought into form" a work of "such Magnitude And beauty."[2] Seeing and appreciating one's own God-anointed country made it all the more important not to give it up to secession and rebellion.

But all bounty was not due to nature's gifts. Again, like so many of his contemporaries, Fulton weighed the worth of the land in terms of what man might, even ought, do with it. Whatever the contradiction, the sublimity and utility of the land went hand in hand for Fulton and many of his generation, much as in the nineteenth-century writings of government-sponsored explorers and the landscape paintings of men venturing westward to find a new land. Fulton's own agricultural interests also led him to assay the potential of river valleys, foothills, and tidewater for growing and reaping what the land would surely yield with hard, honest labor.[3]

In Fulton's mind, such promise was always conditional. The providence the land offered depended on man's purposeful and productive labor. Such belief was a constant refrain in the English promotional literature beckoning colonists to cross the ocean during the seventeenth century to grow and harvest in a new Eden and repeated in the mid-nineteenth-century-era call of a Manifest Destiny for Americans to occupy the whole of the continent and make even the desert bloom. Realizing such promise was God's command.

That thinking underscored the free-soil ideology of the Republican Party that celebrated the American ideal of the simple yeoman republican farmer being free by owning land and keeping the full value of the unfettered, honest labor he earned with his own hands—in effect, by owning himself. That free-soil ideology was rooted in a political and moral economy that made possible what Abraham Lincoln, among others, insisted was the "right to rise" as the essence of liberty and the surety for a democratic polity. America's place in God's grand design and the hope for freedom anywhere and everywhere thus hinged on securing such liberty in America. Slavery posed a clear and present danger to such aspiration and obligation.[4]

Republicans argued that the contrast between a free society and a corrupted and corrupting one was there for all to see, and it was close at hand. One did not need to go to faraway lands in Mississippi or Louisiana to see slavery's baneful consequence. Indeed, the proximity between the prosperity of a free people north of the Mason-Dixon Line and the misery of those in slavery's thrall below it made the contrast all the more telling. So it was that in his travels through Virginia before the war, William Henry Seward spoke for many free-soilers when he observed firsthand what slavery wrought. In Virginia, he found that "the land was sterile, the fences mean, and a universal impress of poverty [was] stamped on all around me."[5] Other Republicans before and during the war made similar indictments of the Old Dominion, and blamed its exhausted soils, poor crops, rundown buildings, and unhappy state on the crippling effects of slavery, which discouraged initiative and improvement and dragged down nonslaveholder and slave alike.

Thus, the Republican Party opposed any extension of slavery into the territories during the 1850s. That issue defined the Republican Party, fractured the ordinary politics of the day, and enraged the slaveholding Southerners who insisted on their right to carry their slaves anywhere into the territories. Secession followed, and the war came. During the war, the Republican-controlled Congress acted on the party's ideology and interest by closing the territories to slavery and organizing them on a free-soil basis, proposing a transcontinental railroad to open the trans-Mississippi West to settlement, and promising education and improvement in agriculture and the mechanical arts through public-supported universities. Congress thus passed the Homestead Act that offered 160 acres of public land to any adult, head-of-household free person who would build a habitation on it, farm it, and live on it for five years. The survival and success of a democratic society demanded it.[6] Fulton surely knew of such actions as he moved south with the Union army. And he surely knew that many Union soldiers and civilians alike believed that such promise was worth fighting for.[7]

As Fulton moved from Pennsylvania through Maryland and into Virginia, he contrasted the well-ordered and productive farms of Pennsylvania with the increasingly disordered and unproductive ones farther south. Riding the train to Harrisburg from Philadelphia in August 1862, he observed that "the most prominent object of attraction on the way being the great Chester Valley the broad Expanse of highly cultivated and fertile land Stretching for Miles before the Entranced Vision of the beholder—the highly cultivated farms with Excellent buildings finely fenced making me feel if possible still more [ap]preciative of my native Country."[8]

In winter encampment at Belle Plain, Virginia, in 1863, Fulton assayed the land and people and condemned the debilitating effects of slavery. He noted that although "the surface of the country is poor," with "proper Management" the country "would be easily cultivated" and "would make a beautiful country." But to do that, "there must be a great change not only in the country but in the people." By his reckoning, the nonslaveholding whites "that now occupy the country are not only poor but ignorant in the Extreme" to the point of even "being below the Negro Slave in point of Gentili[ty]." Whether Fulton's assessment of nonslaveholding whites came from his observation alone or was prejudiced by Northerners' common, especially antislavery, depiction of such people as poor, ignorant, and miserable due to slavery's drag on them, Fulton recited the standard free-soil, antislavery axiom that such people would "never raise as long as that institution [slavery] exists."[9] Fulton repeated such assessments as he traveled through Virginia. In April 1863, for example, he noted that there were some "fine farms" along the Rappahannock River but the corn had not been husked there, and "this country would be beautiful if it was only properly cultivated—but all this is left to the negroes."[10] The towns in Virginia revealed the same lack of energy. In commenting on Culpeper, Virginia, for example, Fulton dismissed its public buildings as inferior to those in the North and thought its "Narrow and dirty" streets "about Equal [to] our Mud Lanes in the Country, but that is the general Characteristic of the towns of Virginia."[11]

And again in June 1863, he added that in returning to Pennsylvania from Virginia, he saw several fine farms but that few compared to those in Pennsylvania, because the Virginia places lacked for "care and cultivation" to improve them. At the same time, he contemplated what opportunities existed there for the right kind of farmer, an inkling of what he, like so many other soldiers, felt when surveying the land before them.[12] In June 1863, he commented favorably on the farms in Loudon County, which "Seemed to have been Kept in a good Condition," but was most impressed by the good land, "Covered with rich grass with fine Springs of water Showing that it was a country well Calculated for Grazeing And in fact would Sent me well to live in having much the appearance of Chester County," including stone spring houses that made the country "looking like as if it was inhabited by a Civilized people." The explanation for its good condition was ready at hand. Fulton opined that most of the people there "have Emigrated from the Northern States there is one settlement near this composed of Emigrants from New Jersey, And they have things in good order And live in a degree of comfort And happiness unknown to the old settlers" there.[13]

Fulton made his conclusions about the land and the people emphatic when he crossed from Virginia north into Maryland.[14] He immediately noted "how different the look of things it seemed as though we had got into another country Entirely—the fences were generally good and we soon began to see fields having crops of grass and grain growing—something that we had not Seen since we had been in the State of Virginia." Part of the reason Virginia fared so poorly in the comparison was the trampling of armies and fighting that drove landholders from their farms, but more fundamentally to Fulton was the people themselves. Upon entering Maryland, he felt "Some thing that made us feel as though we had left the land of Barbarians and got into one of civilization." The proof came soon enough when Fulton "Saw a sight that did us good and made us feel as though we were getting home—the first School House that I had Seen since I left Washington having School in it."[15]

Fulton exulted in what a free people did as he surveyed Maryland. He likened his movement to Maryland to entering "the garden of Eden itself," with "Fields of grain of the very best quality covering the Broad Expanses varigated [variegated] here and there with fields of corn and grass all being well fenced—the wheat I think I never saw Excelled for beauty and Luxuriance." Such beauty and bounty led Fulton to confess that "I had been rather prejudiced against Maryland but this part of it at Least was Equal to any land that I had Ever seen in Chester or Lancaster Counties of Penna." What struck him too was that "the farms had the appearance that they have in Penna the building outhouses and every thing about them giving an air of comfort and plenty seen only in Northern States."[16] This was a land worth fighting for.

SLAVERY AND ABOLITION

Fulton's observations and assessments of the poorly cultivated and poorly managed farms thus constituted a moral indictment of the slaveholding class, and by implication of slavery itself. After all, how one ran his farm attested to his moral worth; bad fences meant bad morals. In that critique of Virginia, Fulton was echoing the free-soil ideology of the Republican Party.

Fulton was less clear about his commitment to abolition. In his diary, Fulton wrote little about the moral wrong of slavery and the need to cleanse the nation of the evil.[17] He did once allude to such after the Emancipation Proclamation went into effect in January 1863, when he remarked that "the Nation seems to be undergoeing a great Struggle and it certainly will not be long untill there will be something decisive known in regard to our countrys future—and it is to be hoped that our nation [is] punished Enough for her many transgressions."[18] Otherwise, Fulton's expressed interest in freeing blacks during and because of the war was practical rather than principled. In 1864, he applauded the move of blacks fleeing bondage with "quite a Notion of goeing into the Army And Making Bold Sojer Boyes." Doing so, Fulton concluded, would "weaken the Rebels And strengthen us," which was one of Lincoln's arguments in drafting the Emancipation Proclamation. At the same time, he did insist, at least to himself, that while some of his fellow soldiers, who he dismissed as Copperheads, resigned due to the Emancipation Proclamation, he stayed to continue in the good cause.[19] Such sentiments about accepting emancipation as a war measure and enlisting blacks into the army were shared by many Union soldiers, whose experience in seeing slavery firsthand, coming to hate the slaveholding rebels, and needing more manpower to win the war all led them to become reluctant abolitionists.[20]

Whatever his personal views on slavery, Fulton did not hide his hatred of slaveholders. Fulton blamed slaveholders for the war and the misery, suffering, and destruction caused by their selfishness and arrogance, and he gloried in their loss during the war. Such was just retribution for their sin of rebellion against God's anointed nation. In Virginia in April 1863, for example, Fulton had only contempt for one unlovely secessionist plantation mistress who "told us her tale of Sorrow which was in the usual Strain" as she "greatly complained of the yankees for coaxing her Nigs to run away from her."[21] After taking a musket ball out of neck of a wounded Confederate soldier and thinking the young man would not survive to see his mother again, Fulton scored the slaveholders for the hard lot of the common soldiers, "many of them forced into the army against their will to be killed and leave their widowed Mothers [to] suffer want." For that, hypocritical slaveholders deserved special condemnation. He thought it "sad the tales of Sorrow that many a poor woman has to relate more pitiful far than those related by the negro drivers [slaveholders] before the rebellion broke out about the running away of their negroes and the taking of their rights by the northern abolitionists." Slaveholders could not suffer enough, in Fulton's estimation: "How much of pain and Remorse must those that did so much toward Bringing about this unhappy strife have if any conscience they have to be goaded into remorse."[22]

The deserved suffering of the slaveholders led Fulton to reflect on the causes and costs of the war. With the Union success at Gettysburg in early July 1863, the Union army's move into Virginia in fall 1863, and prospects for victory seemingly favorable, Fulton again pointed to the sin of secession and rebellion needing retribution, but he also suggested a degree of complicity on Northerners' part for letting slaveholders tear the nation asunder. With the army ready to "strike a Speedy and Effective Blow—that will be felt by the

Enemy with Crushing Effect And that will cool their Audacity And Lead
them to feal that it is futile in them to Still persist in their Efforts to build up
an Aristocracy within the United States," Fulton believed it was now "time
for them to humble themselves And Submit to the fact that they are Nothing
more than Men And that it is useless to Strive against God, who in his all wise
providence has determined to humble them And bring them with ourselves
to Confess our great sin that we have committed in his sight."[23]

ENDURANCE AND DESTRUCTION

War hardened Fulton. Like other soldiers who had served through 1863,
Fulton hardly blinked when the Union army brought the war directly to
civilians and made them pay for supporting the rebellion. This was "hard
war" necessary to win the day.[24] Thus, Fulton was unmoved at the destruction of farms, such as one in Virginia that left only "a few negroes" as "the only
remnant of once departed fortune" with the main house "a perfect wreck,"
the fences "all down," and "things in General looked as though some devastating Pestilence had Swept through the place Leaving nothing in its wake
that had been good or nice."[25] At the same time, he expressed sadness over
personal losses. In one case, in Virginia, for example, Fulton hoped that one
rebel sympathizer who died might "get forgiveness for his Sin . . . though
his poor wife must feel Lonely And Sad Leaving her friends in Penn[a]. the
spring the Rebellion broke out And Seeing three of her family buried in
Virginia with her only Remaining son in the Rebel Army." Fulton thought
to write a letter of consolation to her, but did not find the time.[26] But the war
continued, and with it the "work of destruction still goes on." Deservedly so,
Fulton thought, for "had the people only have stayed at home their property
would not have been burned—still if they had not been traitors they would
have seen no danger." The rebels brought destruction on themselves.[27] Thus,
Fulton could not pity those who "Lived in Comfort before the war broke out"
but now "hardly know one day what they will get to eat the Next." He continued that they "as usual Curse the Yankees for all their trouble And think that
their want and destruction of their property is all to be blamed upon—them,"
but for Fulton it was "Strange to see with what pertinacity they hang on to
their old Notions about the war." Such notions had to be crushed, and hard
war would do so.[28] Fulton thought so, as did many Union soldiers by 1863.

DISLOYAL WOMEN

Especially galling to Fulton, as for many Union soldiers, was the behavior of women who supported the rebellion. The war politicized everything, including the home, and women were expected to support their men and their country in a noble cause. But Union soldiers could not abide what seemed to them a stridency and thus indecency in Southern white women's behavior. Fulton was no different in his responses to "secesh" women or to Northern women "traitors" who opposed the Union war effort.[29]

Fulton had no sympathy for the suffering of a group of seventeen women who were crowded into a house after failing to escape the Union army entering Virginia after the battle of Gettysburg. Fulton dismissed their miserable condition as their due, "Showing that they were willing to live pretty thick rather than give up their treasonable and worthless opinions which I trust they will be compelled Soon to give up by force of surrounding circumstances." He added that "they have held and preached their doctrines of treason long Enough for their own good as well as the good of the whole country—they are not all Backward in Saying that they are Rebs and Showing their proclivities for the cause of Rebellion."[30] The persistence of Southern women's resistance angered Fulton, and he set out to correct them in their belief that the Confederacy would and should succeed. One Mrs. Graves, whose family had eight hundred acres of land and "quite a number of negroes" near Culpeper Court House, Virginia, was one who insisted to Fulton that the Confederacy would "ultimately gain" its independence and that accordingly the Union army should give up the fight. Fulton, though surprised by her confidence and arrogance, argued that she must see that the Confederacy's and her cause were "hopeless" and that the rebels were "Certainly beginning to See the folly of their course."[31] Such women would get no helping hand from Fulton or men like him, and the army would continue to prosecute the war vigorously. Also contemptible to Fulton was the hypocrisy of the "Secesh Ladies of Culpepper" who would dance and flirt with Union officers occupying the town while privately making "fun of the green and awkward Yankees as is their Custom."[32] To Fulton, Northern women who opposed the Union effort were no better, and perhaps worse, than Southern "traitors." Indeed, Fulton seemed pleased that one "young Lady or at Least calling herself such" who "had Strong tendencies to the

Copperhead persuasion" was killed at Gettysburg. She had betrayed a supposed abolitionist to the invading Confederates and so deserved her fate. The Confederates only got the abolitionist's horse, but the woman earned Fulton's complete contempt.[33]

All this was in contrast to the loyal women of Maryland, who exhibited much patriotism "by the waving of Flags And singing of Patriotic Songs." By Fulton's reckoning, such demonstrations "Seemed to do the Boys much good," with the "cheering of the Ladies in particular." The women also handed out apple butter, "good Bread," and other items that "Strengthened up the Boys And Kept their Spirits good And made them think that they were getting among friends again." This was the true calling of women.[34] Likewise, Fulton admired a Mrs. Powers, who after the third day of the battle of Gettysburg went out to the battlefield to "See if there was not some poor men there who were Suffering for the want of attention." After finding two in need, she gave them both water and brought one back to town, where she and "her girls" did "all in their power for the comfort of the poor fellows."[35] And he noted that while the cowardly men of Gettysburg snuck off to hide and refused to help bury the dead still in the field after the first day of battle," the town's patriotic "Ladies Showed a commendable disposition many of them manifesting a disregard of danger" to bury the dead whose "swollen black and hideous forms [were] Exposed to the gaze of all."[36] The war taught that women could be braver than men.

PATRIOTS AND TRAITORS

For Fulton, there were not enough such patriots and too many Northern "tories" whose "treason" kept the war going for the Confederates and corrupted the nation. Fulton hated the "tories" as much as he did Southern "traitors." From the beginning of his military service, he fulminated against them. In January 1863, for example, he complained of deserters, no pay, and poor prospects hobbling the war effort, but especially blamed "the Democrats as a party doeing all in their power to cripple the administration in putting down the Rebellion." Indeed, in Fulton's calculation, "had it not been for the tories in the North the war would have been well nigh Ended by this time." Like many Union soldiers and the Lincoln administration, Fulton thought that Northern opposition to the war and sympathies for the South encouraged the rebels and divided the Union. Like other Union soldiers and the Lincoln administration, he singled out Ohio Democratic Congressman Clement Vallandigham as especially treasonous for his speeches discouraging enlistments and encouraging opposition to Lincoln's wartime measures.[37] Vallandigham became a cause célèbre when the Lincoln administration had him arrested and eventually banished for his antiwar speeches and activities, and seemingly Fulton did not object to such strong measures.[38] Indeed, Fulton excoriated Vallandigham and his ilk for "their treasonable declarations" and willingness to "use E[ver]y. means to injure the cause of the Union." He hoped "hard" that "soon such Men May be silenced And go sneaking to their dens of infamy unnoticed—and unheeded their names handed down to posterity an Everlasting disgrace." The nation, "tried as by fire," needed to win the war at home as much as on the battlefield, a feeling shared by many soldiers.[39] The Union also needed to rid the army of Copperheads, for Fulton suspected that the failures of some generals were due to their disloyalty.[40]

During his capture at Gettysburg, Fulton discovered both the cowardice of many people in the face of the Confederate occupation of the town and the treason of some who sought favor with the enemy.[41] While his captors afforded him supplies and movement enough to tend to wounded soldiers, the "mean town" "had but one citizen that had patriotism," while the rest of the men fled or cowered in cellars. A disgusted Fulton wrote that Gettysburg had "more of copperheadism and . . . less of Patriotism than Any place of the Size that I have Ever been in." He was particularly outraged by one Judge Zeigler, who refused to give him tea for wounded soldiers "for fear that he would not get paid for it," but also, Fulton thought, because Zeigler was "intimate with Some of the Rebel officers" and thought and hoped the rebels would prevail. Fulton likened Zeigler's self-serving duplicity to the hypocritical "character of many men calling themselves Democrats" who "Blow about the persecution of Democrats saying this is no longer a free country that the press is no longer free the freedom of speech has been taken from the American people" while such traitors freely gave the enemy information and went about undermining the war effort. Fulton regretted that "we have not been Sharp Enough on such men" at the same time he was sure that "future history will certainly place such men where they belong"—in infamy.[42]

COURAGE, COWARDICE, AND MANLINESS

Fulton's disgust with "tories" extended to cowards. As noted above, the failure of the men of Gettysburg to stand up to the rebels appalled him. But for soldiers, Fulton was less judgmental about their actions. He thought some soldiers cowardly by nature, and perhaps as a result of their ethnic identity, but it was circumstance more than character that led men to fight or flee. The nature of courage fascinated Fulton as he observed soldiers and civilians confront war. He was not alone in such interest, for the question of courage stood at the center of American concepts of manhood, duty to country, and faith in God.[43] Fulton never seemed to doubt his own courage, though he confessed that the vagaries of courage and cowardice were impossible to predict and perhaps even control. At Warrenton Junction, Virginia, in 1863, he especially reflected on how a single rebel guerrilla came to the Union army picket line and, one by one, got seven soldiers to surrender without any resistance. The guerrilla captor seemed almost engaged in an act of derring-do rather than military purpose, for he marched the men two miles "double quick" to a farmhouse "where he got a woman to hold his pistol to them while a young Lady Kissed him Several times and he wrote them paroles." The wonder of it all was that the seven men so easily captured were regarded by their captain as among the bravest in the company. Fulton surmised that "one of the Mysterys of war that cannot be accounted for" was that "Men Sometimes get panic Stricken when no Reason can be assigned or imagined and they will fly as though pursued by some Demon incarnate." It was as difficult to understand the circumstance of the seven men as the Union army's panic at the battle of Bull Run in 1861, when the otherwise stout soldiers suddenly fled ignominiously, trampling civilians in their rush to escape the charging Confederates. Fulton concluded that "Such is Man at times particularly when Congregated together the rustling of a leaf the Ripple of a Stream will Strike terror to their hearts And Send them flying as a flock of sheep pursued by wolves."[44]

Fulton's views on courage colored his judgment about the worth of men and their place in the Union. Surprisingly, he made no references to blacks as soldiers. He did speculate on the character of immigrants, especially Germans. Indeed, tinges of nativism ran through Fulton's diary. Such thoughts were common in his day. Many Northerners worried about the social, cultural, and political implications of large numbers of immigrants coming into the United States in the late 1840s through the 1850s, wondering if the country could, or even should, absorb so many new and different people at the risk of losing its own essential character. The Catholicism of many of the Irish and Germans entering the United States added to the concerns about maintaining the integrity and vitality of the Protestant-ruled America. Antebellum nativism and anti-Catholicism usually went hand in hand and defined political categories; they even threatened the two-party system during the 1850s, until the slavery issue consumed everything, including nativist political ambitions.[45] To be sure, Fulton never expressed any full-blown nativism, but he did harbor doubts about German immigrants, as his comments about the supposed cowardice of the Germans in battle suggested. For him, as for others, the performance of any people demonstrated their true character and trustworthiness. For Fulton, the Germans came up short.

Germans had a poor reputation among Union soldiers for a want of manliness, but it was their failure at the battle of Chancellorsville, on May 2, 1863, that convinced Union men that such prejudices were true. On that day, Thomas "Stonewall" Jackson's men rolled up the 11th Corps of the Army of the Potomac. The 11th Corps, which had many Germans in its regiments, was caught unawares when Jackson attacked, and the Union soldiers fled the field in disarray. Or so it was reported. Many critics in and out of the army blamed the Union army's humiliating defeat at Chancellorsville on the Germans, and German soldiers and civilians spent the rest of the war denying the charge and trying to repair their reputations.[46] Fulton believed the worst about the Germans at Chancellorsville; indeed, he charged them for having "lost for us the fortunes of that Campaign." He later disparaged Carl Schurz, the prominent German American and Republican political leader, as undeserving of his appointment as a major general to lead the benighted 11th Corps after the battle because Schurz was not native-born. Fulton preferred that men of such rank "be occupied by men more deserving of American birth," though he hoped Schurz might do well enough to undo the "bad odor" of the Germans and the 11th Corps.[47] At Gettysburg, Fulton witnessed the easy capitulation of a group of soldiers when the Confederates advanced into the town on July 1; they were "duch from the 11th Corps" who offered "no resistance whatever—Showing that they were a couwardly Set."[48] Later, in commenting on Union soldiers captured at Gettysburg and forced to work for the Confederate soldiers there, Fulton singled out the Germans among them, admitting that it "pleased me to see the 11ᵗʰ Corps duchmen tugging away at the guns and carrying them about a mile to the rear."[49] Again, while staffing a hospital in winter quarters in Virginia, Fulton showed little sympathy for the plight of a very sick "black Duchman" who "had been Laying on a trash pile for several days and Nights without any Shelter" and was "So dirty and Lousy that no one will take him into their quarters." For this, Fulton blamed "the poor fellow" because "his Laziness made himself sick."[50] So it was for Germans in Fulton's eyes.

RELIGION

Interestingly, Fulton's disparagement of Germans did not extend to criticism of Catholics (see chapter 11). The wartime experience of Catholic nuns, working as "angels of mercy" on battlefields and in hospitals and tendering care to any soldier regardless of rank or loyalty, mitigated anti-Catholic feeling among Union soldiers, at least for a time, though it was conditioned by Catholics' seeming willingness to serve the national cause and not push their own religion on non-Catholics.[51] In his own encounter with Catholics, Fulton remarked favorably on St. Mary's College in Emmitsburg, Maryland, for the "imposing appearance" of its buildings and its "Seclusion and retiredness from all the bustle and din of Society" that might lure the students "from the holy calm of their religious Exercises" in preparing them for the priesthood. He praised the college as "ranking with those of any other in the depth of Learning and Erudition." He continued on this theme when surveying St. Joseph's College for women in Emmitsburg. He praised the school's principal building as "not ostentatious" in appearance and as a "plain white Structure." He appreciated the "fine farm" the nuns ran to support themselves and to care for orphan children there. Such assessment of the physical character of the college and farm reflected a respect for their modesty, which cast the good Catholic nuns in a favorable light. They seemingly posed no danger such as anti-Catholic and nativist Americans saw in the increasingly self-confident Catholic Church asserting its power and place in cities by building majestic cathedrals and substantial churches and other structures.[52]

Fulton wrote little about religion in the army per se. He did note that "the Army cannot be Said to be religious though all Seem to have a profound

Respect for religion." Men talked "of death as a something not . . . unlikely to cross their path and stop their Earthly cares but with little fear." Fulton admired the soldiers' "calusness and resignation" in facing death and thought it "well worthy of imitation." He concluded that "As it is Expected the true and humble Christian dies so due they with a feeling of honorable pride that in their death much has been done for the future freedom and happiness of Millions."[53] What Fulton described was more than giving up one's life for love of country; what the brave soldier wanted was to die a "good death." That meant dying with honor, noble purpose, and Christian faith. Knowing that the good soldier had died in such a way would reassure his family and community that the soldier away from home had not been corrupted by war and that his life counted both in this world and the next. Or so many soldiers and civilians thought and hoped during the war.[54] Without saying so, Fulton likely did too.

PURPOSE AND PERSEVERANCE

He surely wanted such men remembered and honored. For that reason, he took special notice of the dedication of the Gettysburg national cemetery on November 19, 1863. The establishment and dedication of the cemetery was "a step highly to be commended as a testimonial of Respect to the Many departed heroes that fell upon that Blood Stained" battlefield and whose ashes would now be entrusted to Mother Earth. From that, Fulton hoped that "our Country will make No human thing of it but that in appearance it will be Something to attract visitors from Every Nation Every clime to the great Battlefield of America—And there do homage to the heroism of her Departed great."[55] The nation must not forget what the soldiers did there or why. Fulton did not have Lincoln's Gettysburg Address at hand, but he already understood its essential meaning.

What impressed Fulton the most in his time with the army was the steadfastness and purposefulness of the soldiers, who slogged through the mud and rain and then under the hot sun in "long and toilsome" marches, "Showing that they were good Soldiers And had the good of their country at heart and are willing to do anything in their power for that country."[56] To be sure, there were officers petty enough to intrigue about rank and advantage and soldiers unhappy about poor or no pay, incompetent commanders, and the frustrations of a long war. Men resigned, refused to re-enlist, and deserted, and they sought Fulton's help in getting furloughs and discharges, which requests Fulton often refused. Fulton, like other junior officers, was the victim of status-climbing and selfish officers, and he was witness to the suffering of the soldiers. Through it all, he became more the soldier and more steeled to stay the course. He admired such men, whether Union or Confederate, who did so. Indeed, in assessing his experience with Confederates, he respected them for their commitment to their cause, however unjust he thought the Confederacy was, and for their brave and honorable dedication to duty. Fulton was pleased that the Confederates lost at Gettysburg, deflating all their "Blow and Bragadocio," even as he thanked the officers for good treatment of him and wounded soldiers carried into the town.[57] The Confederates were "a brave and in many Respects a noble Enemy," who "Showed to our men many acts of Kindness and Generosity in Bringing them water and caring for them in many ways true." An ignoble cause might have noble men. As a captive at Gettysburg, Fulton was accorded respect and responsibility as a man of honor and a physician who could be trusted to do his duty. Fulton reciprocated by doing just that. This respect for others as good soldiers would provide the basis for some degree of sectional reconciliation after the war, as soldiers placed wartime service and conduct ahead of party politics and issues of racial justice in reaching out to heal the nation's wounds. Where Fulton came out on such matters, his diary does not suggest.

During the war, however, there was still a fight to win, and Fulton did not fool himself as to who was his enemy. When a group of captured "Jonnies" were brought in, barefooted, "Ragged and dirty as usual," Fulton pitied them and helped fill their haversacks with "Broken hard Bread that had been thrown out." Fulton concluded that "it did me good to be able to help them. Notwithstanding they are the sworn Enemys of our country."[58] Fulton wanted to be part of that fight.

In the end, Fulton realized his true purpose during the war. He did not resign or even seek a furlough, as many soldiers were doing in 1864, except to visit his sick wife. As he explained to himself, and perhaps to his wife, he had work to do as a soldier and surgeon, and he preferred that to anything else.[59] There was always the need to explain to others, and to oneself, why one stayed as the war dragged on, as the casualties mounted, and as the people at home suffered for want of their men's skills, good counsel, and love. Fulton, like others, decided that the great cause of preserving American democracy and realizing the promise of the land counted most. Soldiering also gave him purpose.

Fulton came to identify with the nation and the land because of the war. The public buildings in Washington had impressed him in their majesty, with the unfinished dome of the Capitol especially symbolizing for him, as for Lincoln, that there was work to do, that the Union must go on.[60] The history of America also impressed Fulton with the obligations of defending the great experiment in self-government the Revolutionary generation had entrusted to his generation.[61]

Most of all, it was nature and the land that made Fulton understand why he must persist and the nation must endure. On an Indian summer day in November 1863, in Virginia, Fulton took a walk in the woods to "get away from the turmoils and troubles of camp" and "commune with Nature with all its Lovliness." He was drawn there by the smells, colors, and variety and beauty of oak, hickory, and other trees and the abundant foliage, and most of all by the power of being "with something natural And that is in accordance with the will and wish of the Creator—war in all its Bearing And in all Connexion being foreign to the will of him who wishes . . . all things pure And good." The land refreshed and renewed him, as it could a people. There he found the hope that "instead of wounds And Sickness health And happiness Might be the happy lots of thousands that are now Suffering" and that "God in his own good time will cause the wrath of Man to praise him And the remainder of wrath will he restrain"—a thought that anticipated Lincoln's bow to God's purpose for the people and the nation as expressed in his Second Inaugural Address in March 1865. And Fulton continued in his reflection that the God-endowed land summoned up. In a rare mention of the physical suffering and death he saw, Fulton hoped that God's favor would bring the men home to "there remain the remainder of our days Secure from the new alarm of war" and no more to have "the Ear pained with the groans And Shrieks of the Wounded and dying—but that the course of us An[d] our Country May be onward from prosperity until the Sun Shall Shine upon a people no more free no No More happy in his wide domain."[62] Such was a promise worth living for, fighting for, even dying for. Just so for Fulton.

RANDALL M. MILLER, PhD, is the William Dirk Warren '50 Sesquicentennial Chair and Professor of History at Saint Joseph's University in Philadelphia. He is author or editor of more than twenty-five books on subjects as varied as the Civil War and Reconstruction, slavery and the South, religion, race and ethnicity, and politics. His most recent book, with Paul Cimbala as co-author, is *The Northern Home Front during the Civil War* (2017).

NOTES

1. James Fulton, Diary, 1862–1864, entry for June 26, 1863.

2. Ibid., January 1, 1864.

3. On the contrasting and even contradictory aspects of viewing and assessing nature, see William Cronon, "The Trouble with Wilderness, or, Getting Back to the Wrong Nature," in *Uncommon Ground: Rethinking the Human Place in Nature*, ed. William Cronon (New York: Norton, 1996), 69–90; Angela Miller, *The Empire of the Eye: Landscape Representation and American Cultural Politics, 1825–1875* (Ithaca, NY: Cornell University Press, 1993); Anne Farrar Hyde, *An American Vision: The Western Landscape and National Culture, 1820–1920* (New York: New York University Press, 1990), 1–80; and Roderick F. Nash, *Wilderness and the American Mind*, 4th ed. (New Haven, CT: Yale University Press, 2001).

4. On the concept of free soil and free man, and the Republican Party, see especially Eric Foner, *Free Soil, Free Labor, Free Men: The Ideology of the Republican Party before the Civil War* (New York: Oxford University Press, 1970), 40–72, and *passim*; on Lincoln and the Republicans' belief in the "right to rise," see Gabor Boritt, *Lincoln and the Economics of the American Dream* (Champaign: University of Illinois Press, 1994).

5. Seward quoted in Foner, *Free Soil, Free Labor, Free Men*, 41.

6. On Republicans' wartime actions and legislation that extended the free-soil ideology, see Heather Cox Richardson, *The Greatest Nation of the Earth: Republican Economic Policies during the Civil War* (Cambridge, MA: Harvard University Press, 1997), especially 8–30 and 139–208.

7. The literature on why many white Northern men fought for the Union is large. For excellent surveys of the reasons, see Gary W. Gallagher, *The Union War* (Cambridge, MA: Harvard University Press, 2011), especially 1–6 and 33–74, who emphasizes commitment to maintaining democratic government, and James M. McPherson, *What They Fought For, 1861–1865* (Baton Rouge: Louisiana State University Press, 1994), who emphasizes patriotism and duty, for Northerner and Southerner alike, as animating forces.

8. Fulton, August 19, 1862.

9. Ibid., February 19, 1863.

10. Ibid., April n.d., 1863.

11. Ibid., December 24, 1863.

12. Ibid., June 1[2?], 1863.

13. Ibid., June 17, 1863.

14. Fulton's characterizations of Virginia were similar to those of other Northerners. In letters home, soldiers commented on the condition of the land, the towns, and the people. The rundown qualities of Virginia became a metaphor for a lack of care. To cite one example, one Connecticut soldier cautioned his wife not to exert herself too much to keep up

the home place while he was away, writing that he "would rather the whole Place was like a Virginia House than that you should hurt yourself." See Robert L. Bee, ed., *The Boys from Rockville: Civil War Narratives of Sgt. Benjamin Hirst, Company D, 14th Connecticut Volunteers* (Knoxville: University of Tennessee Press, 1998), 122.

15. Fulton, June 25, 1863.

16. Ibid., June 26, 1863.

17. Fulton's silence on slavery and antislavery surely did not come from ignorance about the subject and the history of it, especially efforts by fugitive slaves to flee their bondage and slaveholders' efforts to capture them in southeastern Pennsylvania. The region was contested ground for slavery during the 1850s, with several highly publicized incidents of slaves' escapes and even violent encounters between fugitives and slavecatchers and the persistent work by antislavery groups to encourage and help such fugitives. On the ongoing and very visible activity in Fulton's backyard, see, for example, Lucy Maddox, *The Parker Sisters: A Border Kidnapping* (Philadelphia: Temple University Press, 2016), about a kidnapping in Chester County; William C. Kashatus, *Just Over the Line: Chester County and the Underground Railroad* (West Chester, PA: Chester County Historical Society, 2002); James Oliver Horton, "A Crusade for Freedom: William Still and the Real Underground Railroad," in David W. Blight, ed., *Passages to Freedom: The Underground Railroad in History and Memory* (New York: Harper Collins for the Smithsonian Institution, 2004), 175–93; David G. Smith, *On the Edge of Freedom: The Fugitive Slave Issue in South Central Pennsylvania, 1820–1870* (New York: Fordham University Press, 2013); and more generally, R. J. M. Blackett, *Making Freedom: The Underground Railroad and the Politics of Slavery* (Chapel Hill. University of North Carolina Press, 2013).

18. Fulton, January 16, 1863.

19. Ibid., January 7, 1864.

20. On the process whereby many Union soldiers came to accept emancipation as a necessary and useful war measure, and even to sympathize with the plight of slaves, see Chandra Manning, *When This Cruel War Was Over: Soldiers, Slavery, and the Civil War* (New York: Alfred A. Knopf, 2007); and Ira Berlin, *The Long Emancipation: The Demise of Slavery in the United States* (Cambridge. MA: Harvard University Press, 2015), 165–70.

21. Fulton, April n.d., 1863.

22. Ibid., May n.d., 1863.

23. Ibid., November 14, 1863.

24. On hard war as policy and practice, see Mark Grimsley, *The Hard Hand of War: Union Military Policy Toward Southern Civilians, 1861–1865* (Cambridge, UK: Cambridge University Press, 1995); and Gerald F. Linderman, *Embattled Courage: The Experience of Combat in the American Civil War* (New York: The Free Press, 1987), especially chapters 9–10.

25. Fulton, June 25, 1863.

26. Ibid., October 21, 1863.

27. Ibid., December 10, 1863.

28. Ibid., December 24, 1863.

29. On soldiers' attitudes toward women and their proper role in the war, see, for example, Reid Mitchell, *The Vacant Chair: The Northern Soldier Leaves Home* (New York: Oxford University Press, 1993), chapter 6.

30. Fulton, July 6, 1863.

31. Ibid., December 27, 1863.

32. Ibid., December 25, 1863. Interestingly, Fulton did not comment on or suspect the possibility that such women's flirtations were efforts to win the trust of the Union soldiers

in order to get information about Union military interests and movements. Accusations of Southern women thus "spying" on soldiers, related in soldiers' letters and in the Northern press, were to the Northern mind another example of "secesh" women's duplicity.

33. Ibid., July 3, 1863. Fulton's "young Lady" was Jennie Wade, the only civilian to be killed at Gettysburg during the battle. See chapter 7.

34. Ibid., June 29, 1863.

35. Ibid., July 3, 1863.

36. Ibid., July 3, 1863.

37. Ibid., January 16, 1863.

38. On Vallandigham, soldiers', and Republicans' responses to his and antiwar Democrats' opposition to wartime recruitment and other pro-war measures, soldiers' belief that the home front was rife with disunion and lack of support for the war, and the Lincoln administration's crackdown on perceived antiwar publications, see, for example, Steven J. Ramold, *Across the Divide: Union Soldiers View the Northern Home Front* (New York: New York University Press, 2013), chapters 4–5 and *passim*: Linderman, *Embattled Courage*, chapter 11; and Mark E. Neely Jr., *The Fate of Liberty: Abraham Lincoln and Civil Liberties* (New York: Oxford University Press, 1991), chapter 9.

39. Fulton, January 16, 1863.

40. Ibid., February 8, 1864.

41. On the behavior of the townspeople during and after the battle, see Margaret S. Creighton, *The Colors of Courage: Gettysburg's Forgotten History, Immigrants, Women, and African Americans in the Civil War's Defining Battle* (New York: Basic Books, 2005), especially chapters 5 through 7.

42. Fulton, July 2, 1863.

43. On courage and cowardice, see especially Linderman, *Embattled Courage, passim*; and Earl J. Hess, *The Union Soldier in Battle: Enduring the Ordeal of Combat* (Lawrence: University Press of Kansas, 1997), chapter 4.

44. Fulton, November 8, 1863.

45. On Northern nativism and anti-Catholicism, and Catholic responses to such, see Tyler Anbinder, *Nativism and Slavery: The Northern Know Nothings and the Politics of the 1850s* (New York: Oxford University Press, 1992); Jon Gjerde, *Catholicism and the Shaping of Nineteenth-Century America*, ed. S. Deborah King (Cambridge, UK: Cambridge University Press, 2012); and William B. Kurtz, *Excommunicated from the Union: How the Civil War Created a Separate Catholic America* (New York: Fordham University Press, 2016), 20–9, 45–51, and *passim*.

46. On the Germans' reputation, before and after the battle of Chancellorsville, and German efforts to overcome the disparagements, see Christian B. Keller, *Chancellorsville and the Germans: Nativism, Ethnicity, and Civil War Memory* (New York: Fordham University Press, 2007); and Mischa Honeck, "Men of Principle: Gender and the German American War for the Union," *Journal of the Civil War Era* 5 (March 2015): 48–52.

47. Fulton, June 29, 1863.

48. Ibid., July 1, 1863.

49. Ibid., July 9, 1863.

50. Ibid., December 18, 1863.

51. On Union soldiers' thinking about Catholics, especially their experience with Catholic nuns, see, for example, Kurtz, *Excommunicated from the Union*, 80–8; and Sister Mary Denis

Maher, *To Bind Up the Wounds: Catholic Sister Nurses in the U.S. Civil War* (New York: Greenwood Press, 1989), especially chapter 5.

52. Fulton, June 29, 1863.

53. Ibid., November 18, 1863.

54. On "the good death," see Drew Gilpin Faust, *This Republic of Suffering: Death and the American Civil War* (New York: Alfred A. Knopf, 2008), chapter 1 and *passim*; and George C. Rable, *God's Almost Chosen Peoples: A Religious History of the American Civil War* (Chapel Hill: University of North Carolina Press, 2010), chapter 9.

55. Fulton, November 19, 1863.

56. Ibid., June 25, 1863.

57. Ibid., July 2, 1863.

58. Ibid., November 8, 1863.

59. Ibid., January 1, 1864, and January 8, 1864.

60. Ibid., October 14, 1862.

61. Ibid., July 2, 1863.

62. Ibid., November 14, 1863.

Appendix A

*Rules for the Examination of Assistant Surgeon
Candidates and Examination Questions (1862)*

The Health and lives of the troops being of the first importance to the State, the best professional talent will be demanded of those entrusted with their care. The examination by a Board of Surgeons, as directed by law, is intended to test the fitness of the candidate for this special military duty, and to establish a *Merit Roll* from which the Governor may select the officers of the "Hospital Department." It is not to decide on his professional qualifications as a general practitioner.

RULES FOR THE EXAMINATION OF CANDIDATES

The Examination will be conducted as follows:—

The Candidate will write out his answers to the printed questions, number them to correspond with the numbers of the questions, and sign his address in full (stating post-office), and hand them and the questions, in an envelope, to the Board as soon as called for.

He will also write on the envelope the name of the school and the year in which he graduated—his age at present, and any hospital or other practical experience he may have enjoyed—thus:—

Presented by _____

a graduate of _____

aged_____years.

A Surgeon (or Resident) of _____Hospital during _____years.

In [illegible] practice _____ years.

Promptness in answering the questions, together with the handwriting of the candidate, and the evidence which he exhibits of general education, will all be regarded by the Board and enter into their estimate of his fitness.

After carefully inspecting the essays as handed in, the Board will report in writing to the Governor, the relative order of the merit of such as they deem worthy of a commission. Notice will then be given by the Governor to all candidates who are approved by the Board, and orders for duty issued by the Surgeon General as soon as regiments require medical officers. The successful candidate must in all instances await his commission in the order established by the Board. Personal solicitation for appointments will not be noticed. Delay in obeying an order to join a regiment will deprive the candidate of his right to an appointment. Promotion in the order of seniority of service will be given to Assistant Surgeons who prove themselves worthy of it.

A: SURGERY

1.—What are the symptoms of a wound of the Lung—and how would you check Pulmonary Hemorrhage?

2.—How would you Trephine the Skull—and what fills up the opening made by the Trephine?

3.—What is a Hydrocele—what an [sic] Haematocele, and what is Varicocele?[1]

4.—Describe the circular operation for Amputation of the Thigh.

5.—Describe the dressing usually applied to a Fracture of the Femur.

6.—Describe the method of reducing a Luxation of the Head of the Femur on the Dorsum Ilii.[2]

7.—How many ways may Hemorrhage be arrested?

8.—Name the best styptics for the arrest of Venous Oozing.

9.—Why are Gunshot Wounds tedious in healing, and what are their chief dangers?

10.—How would you treat a Gunshot Fracture of the Humerus?

B: ANATOMY AND PHYSIOLOGY

1.—How many Spinal Nerves are there, and how do they escape from the spinal canal?

2—Name the bones composing the Head.

3.—Describe the portions of the Intestinal Canal.

4.—Name the regions of the Abdomen, and state their relative positions.

5.—What is the composition of the Wrist-joint?—stating its bones and ligaments.

6.—Describe the origin, course, and relations of the Iliac Arteries.

7.—Where is the Thoracic Duct, and what is its function?[3]

8.—Describe the process of Digestion.

9.—How is Respiration accomplished, and what is its object in the economy? What part is performed by the Lungs?

10.—Where are the Kidneys situated? State the name and course of their ducts, and where they empty.

A: MATERIA MEDICA

1.—What preparation of Arsenic is most convenient for medical use?

2.—Write its composition and dose.

3.—What is the composition of the Compound Extract of Colocynth?[4]

4.—What is the difference between Compound Extract of Colocynth and Compound Cathartic Pills?

5.—What Purgatives are given in very small doses?

6.—What medicines can be used as Purgatives, what as Diuretics, and what as Sudorifics?[5]

7.—How ought a Blister to be treated for Endermic Application?

8.—How would you prevent Strangury, and how treat it?[6]

9.—Name some of the indigenous substitutes for Peruvian Bark.[7]

10.—Name some of the indigenous Diaphoretics and Emetics.[8]

11.—Write a prescription for a Mixture for the arrest of Diarrhoea.

12.—Write the formula for the composition of Hope's Mixture as employed in Dysentery.[9]

D: PRACTICE OF MEDICINE

1.—What are your ideas of the responsibilities of an Army Surgeon?

2.—What would you desire to guard against and provide for, in the selection of a Site for a Hospital or Encampment?

3.—Describe the symptoms and treatment of Small Pox.

4.—What conditions most predispose to Typhoid Fever?—and state its pathology and treatment.

5.—Describe the causes, symptoms, pathology, and treatment of Pernicious Fever.[10]

6.—Describe the causes, symptoms, and treatment of Dysentery.

7.—Describe the symptoms, causes, and treatment of Scorbutus.[11]

8.—What is Intussusception—what are its symptoms—what may it be confounded with, and how would you treat it?[12]

9.—What are the causes of Ascites—and how would you treat it?[13]

10.—What are the symptoms, stages and treatment of Pneumonia?

11.—Write a formula for a Cough Medicine.

12.—Describe the symptoms, diagnosis, and treatment of Scabies.[14]

SOURCES

"1862 Rules for the Examination of Candidates (unsigned)," 19.167 Medical Examinations, Roll 6810, Pennsylvania State Archives.

Examination questions found in file 19.167 Medical Examinations, Roll 6803, Pennsylvania State Archives.

NOTES

1. Hydrocele refers to swelling of the testicles due to fluid buildup; haematocele is swelling because of blood accumulation in body cavities; variocele is the swelling of a vein in the scrotum.

2. The pelvis has two illii (singular, illium), bony flanges that constitute the hips.

3. The largest lymphatic duct in the body through which all lymph passes.

4. Colocynth is an herb with purgative properties, commonly used throughout the nineteenth century.

5. Diuretic substances promote the flow of urine; sudorifics promote perspiration.

6. Strangury is a blockage of the bladder causing a painful urge to urinate.

7. Peruvian bark was a common name for cinchona, a natural source of quinine.

8. Diaphoretic substances induce perspiration; emetics induce vomiting.

9. A nineteenth-century compound for the relief of diarrhea consisting mainly of nitric acid, opium, and camphor.

10. Medicine of the Civil War era recognized some fevers as diseases in their own right. Pernicious fever, not easy to identify in practice, usually referred to extreme and prolonged fever that progressed to a comatose condition.

11. Scurvy.

12. Intussusception refers to a prolapse of the rectum and extrusion of the intestines into the bowels.

13. Fluid buildup in the peritoneal cavity, today recognized as related to liver dysfunction.

14. A contagious skin infection due to a mite. Very common in Civil War camps.

Appendix B

*Gettysburg Reminiscences: A Surgeon's Story
of the Battle on Pennsylvania's Soil.*

"GOING IN"—AMONG THE WOUNDED.
IN GETTYSBURG—TAKEN PRISONER.
INCIDENTS OF THREE TERRIBLE DAYS.

BY JAMES FULTON. M. D.

While on the march to Gettysburg, Jan 27, 1863, we stopped on Mason and Dixon's Line. This day the Quartermaster had supplied our command with shoes, for many of the men during their long march had worn out theirs and were nearly barefoot; weary and footsore, they had borne their burdens with little complaint.

The next morning we took up the march in Pennsylvania, moving along until about noon. We halted in a grove on the banks of Marsh Creek. Soon after getting into camp we learned that a church nearby had been visited the previous Sunday during service by the rebs, and the horses taken from the carriages and appropriated to the Johnnies' own special use. From a few such incidents as this we learned that our coming into Pennsylvania was not mere holiday pastime, but a work of necessity to protect our homes and those left behind by us when we entered the service.

Many of us had been born and reared on Pennsylvania's soil. My regiment was the 143d Pa. Our brigade, the Third, was composed of the 143d, 149th, and 150th Pa. Our division, the Third, was commanded by Doubleday; and our corps, the First, by Gen. Reynolds.

Early in the morning of July 1 we broke camp, and took up the line of march for Gettysburg, the distance being about four miles. We had not passed over more than half the distance when we heard the sound of artillery. The impression made by this upon us is beyond the power of pen to describe; but on we went. It was exceedingly warm, a heavy mist falling at the time, wetting us to the skin. The ground was wet and slippery, making it very hard for the men, loaded as they were with their full equipment. No complaint was offered; there was no straggling to speak of.

Needed at the Front

About this time orders came for us to hurry up, as we were needed at the front. We immediately started at a double-quick. When within short distance of the town we left the Emmitsburg road; turning to the left, we passed through the fields until we came to Seminary Ridge.

We crossed the Fairfield road into a grove just back of the Seminary and skirting the ridge. The timber was composed mostly of white oak of natural growth. The men passed through this grove and down a gentle declivity to the level space or valley below. In this valley they threw away their knapsacks, never to see them again, the enemy getting possession of them and appropriating everything useful.

After relieving themselves of all possible incumbrances [sic] they crossed the small valley up an ascent to the top of the next rise, then down again into a narrow valley to the left of the Chambersburg turnpike, there lying down in line in a peach orchard; this being on the McPherson farm. We formed the right of the line, extending to the turnpike.

As we went over the ridge to take position we saw a battery stationed on the summit just to the left of the turnpike. Many of the horses had been killed, the guns silenced, and the wounded had been taken into a small stone house to the left of the pike, also on the McPherson farm. The house is not standing at this time, having been burned since the battle.

Just after going into line one of our men was wounded. Capt. Blair, of our regiment, helped him over the fence to me. I took him into the house spoken of.

A Sad Spectacle

There was presented a sad spectacle. Spread over the floor the men of the battery lay, wounded and bleeding. There was no one to care for them. I looked around for my Orderly. He was nowhere to be seen. His duty was to carry the instruments, bandages and medicines. I had nothing to work with, consequently could do nothing without those things.

On going back to Seminary Ridge I found him, but while there received orders to go into town to work.

I had left things at the small house on the line, so had to go and procure them before I could go into town.

Finding the Orderly and Hospital Steward, we went into town. Our division had already appropriated the Seminary for hospital purposes. In Gettysburg we found they had taken possession of the Catholic church, the Courthouse and a great many private houses for the wounded. At the church, we had no means of heating or cooking. It became necessary that we have fire, in order to prepare beef tea. In looking around we went into the house of a Mr. Meyers, where we had full permission to use the stove.

Eleventh Corps Men

Being busy we took no note of time until the ladies of the house, who had gone to the cellar for safety, came to me, saying that our men were crowding in upon them, and wanted me to drive them out. I tried to get the poor follows [sic] (Eleventh Corps men) to go on and make their escape to our lines, they being on the retreat. But I could not get them to move, and many were taken prisoners that night who could easily have made their escape. They had, however, done good work; for had the Eleventh Corps not come up and supported the right of the First Corps in that first day's fight, when Gen. Gordon was trying to get around our right flank, the left being slowly turned all day toward the right, the rebels certainly would have captured a large portion of our corps. But in helping us the Eleventh Corps suffered severely.

About this time the commotion outside seemed to be very great. I went to the front into the street to see what was really going on. The first thing I knew a Confederate Major tapped me on the shoulder and said I was his prisoner. I asked him what was to be done. He told me where I would find Gen. A. P. Hill, and to report to him. I did so. The General asked me if we did not have a good many sick and wounded. I told him we had, not only of our own men but of theirs also. He politely told me to go back and do the best I could for them.

Very glad to get away so easily, I again went to duty and hard duty it was with the means we had at our command. The place had been ransacked by the enemy before we came, and at this time was in their possession, and most all the provisions given by the people or taken by the enemy that was to spare. We had nothing upon which to feed our wounded save such as we begged from house to house; that being an exceedingly slow proceeding, the women of the city being so frightened they kept in their cellars, out of the way of the shot and shell; they consequently could cook nothing for their own families, to say nothing about us.

Working Under Hardship

We were reduced to sad straits. Our provision-train was far to the rear, and might just as well have been a thousand miles away for all the good it was to us. We had a little beef extract, and but little of it. We could by going to the houses get a little apple-butter, sometimes a little rusk or bread. In this condition we worked along the first and part of the second day.

However, in looking around I found a bakery. The proprietor told me if we could get flour, bakers could be procured and bread furnished in sufficient quantity to supply our present necessity. I talked with the officers of the enemy on the street, telling them our situation and what I could do if I could only get flour. They said they had plenty of flour in their trains, and for me to go and see Gen. Hays. I did so. He sent me to Gen. Ewell, out to the east of Gettysburg on the Poorhouse road. I found the General eating his breakfast on the bridge-way of a small Pennsylvania barn. I saluted him as politely as I knew how. After looking me over he wanted to know my business. I stated it in as few words as possible. He wanted to know how many sick and wounded we had to feed. I told him I could not tell, owing to the confused condition of things incident to the battle; the wounded were constantly coming in; we had no record, and it was impossible to keep one; but I thought about 2,000. If we could get provisions for that many I believed we could get along.

He replied in a sharp manner that it was a queer way of doing business, wanting bread, to feed people and not knowing how many there were to feed. However, he directed me to go back, and the flour would be there. I did go back, feeling fairly good, thinking I had found the way out of a very trying position. The flour never came.

Food At Last

On going back to the bakery and telling the baker what I had done, the baker asked me in a quiet way if there was any assurance a person would be paid, provided any provision could be obtained. I answered there was just as much certainty that the Government would pay its debts as there was that it would be able to maintain its integrity against the foe with which it was contending. As for me, I had full faith in its ability to do so, notwithstanding the sad condition in which we seemed to be placed at that time. I had full faith in the justice of our cause, and fully believed in the end we would be victorious.

Either my argument or the presence of the enemy all around us made an impression on him, for after thinking a short time he said he had some crackers and would let me have them. I gave him vouchers. He procured his money, as he never troubled me afterward.

A Confederate officer gave me a guard. The baker took up his garret floor, and from a hiding-place brought out 13 barrels of crackers. The greater portion of the floor had been carefully nailed down. If the enemy had only known of this receptacle but little good they would have done us; but as it was, we got the crackers out safely.

They were distributed among the different hospitals and some among private households where wounded men were placed for the time. I well remember of Mrs. Catharine Powers, one of the heroines of Gettysburg, coming, and getting an apron full for her "poor fellows," as she styled them. Well were they cared for who had the good fortune to get into her house. Her whole family gave their undivided attention to the wounded under their care, without reward or expectation of any. When Winter came on, and Mr. Powers wished, to put on his Winter clothing, he had none; all had been used for the benefit of the sick and wounded. They had during the time about 30; one dying, the rest, recovering. Mr. Powers died first; Mrs. Powers died later, at a ripe old age, receiving the blessings of those for whom she cared.

Gen. Ewell's Manner

My intercourse with Gen. Ewell did not give me a very exalted opinion of the man. His bearing toward me was that of great superiority, giving the impression that it was to him a great condescension to enter into conversation with an ordinary Yank. I never saw him afterwards, and am unable to say whether the two days following knocked any of the nonsense out of him or not. I had met quite a number of the rebel officers on the streets. They were cordial and gentlemanly. Several times the pickets stopped me. They were reprimanded, and told I had the right to go where I pleased inside of their

lines. I accordingly did use the privilege when there was a prospect of getting anything, for our sick and wounded, or those of the enemy in our care.

I had noticed when visiting Gen. Ewell that large quantities of guns and
other warlike material were being gathered, and that the Eleventh Corps
men taken prisoners had that unpleasant duty to perform, carrying it from
the field, storing it up carefully prior to its removal.

In the afternoon, or towards evening of July 2, as the cannonade was
progressing, an old Confederate officer with his staff came along by our
hospital, the Catholic church. He said "We must go up here," meaning the
cupola of the church. The young men looked up, and did not seem to admire
the undertaking; they did not make any move toward going. The old gentleman said:

"Young men, dismount and give your horses to the Orderly." They did so,
and all went up into the gallery of the church, thence to the ladder into the
cupola, I alone of our men going with them. At that time a splendid view was
to be obtained of the left of our line as far as Big Round Top.

At this time little or nothing can be seen. When we looked out upon the
broad expanse laid before us a beautiful but terrible spectacle was presented.

Longstreet's Advance

Gen. Longstreet's Corps had left its position behind the long range of hills
extending from the Seminary south towards Emmitsburg, and was advancing to attack Sickles, that General occupying the extreme left on our line, as
there formed, but not reaching to Little Round Top by nearly the eighth of a
mile, leaving this important part of the line unprotected.

Gen. Longstreet had seen the weak point; also the, importance of the
hill to the position. He was not only advancing the main portion of his corps
against Sickles, but sending a portion of his command around our left to pass
through the wood and undergrowth between the Little and Big Round Tops
to gain the rocky hights [sic] of the former.

Just before Gun. Sickles advanced, Gen. Berdan came to him and asked if
he had not better take his regiment of sharpshooters and go around there and
see what was going on. Sickles said he did not think it worth while, but told
him to do as he chose, and if he went he could take a Massachusetts regiment
of 700 men: these, with his own, made a command of 1,400. Berdan went
around to the ravine and found the woods full of the enemy. He located his
men on the side of the hill and among the rocks. They kept up such a fusillade

that Gen. Longstreet stated during his visit in 1888 that the rebels were held about 40 minutes. He said that from the racket our men made he thought that a division was fighting them.

When the rebs finally routed our forces and reached the hight [*sic*] above they were just in time to meet the Pennsylvania Reserves, when they were pushed, down the rocky sides of Round Top to the Valley of Death, to the Den, to the woody space beyond, where fell Fred Taylor, the gallant Colonel of the Bucktail regiment.

Gen. Longstreet said that had they been held not more than 10 minutes, or even not more than 20 minutes, the Confederates would have had Little Round Top, the key to the position. Longstreet was certainly a General of keen perception and great military sagacity. But such is war. Momentous events turn on very small points. His plans failed almost by accident.

Gen. Longstreet had advanced quite a distance when Gen. Sickles came from behind a slight barricade of stones and advanced to meet him. The enemy advanced in elegant formation, the finest military movement I have ever seen made.

The Third Corps did well, advancing in good shape until they were almost within gunshot of the enemy, when the line began to have somewhat the appearance of a worm-fence; they broke and ran; were reformed and advanced again, and came up finely, until within about the same distance of the enemy, when they again broke and away they went.

My friend, the General, and his staff were highly elated; the young men cheered; I was correspondingly depressed. Sick at heart, I left the lookout, went down into the gallery, and lay down upon a bench.

After some time the Confederates came down looking crest-fallen, showing that things were not going quite to their liking. They hurried away, possibly to give information of the knowledge obtained from the top of our hospital. It afterward proved that those men, at first faltering, afterward went into and made one of the grandest contests for civil liberty the world has ever witnessed; not like the hosts of Napoleon, fighting without an aim, but for principles grander, more weighty than had ever been assigned to the arbitrament of the sword. Gloriously did they perform their part. All honor to them.

The evening and night of July 2 are not readily blotted from the memory of those engaged in the fight of that day. Beaten back with fearful loss in killed, wounded, and prisoners, I had seen the streets raked with grape and canister after our retreating comrades; the dead, swollen to three times their natural size, lying as they fell upon the thoroughfares of that small town, and many of the Eleventh Corps captured. The hosts of the exultant enemy were around us, declaring that on the morrow they would "clean us out" and go on their way rejoicing to Baltimore and Washington, there to dictate terms of peace of abject submission on our part.

The Third Day

At this time little we knew of how much force we had—how many of our men had reached the scene of action. We knew they had long, hard marches to get there, oppressed with heavy burdens and intense heat. Rebel enlisted men told me how much force they mustered, and what they were going to do on the morrow. I thought it idle boasting, not believing it possible that the men of the rank and file knew so much of movements to be made. The officers had nothing to say. After events, however, proved the truth of the assertions in regard to their plans of action.

With the morning came renewed strength on our part; also on the part of the enemy. At early dawn our men attacked them fiercely, driving them back. The contest was sanguinary, the enemy losing heavily, Ewell's Corps being the one engaged on the part of the enemy.

The enemy losing in the morning what they had gained the evening of the second, it is not hard to see they had little to encourage them. They, however, held to the idea that our lines could be broken; hence the insane charge of Pickett, resulting; so disastrously to them.

Gen. Kemper, of the enemy, said to me that one of the officers in that charge was thrown upon the ground, wounded. After the smoke and dust had cleared a little he raised himself to look for his command. It had disappeared as though the wind had blown it away.

Gen. Kemper told me of another officer who came to Gen. Lee after the charge with tears in his eyes, saying: "General, my men have been all destroyed." The General sympathized with him but said: "Such is the fortune of war." The evening of the 3d of July those of us in the enemy's lines could only surmise as to how things were going. we [sic] had but little to cheer us; though the enemy had gone through our hospitals and paroled the sick and wounded.

After the Battle

Early in the morning of July 4 I was called and told that the enemy had gone, and we were left to pleasant reflections as to the results. After the battle provisions poured in from every quarter. Soon the Catholic church was wanted for service. We sent our patients some to one place, some to another. I went to the Courthouse for duty. It was soon wanted for the purpose of meting out justice. I then went to the Seminary. We there had Gens. Kemper and Trimble, with a number of other Confederate officers, Kemper being the only brigade commander of Pickett's Division left after that fearful slaughter caused by his charge on our left-center.

These Confederate officers had scores of friends to visit them, particularly Trimble, who had lost a foot in the fight. Ladies from Baltimore came and brought to him an abundance of good things to eat.

Kemper liked to have me talk with him, no doubt feeling lonely. We sometimes had it pretty warm, neither hesitating to utter his sentiments fully and frankly. A warm friendship sprang up between Kemper and me. He was a gentleman of whom I learned to think highly before we were separated by the fortunes of war.

SOURCE

The National Tribune (Washington, DC), October 20, 1898. Library of Congress collection.

Bibliography

American Philosophical Society, Philadelphia, Pennsylvania
Keen, W. W. "An Autobiographical Sketch by W. W. Keen," Reminiscences for His Children,
   1912, with additions 1915. Unpublished draft.
LeConte, John. Papers.
Chester County Historical Society, West Chester, Pennsylvania
Carlson, Robert E., ed. and comp. "Chester County (Pennsylvania) Medical Practitioners to
   1940." Unpublished manuscript, 1986.
Chester County maps.
Jordan Bank Academy Exhibition Program 1852–53, East Nottingham.
Jordan Bank Academy Newspaper Reference, Box 88.
Newspaper clippings files [*Daily Local News* (West Chester); *American Republican*
   (West Chester); *Chester County Times* (West Chester); *Village Record* (West Chester);
   Oxford Press; Coatesville Record].
Jefferson Medical College Historic Collections
Register Book and Catalogs
National Archives and Records Administration (NARA), Washington, DC
Military service record, James Fulton.
Record Group (RG) 19: Record Book of Candidates Examined by the Pennsylvania Medical
   Board, 1862, #19.168.
RG 94: Records of the Adjutant General's Office, 1780s–1919.
   Entry 621, Medical Records: Reports of Diseases and Individual Cases, 1841–93, file A and
      bound manuscripts.
   Entry 623, Medical Records, 1814–1919, D file.
RG 112: The Records of the Office of the Surgeon General.
   Entry 2, Central Office Correspondence, Letters and Endorsements Sent, 1818–1946.
   Entry 63, Central Office Issuances and Forms: Circulars and Circular Letters of the Sur-
      geon General's Office, 1861–1865.
National Museum of American History/Smithsonian Institution
Matthew A. Henderson, Diary, 1863. #MG*M-09670.

Otis Historical Archives, National Museum of Health and Medicine, Bethesda, Maryland
RG 28, Joseph Woodward Letterbooks, 1864–1883.
RG 83, Joseph Woodward's Photomicrographs, 1860s–1880s.
RG 363, Joseph Woodward Papers.
Pennsylvania State Archives
Medical Examinations, Roll 6802–6803, #19.167.
Medical Examinations, Roll 6810, #19.167.
Reports of Examination, Roll 6835, #19.174.
Record Book of Candidates Examined by Pennsylvania State Medical Board, 1862, Roll 6835, #19.168.
Registers, 143rd Pennsylvania Volunteers, Roll 6836, #19.172
Union League of Philadelphia Archives
124th Pennsylvania Volunteers Orders Book, MSS1805.040.

MEMOIRS, DIARIES, OR COLLECTIONS OF CORRESPONDENCE
BY PHYSICIANS AND OTHER HEALTH WORKERS

Belcher, Dennis W., ed. *"This Terrible Struggle for Life": The Civil War Letters of a Union Regimental Surgeon* [Thomas S. Hawley]. Jefferson, NC: McFarland & Company, Inc., 2012.
Broadhead, Sarah. *The Diary of a Lady of Gettysburg, Pennsylvania, from June 15 to July 15, 1863.* Privately published, no date.
Chesson, Michael B., ed. *The Journal of a Civil War Surgeon* [J. Franklin Dyer]. Lincoln: University of Nebraska Press, 2003.
Child, William. *Letters from a Civil War Surgeon: The Letters of Dr. William Child of the Fifth New Hampshire Volunteers.* Transcribed by Merill C. Sawyer, Betty Sawyer, and Timothy C. Sawyer. Solon, ME: Polar Bear & Co., 2001.
Ellis, Thomas T. *Leaves from the Diary of an Army Surgeon.* New York: John Bradburn, 1863.
Fatout, Paul, ed. *Letters of a Civil War Surgeon* [William Watson]. Purdue, IN: Purdue Research Foundation, 1961.
Fulton, James. Diary, 1862–1864. Garrett and Brenda Hollands family.
———. "Gettysburg Reminiscences. A Surgeon's Story." Washington, DC. *The National Tribune*, October 20, 1898.
Greiner, James M., Janet L. Coryell, and James R. Smither, eds. *A Surgeon's Civil War: The Letters and Diary of Daniel M. Holt, M.D.* Kent, OH: Kent State University Press, 1994.
James, W. W. Keen, ed. *The Memoirs of William Williams Keen, M.D.* Doylestown, PA: privately published, 1990.
Johnson, Charles Beneulyn. *Muskets and Medicine or Army Life in the Sixties.* Philadelphia: F. A. Davis, 1917.
Josyph, Peter, ed. *The Wounded River: The Civil War Letters of John Vance Lauderdale, M.D.* East Lansing: Michigan State University Press, 1993.
Keen, W. W. "Surgical Reminiscences of the Civil War," in *Addresses and Other Papers.* Philadelphia: W. B. Saunders and Company, 1905.
Letterman, Jonathan. *Medical Recollections of the Army of the Potomac.* New York: D. Appleton, 1866.
Loperfido, Christopher E., ed. *A Surgeon's Tale: The Civil War Letters of Surgeon James D. Benton, 111th and 98th New York Infantries 1862–1865.* Gettysburg, PA: Ten Roads Publishing, 2011.

Lowry, Thomas P., ed. *Swamp Doctor: The Diary of a Union Surgeon in the Virginia & North Carolina Marshes* [William Mervale Smith]. Mechanicsville, PA: Stackpole Books, 2001.

Perry, John Gardner. *Letters from a Surgeon of the Civil War.* Compiled by Martha Derby Perry. Boston: Little, Brown, 1906.

Priest, John Michael, ed. *One Surgeon's Private War: Doctor William W. Potter of the 57th New York.* Buffalo, NY: White Mane Publishing Company, 1996.

Reid, Richard M., ed. *Practicing Medicine in a Black Regiment: The Civil War Diary of Burt G. Wilder, 55th Massachusetts.* Boston: University of Massachusetts Press, 2010.

Smith, Edward Parmelee. *Incidents of the United States Christian Commission.* Philadelphia, PA: J. P. Lippincott, 1871.

Winsor, Frederick. "The Surgeon at the Field Hospital." *Atlantic Monthly* 46 (August 1880): 183–88.

Woolsey, Jane Stuart. *Hospital Days.* New York: D. Van Nostrand, 1870.

PUBLISHED PRIMARY SOURCES

Bartholow, Roberts. *A Manual of Instructions for Enlisting and Discharging Soldiers.* Philadelphia: J. B. Lippincott & Co., 1863.

"The Battle of Gettysburg and the Pennsylvania Campaign. Extract from the Diary of an English Officer present with the Confederate Army." *Blackwood's Edinburgh Magazine* 94 (September 1863): 365–94.

Beach, W. *The American Practice of Medicine, Revised, Enlarged, and Improved: Being a Practical Exposition of Pathology, Therapeutics, Surgery, Materia Medica, and Pharmacy, on Reformed Principles.* New York: Charles Scribner, 1855.

Bee, Robert L., ed. *The Boys from Rockville: Civil War Narratives of Sgt. Benjamin Hirst, Company D, 14th Connecticut Volunteers.* Knoxville: University of Tennessee Press, 1998.

Bennett, John Hughes. *Clinical Lectures on the Principles and Practice of Medicine.* 2nd ed. New York: Samuel S. and William Wood, 1858.

Billings, John D. *Hardtack and Coffee or The Unwritten Story of Army Life.* Reprint of 1887 edition. Lincoln, NE: Bison Books, 1993.

Budd, William. *On the Causes and Mode of Propagation of the Common Continued Fevers of Great Britain and Ireland (1839).* Edited by Dale Smith. Baltimore: Johns Hopkins University Press, 1984.

Calhoun, J. Theodore. "Rough Notes of an Army Surgeon's Experience during the Great Rebellion: Camp Diarrhoea—Continued." *Medical and Surgical Reporter,* n.s. 10 (May 30, 1863): 68–70.

———. "Rough Notes of an Army Surgeon's Experience during the Great Rebellion: The Dispensary or Hospital Steward's Department." *Medical and Surgical Reporter,* n.s. 9 (November 1, 1862): 123–4.

———. "Rough Notes of an Army Surgeon's Experience during the Great Rebellion: A Sick Call." *Medical and Surgical Reporter,* n.s. 9 (October 25, 1862): 99–100.

Chamberlin, Thomas. *History of the One Hundred and Fiftieth Regiment Pennsylvania Volunteers, Second Regiment, Bucktail Brigade.* Philadelphia: J. B. Lippincott, 1895.

Clements, Bennett A. "Memoir of Jonathan Letterman, M.D." *Journal of the Military Service Institution of the United States* 4 (September 1883): 250–87.

Confederate States Medical and Surgical Journal. 1864.

Fulton, Hugh R., ed. *Genealogy of the Fulton Family.* Lancaster, PA: privately printed, 1900.

Grace, William. *The army surgeon's manual: for the use of medical officers, cadets, chaplains, and hospital stewards: containing the regulations of the Medical Department, all general orders from the War Department, and circulars from the Surgeon-General's Office from January 1st, 1861, to July 1st, 1864.* New York: Baillière Bros., 1864.

Gross, Samuel D. "An Inaugural Address Introductory to the Course on Surgery in the Jefferson Medical College of Philadelphia, Delivered October 17, 1856." Philadelphia: Joseph M. Wilson, 1856.

———. *A Manual of Military Surgery.* Philadelphia: J. B. Lippincott, 1861.

———. *System of Surgery; Pathological, Diagnostic, Therapeutic and Operative.* 2nd ed. Philadelphia: Blanchard and Lee, 1862.

Gross, Samuel W., and A. Haller Gross, eds. *Autobiography of Samuel D. Gross, M. D.* Philadelphia: George Barrie, 1887.

Harris, Elisha. *Hints for the Control and Prevention of Infectious Disease in Camps, Transports and Hospitals.* New York: United States Sanitary Commission, 1863.

———. "Vaccination in the Army—Observations on the Normal and Morbid Results of Vaccination and Revaccination during the War, and on Spurious Vaccination." In *Contributions Relating to the Causation and Prevention of Disease, and to Camp Diseases,* edited by Austin Flint, 137–65. New York: US Sanitary Commission by Hurd and Houghton, 1867.

Hill, A. F. *Our Boys: The Personal Experiences of a Soldier in the Army of the Potomac.* Philadelphia: John E. Potter, 1864.

Hunt, Sanford. "Army Alimentation in Relation to the Causation and Prevention of Disease." In *Contributions Relating to the Causation and Prevention of Disease, and to Camp Diseases,* edited by Austin Flint, 64–94. New York: US Sanitary Commission by Hurd and Houghton, 1867.

Jones, Joseph. "Medical History of the Confederate States Army and Navy," *Southern Historical Society Papers* 20 (1892): 109–66.

———. "Researches upon 'Spurious Vaccination' or the Abnormal Phenomena Accompanying and Following Vaccination in the Confederate Army during the Recent American Civil War, 1861–1865." Nashville, TN: University Medical Press, W. H. F. Printer, 1867.

Lincoln, Abraham. Executive Order—Call for Troops, June 30, 1862. In *The American Presidency Project,* edited by Gerhard Peters and John T. Woolley, accessed March 18, 2016, http://www.presidency.ucsb.edu/ws/?pid=69810.

Merrillat, J. M. "On the Absence of Chlorides in the Urine of Persons affected with Variolous Diseases." *Confederate Medical and Surgical Journal* 1 (May 1864): 69–71.

Myers, Elizabeth Salome. "How A Gettysburg Schoolteacher Spent Her Vacation in 1863." *San Francisco Call.* August 16, 1903.

Mitchell, Thomas D. *Materia Medica and Therapeutics.* Philadelphia: J. B. Lippincott, 1857.

Mulholland, St. Clair Augustine. *The Story of the 116th Regiment Pennsylvania Volunteers in the War of the Rebellion.* Philadelphia: F. McManus, Jr. & Co., 1903.

"On the External Application of Oil of Turpentine as a Substitute for Quinine in Intermittent Fever, with Report of Cases." *Confederate States Medical and Surgical Journal* 1 (January 1864): 7–8.

Pereira, Jonathan. *Physicians' Prescription Book.* 14th ed. Philadelphia: Lindsay and Blakiston, 1865.

Porcher, Francis Peyre. *Resources of the Southern Fields and Forests.* Charleston: Evans & Cogswell, 1863.

Powers, Alice. "Dark Days of the Battle Week." *The Compiler* (Gettysburg). July 1, 1903.

Smith, Stephen. *Handbook of Surgical Operations*. New York: Baillière Brothers, 1863.

Sommé, C. L. "Notes sur l'Emploi Nouveau ou Peu Usité de Queíques Médicamens dans Plusieurs Maladies." *Archives Générales de Médecine* 1 (April 1823): 481–7.

Tomasak, Peter, ed. *Avery Harris Civil War Journal*. Luzerne, PA: Luzerne National Bank, 2000.

Tripler, Chas., and Blackman, George C. *Hand-Book for the Military Surgeon*. Cincinnati, OH: Robert Clarke & Co., 1861.

Triplett, W. H. "Improper Treatment of Wounds in Some of the United States Hospitals." *Boston Medical and Surgical Journal* 71 (September 15, 1864): 136–9.

United States Army. *Revised Regulations for the Army of the United States, 1861*. Philadelphia: J. G. L. Brown, 1861.

United States Surgeon General's Office.

———. Circular No. 5 (publication of the *Medical and Surgical History*), June 9, 1862.

———. Circular No. 2 (monthly sick reports), May 21, 1862.

———. *Directions Concerning the Duties of Medical Purveyors and Medical Storekeepers, and the Manner of Obtaining and Accounting for Medical and Hospital Supplies for the Army, with a Standard Supply Table*. Revised edition of Circular No. 12. Washington, DC: Government Printing Office, 1863.

———. *Directions Concerning the Manner of Obtaining and Accounting for Medical and Hospital Supplies for the Army, with a Standard Supply Table*. Washington, DC: Government Printing Office, 1862.

———. *Medical and Surgical History of the War of the Rebellion*. Washington, DC: Government Printing Office, 1875–1885.United States War Department. *War of the Rebellion: A Compilation of the Official Records of the Union and Confederate Armies*. Washington, DC: Government Printing Office, 1880–1901.

University of Pennsylvania. *Catalog of the Trustees, Officers, and Students of the University of Pennsylvania, Session 1862–63*. Philadelphia: Collins, 1863.

Wood, George B., and Franklin Bache. *The Dispensatory of the United States of America*. 11th ed. Philadelphia: J. B. Lippincott, 1858.

Woodward, Joseph Janvier. *The Hospital Steward's Manual*. Philadelphia: J. B. Lippincott, 1863.

———. *Outlines of the Chief Camp Diseases of the United States Armies*. Philadelphia: J. B. Lippincott & Co., 1863.

Wormeley, Katherine Prescott. *The United States Sanitary Commission: A Sketch of Its Purposes and Its Work*. Boston: Little, Brown and Company, 1863.

SECONDARY SOURCES

Aaron, Daniel. *The Unwritten War: American Writers and the Civil War*. New York: Alfred A. Knopf, 1973.

Adams, George W. *Doctors in Blue: The Medical History of the Union Army in the Civil War*. New York: Henry Schuman, 1952.

Adams, Jedidiah H. *History of the Life of D. Hayes Agnew*. Philadelphia: F. A. Davis Co., 1892.

Anbinder, Tyler. *Nativism and Slavery: The Northern Know Nothings and the Politics of the 1850s*. New York: Oxford University Press, 1992.

Attie, Jeanie. *Patriotic Toil: Northern Women and the American Civil War*. Ithaca, NY: Cornell University Press, 1998.

Bates, Samuel P. *History of Pennsylvania Volunteers, 1861–5*. Harrisburg, PA: B. Singerly, 1870.

Baxandall, Rosalyn, Linda Gordon, and Susan Reverby, eds. *America's Working Women*. New York: Random House, 1976.

Berlin, Ira. *The Long Emancipation: The Demise of Slavery in the United States*. Cambridge, MA: Harvard University Press, 2015.

Bernard, H. Russell, ed. *Handbook of Methods in Cultural Anthropology*. Walnut Creek, CA: Alta Mira Press, 1998.

Blackett, R. J. M. *Making Freedom: the Underground Railroad and the Politics of Slavery*. Chapel Hill: University of North Carolina Press, 2013.

Blair, William, and William Pencak, eds. *Making and Remaking Pennsylvania's Civil War*. University Park: Pennsylvania State University Press, 2001.

Blight, David W., ed. *Passages to Freedom: The Underground Railroad in History and Memory*. New York: Harper Collins for the Smithsonian Institution, 2004.

———. *Race and Reunion: The Civil War in American Memory*. Cambridge, MA: Harvard University Press, 2001.

Blustein, Bonnie Ellen. "To Increase the Efficiency of the Medical Department: A New Approach to Civil War Medicine." *Civil War History* 33, no. 1 (1987): 22–39.

Boatner, Mark. *Civil War Dictionary*. New York: David McKay Company, Inc., 1959.

Bollet, Alfred. *Civil War Medicine: Challenges and Triumphs*. Tucson, AZ: Galen Press, 2002.

Bonner, Thomas N. *Becoming a Physician: Medical Education in Britain, France, Germany and the United States, 1750–1945*. New York: Oxford University Press, 1995.

Boritt, Gabor. *Lincoln and the Economics of the American Dream*. Champaign: University of Illinois Press, 1994.

Boydston, Jeanne. *Home and Work: Housework, Wages, and the Ideology of Labor in the Early Republic*. Oxford, UK: Oxford University Press, 1990.

Brodman, Estelle, and Elizabeth B. Carrick. "American Military Medicine in the Mid-Nineteenth Century: The Experience of Alexander H. Hoff, M.D." *Bulletin of the History of Medicine* 64 (1990): 63–78.

Brown, R. Shepard. *Stringfellow of the Fourth*. New York: Crown, 1960.

Burnham, John. *Heath Care in America: A History*. Baltimore: Johns Hopkins University Press, 2015.

Clarke, Frances M. *War Stories: Suffering and Sacrifice in the Civil War North*. Chicago: University of Chicago Press, 2011.

Clinton, Catherine, and Nina Silber, eds. *Divided Houses: Gender and the Civil War*. New York: Oxford University Press, 1992.

Coco, Gregory A. *A Vast Sea of Misery: A History and Guide to the Union and Confederate Field Hospitals at Gettysburg July 1–November 20, 1863*. Gettysburg, PA: Thomas Publications, 1988.

Crabtree, Benjamin F., and William L. Miller, eds. *Doing Qualitative Research*. 2nd edition. Newbury Park, CA: Sage Publications, 1999.

Creighton, Margaret S. *The Colors of Courage: Gettysburg's Forgotten History, Immigrants, Women, and African Americans in the Civil War's Defining Battle*. New York: Basic Books, 2005.

Cronon, William, *Uncommon Ground: Rethinking the Human Place in Nature*. New York: Norton, 1996.

Dammann, Gordon. *Pictorial Encyclopedia of Civil War Medical Instruments and Equipment*. Missoula, MT: Pictorial Histories Publishing Company, 1983.

Davis, William C. *A Taste for War: The Culinary History of the Blue and the Gray*. Lincoln: University of Nebraska Press, 2003.

Diffley, Kathleen, ed. *To Live and Die: Collected Stories of the Civil War, 1861–1876.* Durham, NC: Duke University Press, 2002.

Dorwart, Bonnie Brice. *Death is in the Breeze: Disease During the American Civil War.* Frederick, MD: National Museum of Civil War Medicine Press, 2009.

Dougherty, James J. *Stone's Brigade and the Fight for the McPherson Farm.* Conshohocken, PA: Combined Publishing, 2001.

Drake, Brian Allen, ed. *The Blue, the Gray, and the Green: Toward an Environmental History of the Civil War.* Athens: University of Georgia Press, 2015.

Dreese, Michael A. *The Hospital on Seminary Ridge at the Battle of Gettysburg.* Jefferson, NC: McFarland & Company, Inc., 2002.

Edmonson, James M. *American Surgical Instruments: An Illustrated History.* San Francisco: Norman Publishing, 1997.

Egle, William Henry. *Notes and Queries Historical and Genealogical Chiefly Relating to Interior Pennsylvania.* Vol. 1. Harrisburg, PA: Harrisburg Publishing Company, 1894.

Faust, Drew Gilpin. *This Republic of Suffering: Death and the American Civil War.* New York: Random House, 2008.

Flannery, Michael. *Civil War Pharmacy: A History of Drugs, Drug Supply and Provision, and Therapeutics for the Union and Confederacy.* New York: Haworth Press, Inc., 2004.

Foner, Eric. *Free Soil, Free Labor, Free Men: The Ideology of the Republican Party before the Civil War.* New York: Oxford University Press, 1970.

Freemon, Frank R. *Gangrene and Glory: Medical Care during the American Civil War.* Champaign: University of Illinois Press, 2001.

Futhey, J. Smith, and Gilbert Cope. *History of Chester County, Pennsylvania.* Philadelphia: J. B. Lippincott, 1881.

Gallagher, Gary W. *The Union War.* Cambridge, MA: Harvard University Press, 2011.

Giesberg, Judith Ann. *Army at Home: Women and the Civil War on the Northern Home Front.* Chapel Hill: University of North Carolina Press, 2009.

———. *Civil War Sisterhood: The U.S. Sanitary Commission and Women's Politics in Transition.* Boston: Northeastern University Press, 2000.

———. "In Service to the Fifth Wheel: Katharine Prescott Wormeley and Her Experiences in the United States Sanitary Commission." *Nursing History Review* 3 (1995): 43–53.

Gillett, Mary C. *The Army Medical Department, 1818–1865.* Washington, DC: Center for Military History, United States Army, 1987.

Gjerde, Jon. *Catholicism and the Shaping of Nineteenth-Century America.* Edited by S. Deborah King. Cambridge, UK: Cambridge University Press, 2012.

Gould, George M. *The Jefferson Medical College of Philadelphia.* New York: Lewis Publishing Company, 1904.

Grimsley, Mark. *The Hard Hand of War: Union Military Policy Toward Southern Civilians, 1861–1865.* Cambridge, UK: Cambridge University Press, 1995.

Guelzo, Allen C. *Gettysburg: The Last Invasion.* New York: Alfred A. Knopf, 2013.

Halttunen, Karen, and Perry Lewis, eds. *Moral Problems in American Life: New Perspectives on Cultural History.* Ithaca, NY: Cornell University Press, 1998.

Handwerker, W. Penn. *Quick Ethnography.* Walnut Creek, CA: Alta Mira Press, 2001.

Harrison, Mark. *Contagion: How Commerce Has Spread Disease.* New Haven: Yale University Press, 2012.

Hess, Earl J. *The Union Soldier in Battle: Enduring the Ordeal of Combat.* Lawrence: University of Kansas Press, 1997.

Holzer, Harold. *The Civil War in 50 Objects*. New York: Viking, 2013.

Honeck, Mischa. "Men of Principle: Gender and the German American War for the Union." *Journal of the Civil War Era* 5 (March 2015): 48–52.

Humphreys, Margaret. *Intensely Human: The Health of the Black Soldier in the American Civil War*. Baltimore, MD: Johns Hopkins University Press, 2008.

———. *Marrow of Tragedy: The Health Crisis of the American Civil War*. Baltimore, MD: Johns Hopkins University Press, 2013.

Hyde, Anne Farrar. *An American Vision: The Western Landscape and National Culture, 1820–1920*. New York: New York University Press, 1990.

Johnson, David A. and Humayun J. Chaudry. *Medical Licensing and Discipline in America* New York: Lexington Books, 2012.

Johnson, Jeffrey J. *Selecting Ethnographic Informants*. Newbury Park, CA: Sage Publications, 1990.

Jolly, Ellen Ryan. *Nuns of the Battlefield*. Providence, RI: Providence Visitor Press, 1927.

Jordan, Brian Matthew. *Marching Home: Union Veterans and Their Unending Civil War*. New York: Liveright Publishing Corporation, 2014.

Jordan, Ewing. *University of Pennsylvania Men Who Served in the Civil War*. Pt. 1: Department of Medicine Classes 1816–1862. Philadelphia, 1900.

Kagan, Neil, ed. *Smithsonian Civil War: Inside the National Collection*. Washington, DC: Smithsonian Books, 2013.

Kalisch, Philip, and Beatrice Kalisch. *The Advance of American Nursing*. 3rd ed. Philadelphia: J. B. Lippincott, 1995.

Kamen, Michael. *Mystic Chords of Memory: The Transformation of Tradition in American Culture*. New York: Alfred A. Knopf, 1991.

Kashatus, William C. *Just Over the Line: Chester County and the Underground Railroad*. West Chester, PA: Chester County Historical Society, 2002.

Keener-Farley, Lawrence E., and James E. Schmick, eds. *Civil War Harrisburg, A Guide to Capital Area Sites, Incidents and Personalities*. Rev. ed. Harrisburg, PA: Camp Curtin Historical Society, 2014.

Keller, Christian B. *Chancellorsville and the Germans: Nativism, Ethnicity, and Civil War Memory*. New York: Fordham University Press, 2007.

Kurtz, William B. *Excommunicated from the Union: How the Civil War Created a Separate Catholic America*. New York: Fordham University Press, 2016.

Leavitt, Judith Walzer. *Typhoid Mary: Captive to the Public's Health*. Boston: Beacon Press, 1996.

Linderman, Gerald F. *Embattled Courage: The Experience of Combat in the American Civil War*. New York: The Free Press, 1987.

Lowry, Thomas P., and Jack D. Welsh. *Tarnished Scalpels: The Court-Martials of Fifty Union Surgeons*. Mechanicsburg, PA: Stackpole Books, 2000.

Ludmerer, Kenneth. *Learning to Heal: The Development of American Medical Education*. New York: Basic Books, 1985.

Lundberg, David. "The American Literature of War: The Civil War, World War I, and World War II." *South American Quarterly* 36, no. 3 (1984): 373–88.

Maddox, Lucy. *The Parker Sisters: A Border Kidnapping*. Philadelphia: Temple University Press, 2016.

Maher, Sister Mary Denis. *To Bind Up the Wounds: Catholic Sister Nurses and the U.S. Civil War*. Baton Rouge: Louisiana State University Press, 1989.

Manning, Chandra. *When This Cruel War Was Over: Soldiers, Slavery, and the Civil War*. New York: Alfred A. Knopf, 2007.

Martin, David G. *Gettysburg July 1*. Conshohocken, PA: Combined Books, Inc., 1995.

Matthews, Richard E. *The 149th Pennsylvania Volunteer Infantry Unit in the Civil War*. Jefferson, NC: McFarland & Company, 1994.

McGaugh, Scott. *Surgeon in Blue: Jonathan Letterman, the Civil War Doctor Who Pioneered Battlefield Care*. New York: Arcade Publishing, 2013.

McNeil, Sister Betty A. "The Daughters of Charity as Civil War Nurses, Caring without Boundaries," *Vincentian Heritage Journal* 27, no. 1 (2007): 133–68.

McPherson, James M. *Battle Cry of Freedom*. New York: Oxford University Press, 1988.

———. *For Cause and Comrades: Why Men Fought in the Civil War*. New York: Oxford University Press, 1997.

———. *What They Fought For, 1861–1865*. Baton Rouge: Louisiana State University Press, 1994.

Meier, Kathryn Shively. *Nature's Civil War: Common Soldiers and the Environment in 1862 Virginia*. Chapel Hill: University of North Carolina Press, 2013.

Miller, Angela. *The Empire of the Eye: Landscape Representation and American Cultural Politics, 1825–1875*. Ithaca, NY: Cornell University Press, 1993.

Mitchell, Reid. *The Vacant Chair: The Northern Soldier Leaves Home*. New York: Oxford University Press, 1993.

Mohr, James. *Licensed to Practice: The Supreme Court Defines the American Medical Profession*. Baltimor: Johns Hopkins University Press, 2013.

Nash, Roderick F. *Wilderness and the American Mind*. 4th ed. New Haven: Yale University Press, 2001.

Neely, Mark E., Jr. *The Fate of Liberty: Abraham Lincoln and Civil Liberties*. New York: Oxford University Press, 1991.

Numbers, Ronald, ed. *The Education of American Physicians*. Berkeley: University of California Press, 1979.

Oates, Stephen B. *A Woman of Valor: Clara Barton and the Civil War*. New York: The Free Press, 1994.

Parish, Peter J. *The American Civil War*. New York: Holmes & Meier, 1975.

Pelling, Margaret. *Cholera, Fever, and English Medicine 1825–1865*. New York: Oxford University Press, 1978.

Pernick, Martin. *A Calculus of Suffering: Pain, Professionalism, and Anesthesia in Nineteenth-Century America*. New York: Columbia University Press, 1985.

Pinkowski, Edward. *Chester County Place Names*. Philadelphia: Sunshine Press, 1962.

Portrait and Biographical Record of Buchanan and Clinton Counties, Missouri. Chicago: Chapman Bros., 1893.

Pryor, Elizabeth Brown. *Clara Barton, Professional Angel*. Philadelphia: University of Pennsylvania Press, 1987.

Rable, George C. *God's Almost Chosen Peoples: A Religious History of the American Civil War*. Chapel Hill: University of North Carolina Press, 2010.

Ramold, Steven J. *Across the Divide: Union Soldiers View the Northern Home Front*. New York: New York University Press, 2013.

Richardson, Heather Cox. *The Greatest Nation of the Earth: Republican Economic Policies during the Civil War*. Cambridge, MA: Harvard University Press, 1997.

Rogers, Henry M., "Henry Shippen Huidekoper, 1839–1918." *The Harvard Graduates' Magazine*, 27 (March 1919): 325–7.

Rosenberg, Charles E. "The Therapeutic Revolution: Medicine, Meaning, and Social Change in Nineteenth-Century America." *Perspectives in Biology and Medicine* 20 no. 4 (Summer 1977): 485–506.

Rothstein, William. *American Medical Schools and the Practice of Medicine: A History.* New York: Oxford University Press, 1987.

———. *American Physicians in the 19th Century: From Sects to Science.* Baltimore: Johns Hopkins University Press, 1972.

Rutkow, Ira M. *Bleeding Blue and Gray: Civil War Surgery and the Evolution of American Medicine.* New York: Random House, 2005.

Sappol, Michael. A *Traffic of Dead Bodies: Anatomy and Embodied Social Identity in Nineteenth-Century America.* Princeton, NJ: Princeton University Press, 2002.

Schultz, Jane E. *Women at the Front: Hospital Workers in Civil War America.* Chapel Hill: University of North Carolina Press, 2004.

Sifakis, Stewart. *Who Was Who in the Civil War.* New York: Facts on File Publications, 1988.

Smith, Dale C. "Austin Flint and Auscultation in America." *Journal of the History of Medicine and Allied Sciences* 33 (1978): 129–49.

———. "Gerhard's Distinction between Typhoid and Typhus and its Reception in America, 1833–1860." *Bulletin of the History of Medicine* 54 (1980): 368–85.

———. "The Rise and Fall of Typhomalarial Fever: I. Origins." *Journal of the History of Medicine and Allied Sciences* 37 (April 1982): 182–220.

Smith, David G. *On the Edge of Freedom: The Fugitive Slave Issue in South Central Pennsylvania, 1820–1870.* New York: Fordham University Press, 2012.

Society of Civil War Surgeons. *James Fulton, Biographical Information.* Unpublished Paper.

Stevens, Rosemary. *American Medicine and the Public Interest: A History of Specialization.* Berkeley: University of California Press, 1971.

Thomas, Keith. "History and Anthropology." *Past and Present* 24 (1963): 3–24.

Trudeau, Noah. *Gettysburg: A Testing of Courage.* New York: Harper Collins, 2002.

Wagner, Frederick B., Jr., and J. Woodrow Savacool, eds. *Thomas Jefferson University— A Chronological History and Alumni Directory, 1824–1990.* Philadelphia: Thomas Jefferson University, 1992.

Wald, Pricilla. *Contagious: Cultures, Carriers and the Outbreak Narrative.* Durham, NC: Duke University Press, 2008.

Wall, Barbra Mann. "Called to a Mission of Charity: The Sisters of St. Joseph in the Civil War." *Nursing History Review* 6 (1998): 85–113.

Ward, Geoffrey C. *The Civil War: An Illustrated History.* New York: Alfred A. Knopf, 1990.

Warner, John Harley. *Against the Spirit of the System: The French Impulse in Nineteenth-Century American Medicine.* Princeton, NJ: Princeton University Press, 1998.

White, Jonathan W. *Midnight in America: Darkness, Sleep, and Dreams during the Civil War.* Chapel Hill: University of North Carolina Press, 2017.

Wingert, Cooper H. *Harrisburg and the Civil War.* Charleston, SC: The History Press, 2013.

Wood, Ann Douglas. "The War Within a War: Women Nurses in the Union Army." *Civil War History* 18 (1972): 197–212.

Index

Page numbers in italics refer to figures.

ROBERT D. HICKS, PhD, is Director of the Mütter Museum and Historical Medical Library of the College of Physicians of Philadelphia, where he holds the William Maul Measey Chair for the History of Medicine.

Lightning Source UK Ltd.
Milton Keynes UK
UKHW020810280419
341677UK00007B/28/P